The Official Guide for Foreign-Educated Allied Health Professionals

Barbara L. Nichols, DHL, MS, RN, FAAN, is the Chief Executive Officer of CGFNS International (Commission on Graduates of Foreign Nursing Schools), which is an internationally recognized authority on credentials evaluation and verification pertaining to the education, registration, and licensure of nurses and health care professionals worldwide. Dr. Nichols served as professor of nursing at the University of Wisconsin School of Nursing and director of nursing for the Wisconsin Area Health Education Center System. Currently, she serves on the Board of Directors for the American National Standards Institute (ANSI) and is on their Conformity Assessment Policy Committee. She held a cabinet position in Wisconsin State Government, is a former International Council of Nurses (ICN) Board Member and a past President of the American Nurses Association. As Secretary of the Department of Regulation and Licensing for the state of Wisconsin, she was responsible for 17 boards that regulated 59 occupations and professions. Dr. Nichols is the author of over 70 publications on nursing and health care delivery, including her most recent contribution as a guest editor, "Policy, Politics and Nursing Practice," in the August 2006 edition of *Building Global Alliances III: The Impact of Global Nurse Migration on Health Service Delivery.* She was a lieutenant in the United States Navy Nurse Corps. Among other accolades, Dr. Nichols was a 2006 Inaugural Inductee into the National Black Nurses Association Institute of Excellence; was named the 2007 Distinguished Scholar, Howard University College of Pharmacy, Nursing, and Allied Health Sciences, Division of Nursing; in 2009 received an Honorary Doctorate of Humane Letters from Drexel University; and is a Fellow in the American Academy of Nursing.

Catherine R. Davis, PhD, RN, is the Director of Global Research and Test Administration for CGFNS International. Dr. Davis provides senior leadership for CGFNS test development activities, research initiatives, and related publications. Prior to joining CGFNS International, Dr. Davis was Associate Professor of Nursing at Hahnemann University in Philadelphia. She holds a PhD in Nursing from Adelphi University and a Master's degree in Child and Adolescent Psychiatric Nursing from the University of Pennsylvania. She serves on the National Editorial Advisory Board of Advance for Nurses and as a manuscript reviewer for Sigma Theta Tau International's *Journal of Nursing Scholarship.* Dr. Davis has authored and edited numerous publications on international nursing issues and has served as a national and international speaker on nurse migration trends and challenges, international testing and test development issues, and certification program development.

The Official Guide for Foreign-Educated Allied Health Professionals

What You Need to Know About Health Care and the Allied Health Professions in the United States

CGFNS International, Inc.
(Commission on Graduates of Foreign Nursing Schools)

BARBARA L. NICHOLS, DHL, MS, RN, FAAN
CATHERINE R. DAVIS, PhD, RN
EDITORS

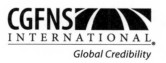

CGFNS
INTERNATIONAL®
Global Credibility

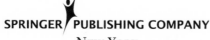

SPRINGER PUBLISHING COMPANY
NEW YORK

Springer Publishing Company, LLC
11 West 42nd Street
New York, NY 10036
www.springerpub.com

Acquisitions Editor: Margaret Zuccarini
Project Manager: Julia Rosen
Cover design: Steve Pisano
Composition: Apex CoVantage, LLC

Ebook ISBN: 978-0-8261-1064-0

09 10 11 12 / 5 4 3 2 1

The author and the publisher of this Work have made every effort to use sources believed to be reliable to provide information that is accurate and compatible with the standards generally accepted at the time of publication. Because medical science is continually advancing, our knowledge base continues to expand. Therefore, as new information becomes available, changes in procedures become necessary. We recommend that the reader always consult current research and specific institutional policies before performing any clinical procedure. The author and publisher shall not be liable for any special, consequential, or exemplary damages resulting, in whole or in part, from the readers' use of, or reliance on, the information contained in this book. The publisher has no responsibility for the persistence or accuracy of URLs for external or third-party Internet Web sites referred to in this publication and does not guarantee that any content on such Web sites is, or will remain, accurate or appropriate.

Library of Congress Cataloging-in-Publication Data
The Official Guide for Foreign-Educated Allied Health Professionals: What You Need to Know About Health Care and the Allied Health Professions in the United States / CGFNS International, Inc. (Commission on Graduates of Foreign Nursing Schools) ; Barbara L. Nichols, Catherine R. Davis, editors.
    p. ; cm.
  Includes bibliographical references and index.
  ISBN 978-0-8261-1063-3 (alk. paper)
  1. Allied health personnel, Foreign—United States.   2. Allied health personnel, Foreign—Vocational guidance—United States.   3. Medical care—United States.
I. Nichols, Barbara L.   II. Davis, Catherine R.   III. Commission on Graduates of Foreign Nursing Schools (U.S.)
  [DNLM: 1. Allied Health Personnel—United States.   2. Delivery of Health Care—United States.   3. Emigration and Immigration—United States.   4. Foreign Professional Personnel—United States. W 21.5 O32 2009]
  R697.A4O44 2009
  610.69'6—dc22   2009033173

Printed in the United States of America by Hamilton Printing

This book is dedicated to all foreign-educated health care professionals whose knowledge, dedication, and deeds live on through their caring spirit.

Contents

Contributors

Virginia C. Alinsao, MBA, MS, RN, has over 30 years experience in health care and was the Director of International Recruitment for The Johns Hopkins Health System in Baltimore, Maryland. Ms. Alinsao has been an active advocate in the ethical recruitment of international nurses and in supporting transition programs to ensure success of foreign-educated nurses in the United States. She has presented locally and internationally on issues related to international recruitment. As a foreign-educated nurse herself, she will continue advocating in this area.

Geraldine Buck, MHS, PA-C, is a senior faculty member at the Drexel University Physician Assistant Program in Philadelphia, Pennsylvania, where she teaches courses in health policy, research, and evidence-based practice. She is a certified physician assistant whose clinical practice has been primarily with uninsured and homeless populations. Ms. Buck is currently completing a doctorate of public health, in community health and prevention. Her professional interests focus on innovative improvements to the U.S. health system for the elimination of health disparities, and enhanced quality of care.

Kathryn M. Doig, PhD, CLS(NCA), CLSp(H), is Professor of Biomedical Laboratory Diagnostics at Michigan State University, where she teaches clinical hematology and an introduction to health professions careers. She is also the Associate Dean for Undergraduate Education in the College of Natural Science. Dr. Doig is a past president of the National Credentialing Agency for Laboratory Personnel and received the Member of the Year Award from the American Society for Clinical Laboratory Science. Her scholarly interests and published papers include workforce and educational issues in medical laboratories.

Julia To Dutka, EdD, is Director of Global Assessment and Professional Services at CGFNS International, a nonprofit organization that provides credential assessment for health professionals educated outside the United States. Educated as a psycholinguist, Dr. To Dutka has served in a variety of faculty and administrative roles in higher education and has worked with educational systems operating under different curricular structures in different world regions. In her prior role as the Executive Director of the Test of English as a Foreign Language (TOEFL) at the Educational Testing Service (ETS), she introduced computer-based testing as a technology platform to transform language assessment and to improve its access to applicants worldwide.

David D. Gale, PhD, FASAP, is Professor and Dean of the College of Health Sciences at Eastern Kentucky University, where he is responsible for administration of the health sciences programs, with nearly 200 full-time faculty and 34 separately accredited degree programs. Dr. Gale holds a PhD from the University of Iowa and completed a postdoctorate at Indiana University School of Medicine. He has taught in the fields of human genetics, preventive medicine, and physiology. Dr. Gale has served on advisory panels and boards and as a consultant for many institutions as well as national and international organizations.

Nicole Gara, MA, is Senior Vice President for Advocacy and Government Affairs at the American Academy of Physician Assistants in Alexandria, Virginia. She is a graduate of Syracuse University and holds a master's degree from New York University. She began her Washington career as a congressional lobbyist for the American Institute of Architects (AIA) in 1972. She also worked on state government issues for AIA, as well as minority medical education issues at Georgetown University School of Medicine, before joining AAPA in 1981. Ms. Gara currently directs a staff of 14 federal and state lobbyists, reimbursement experts, and professional practice experts.

Carolyn Wiles Higdon, PhD, CCC-SLP, F-ASHA, LCP, is a speech-language pathologist, a Fellow in the American Speech-Language-Hearing Association, and an associate professor at the University of Mississippi in Oxford, Mississippi. She owns and operates an international private practice in Communication Sciences and Disorders that is based in Atlanta, Georgia. In addition to her professional areas of specialty (adult and pediatric neurogenics, voice science, and international rehabilitation), Dr. Higdon is a site visitor for accrediting and credentialing teams, and a qualified and published legal expert in the area of rehabilitation. In her free time, Dr. Higdon takes rehabilitation delegations to such countries as China, Russia, Costa Rica, Kenya, and Bosnia.

Jay Lubinsky, PhD, CCC-A/SLP, F-ASHA, is Professor Emeritus in the Department of Communication Disorders at Governors State University, University Park, Illinois. At Governors State he served as professor and, for many years, as department chair/program director. Dr. Lubinsky is certified in both audiology and speech-language pathology by the American Speech-Language-Hearing Association (ASHA) and served as chair of ASHA's Council for Academic Accreditation as well as its Council for Clinical Certification, also serving on ASHA's Board of Ethics. He is currently a member of the International Commission on Healthcare Professions' Speech-Language Pathology and Audiology Standards Committee.

Scott McPhee, DrPH, OTR/L, FAOTA, is a tenured professor of occupational therapy at Belmont University in Nashville, Tennessee. He has worked as an occupational therapy practitioner, manager, and educator for over 30 years, spending 21 years as an army occupational therapist and retiring at the rank of Lieutenant Colonel. Dr. McPhee served as the inaugural Chair for Belmont University's School of Occupational Therapy. He has authored over 20 professional papers on varying health care topics and lectures extensively across the United States on topics relevant to occupational therapy.

Donna R. Richardson, JD, RN, is the Director of Governmental Affairs and Professional Standards for CGFNS International in Philadelphia, Pennsylvania. As Director of Governmental Affairs for the American Nurses Association she directed the legislative and regulatory policies that led to the Nursing Immigration Relief Act and occupational health protections for nurses. A registered nurse and attorney, she is an experienced lecturer on foreign-educated nurses, minority and women's health issues and clinical trials, and legal issues in nursing and health administration.

Barbara Sanders, PhD, PT, SCS, is Professor of Physical Therapy and Associate Dean of the College of Health Professions, Texas State University-San Marcos. She has been a consultant on evaluation of foreign-educated physical therapists for over 10 years. Dr. Sanders has been in clinical practice in Kentucky, Wisconsin, Minnesota, Tennessee, and Texas in acute care, rehabilitation, home health, long-term care, outpatient orthopedics, and sports. For over 20 years at Texas State, she has been responsible for the development of entry-level curricula for physical therapists at the baccalaureate, master's, and doctorate levels.

Nancy C. Sharts-Hopko, PhD, RN, FAAN, is Professor and Director of the Doctoral Program in the College of Nursing at Villanova University, in Villanova, Pennsylvania. As a veteran of nearly 3 years working in Asia, first as a short-term consultant for WHO and then as an Overseas Associate of the Presbyterian Church (USA), she understands the challenges associated with living and working in an international context. She has served as an advisory committee member and consultant for the United States Food and Drug Administration since 1992.

Michael D. Ward, PhD, RTR, FASRT, is the Associate Dean for Student Programs and Professor at Barnes-Jewish College, St. Louis, Missouri. He is a past President and Fellow of the American Society of Radiologic Technologists and serves on the Board of Management for the International Society of Radiographers and Radiologic Technologists. Dr. Ward is a frequent speaker on various topics related to the radiologic sciences and higher education.

Deborah McNeil Whitehouse, DSN, PMHNP-BC, serves as Professor and Associate Dean of Health Sciences at Eastern Kentucky University, Richmond, Kentucky. She is a psychiatric/mental health nurse practitioner. Dr. Whitehouse concentrates on curriculum and accreditation issues in multiple disciplines and is interested in smoking cessation, organizational leadership, and mental health delivery.

Foreword

The current shortage of health care providers in the United States has stimulated a demand for the recruitment of foreign-educated health care workers—audiologists, clinical laboratory scientists, clinical laboratory technicians, nurses, occupational therapists, physical therapists, physician assistants, and speech-language pathologists. This book has been developed with the foreign-educated health care professional in mind. It is a definitive source for information on understanding the myriad of requirements as the health care professional moves through the process of securing an occupational visa, licensure, and employment in the United States.

As a physical therapist educator for almost 30 years, I have had the opportunity to work with many foreign-educated health care professionals and with the legal jurisdictions as the physical therapist strives to meet the challenges and opportunities of licensure. This book has been developed and written by some of the leading health care professionals in the United States today. Their experience and knowledge should provide you with the knowledge and insight needed to maneuver through the complicated visa and licensure systems. It is our intent that this book will serve as a resource to assist individuals as they consider immigration to this country, apply for occupational visas, complete the federal screening and state licensure processes, and meet employment requirements in the United States.

CGFNS International® was named in the 1996 Illegal Immigration Reform and Immigrant Responsibility Act and certified in 2004 by the Department of Homeland Security to certify health care workers in pursuit of practice in the United States. CGFNS International's work includes credentials evaluation and assessment services that are designed to protect individuals seeking licensure and practice in the United States and to protect the U.S. public. The authors of the chapters in this book have worked with CGFNS International over the years and have provided the reader with the most up-to-date information on topics ranging from the U.S. health care delivery system to employment opportunities, from entry into the United States to entry into professional practice.

Why you will want this book? It is unique in that it is the first official guide for foreign-educated health care professionals entering the U.S. health care workforce; it is published by CGFNS International®, Inc., an internationally recognized and respected agency that evaluates the credentials of foreign-educated health professionals seeking employment in the United States; and the contributors are well-known experts in their fields.

Barbara Sanders, PhD, PT, SCS
Associate Dean, College of Health Professions
Texas State University

Preface

In 1996 the debate regarding the Illegal Immigration Reform and Immigrant Responsibility Act centered on the necessity to screen foreign-educated health care professionals seeking employment in the United States. The focused and controversial discussion also raised cogent points regarding the qualifications of an entity to perform such an assessment.

Based on its established track record in providing credentialing services to a variety of health occupations, CGFNS International was named in the Act to provide health professions screening when the law passed. The Congressional mandate acknowledged, then and now, the expertise of CGFNS International to protect the U.S. public, by assuring the integrity of health professionals' credentials in the context of global migration.

In creating this book, CGFNS has attempted to provide a bridge that will foster a successful transition for those whose journey brings them to the United States to work. The book is organized into nine chapters that present information to assist the foreign-educated health care professional who is considering practicing in the United States. No doubt the contents of the book will be viewed differently among a variety of readers, but the authors hope that all will benefit from the perspectives presented.

In chapter 1, "Foreign-Educated Health Care Professionals in the United States Health Care System," Deborah McNeil Whitehouse and David D. Gale present an overview of the current health care professional shortage in the United States and the employment of foreign-educated health professionals to respond to the shortages. The history of foreign-educated health professionals in the U.S. workforce and comparability of their professional education in the United States to education in other nations is discussed.

In chapter 2, "Preparing to Leave Your Home Country," Catherine R. Davis and Donna R. Richardson identify the many reasons that health professionals migrate. The factors that make a host country a favorable destination are depicted. Pitfalls to avoid and ways to reduce the risk of abuse and intimidation also are emphasized. The chapter identifies what should be done in the professional's home country once the decision is made to move to the United States to work.

In chapter 3, "Entry Into the United States," Donna R. Richardson and Catherine R. Davis explain the visa requirements to work successfully as a health care professional in the United States. Tips are offered for successfully navigating the process of obtaining a visa and a VisaScreen® certificate.

Michael D. Ward, in chapter 4, "Employment in the United States," addresses the rights and responsibilities of employees and employers, and describes fundamental issues for work success across a variety of health care settings in the United States.

Nancy C. Sharts-Hopko, in chapter 5, "The U.S. Health Care System," offers a broad overview of the scope and structure of the U.S. health care system, and how individuals access care. She underscores the importance of knowledge of the health care system as a key to successful practice in the United States.

Chapter 6, "Health Care Professional Practice in the United States," presents summarized information about the health care professions of audiology, medical technician, medical technology, occupational therapy, physician assistants, physical therapy, and speech language pathology. Each is presented in terms of education, licensure, and ethical and legal considerations for practice.

In chapter 7, "Communicating in the U.S. Health Care System," Catherine R. Davis and Donna R. Richardson describe the legal basis for English language proficiency requirements and focus on interpersonal skills and challenges that foreign-educated health professionals must face as they enter practice in the United States. They also explore the meaning and impact of English language proficiency and interpersonal skills on the provision of safe care.

Virginia C. Alinsao, in chapter 8, "Adjusting to a New Community," provides useful information for newly arriving immigrants adjusting to a new community in the United States. She addresses major concerns about housing, transportation, and personal safety, all factors that must be considered when adapting to a new country and work environment.

In chapter 9, "Furthering Your Education," Julia To Dutka discusses academic and nonacademic educational programs for foreign health professionals in the United States. This chapter outlines the types of educational programs and the requirements for academic entry, and discusses continuing education programs. The author conveys that a spirit of continuous learning is central to adjusting to working and living in the United States.

The five appendices supplement the primary content and are summarized as follows: Appendix A provides profession-specific excerpts from the Bureau of Labor Statistics Occupational Outlook Handbook, 2008–2009 Edition on audiologists, clinical laboratory scientists and technicians (medical technologists and technicians), occupational therapists, physical therapists, physician assistants, and speech-language pathologists.

Appendix B focuses on what a foreign-educated professional will need when searching for a job in the United States. It contains a sample cover letter requesting an interview, a sample résumé, and a sample letter of thanks following an interview.

Appendix C provides a glossary of common visa terms and their meanings as well as frequently asked questions about admission to the United States.

Appendix D presents additional information on speech-language pathology as far as treatment areas and etiologies. It also provides a comparison of American Speech-Language-Hearing Association (ASHA) certification, state licensure, and state department of education certification.

Appendix E provides communication aids and contains a list of commonly heard idioms, slang, and jargon in the United States and in the U.S. health care system. It also contains a list of abbreviations commonly seen in practice settings.

In creating this book, CGFNS has attempted to provide a bridge that will foster a successful transition for those whose journey brings them to the United States to work. We hope that as each professional reads the chapters that not only will we answer important questions and address relevant inquiries, but also that each reader will find the book both informative and helpful.

Barbara L. Nichols, CEO, CGFNS International
Fall, 2009

Acknowledgments

We thank the authors for not only taking time to prepare the manuscripts but also for their scholarship, diligence, and enthusiasm. We are indebted to each for helping us realize our goal of creating a helpful, readable book.

Special thanks go to Melanie Jones and Amanda Nickerson, whose attention to detail and indefatigable work to meet deadlines made the book possible, and to Donna R. Richardson for her keen eye and professional assistance.

We thank Springer Publishing Company, especially Executive Acquisitions Editor Margaret Zuccarini and Assistant Editor Brian O'Connor, for the trust and support they provided throughout the development of the book. Their thought-provoking questions and skill with words transformed a manuscript into a book.

Our gratitude is extended to our colleagues who helped with their encouragement and conversations. They include the CGFNS International Board of Trustees, CGFNS administrative, managerial, and operational staff, and the health care professionals who shared their migration journey with us.

About CGFNS International

CGFNS International is an internationally recognized authority on credentials evaluation and verification pertaining to the education, registration, and licensure of nurses and health care professionals worldwide. The mission of CGFNS International is to provide expert credentials evaluation and professional development services to promote the health and safety of the public. CGFNS International protects the public by ensuring that nurses and other health care professionals educated in countries other than the United States are eligible and qualified to meet licensure, immigration, and other practice requirements in the United States.

CGFNS International and its divisions provide products and services that validate international professional credentials and support international regulatory and educational standards for health care professionals. The organization focuses on four key objectives:

1. To develop and administer a predictive testing and evaluation program for internationally educated nurses.
2. To provide a credentials evaluation service for internationally educated and/or internationally born health care professionals.
3. To serve as a clearinghouse for information on the international education and licensure of health care professionals.
4. To conduct and publish studies relevant to internationally educated health care professionals.

The major CGFNS programs used by internationally educated health care professionals are the VisaScreen Program®, which is the leading health care worker certification program for immigration and for obtaining occupational visas in the United States; the Credentials Evaluation Service, which provides a course-by-course comparison of international education to U.S. standards for licensure, further education, and employment; and the Credentials Verification Service for New York State, which is required of internationally educated RNs, LPNs, OTs and assistants, and PTs and assistants seeking licensure in New York State.

CGFNS International celebrated its 30th anniversary in 2007. It has reviewed and/or certified the credentials of over 500,000 internationally educated nurses and other health care professionals for U.S. licensure and immigration.

The Official Guide for Foreign-Educated Allied Health Professionals

1

Foreign-Educated Health Care Professionals in the United States Health Care System

**DEBORAH McNEIL WHITEHOUSE
AND DAVID D. GALE**

In This Chapter

Keywords

Accreditation Commission for Audiology Education (ACAE): Organization whose mission is to assure the public that only those programs that have complied with this agency's standards and that graduate competent audiologists trained at the AuD level will be accredited.

Accreditation Review Commission on Education for Physician Assistants (ARC-PA): The accrediting agency that defines the standards for physician assistant education and evaluates physician assistant educational programs within the United States to ensure their compliance with those standards.

Allied health professionals: Clinical health care professionals distinct from those who practice medicine, dentistry, and nursing. Allied health professionals work as part of the health care team.

American Academy of Physician Assistants (AAPA): National professional society, founded in 1968, that represents physician assistants in all 50 states, the District of Columbia, Guam, and the Federal Services.

American Physical Therapy Association (APTA): The national professional organization for physical therapists representing more than 72,000 members. Its goal is to advocate for the advancement of physical therapy practice, research, and education.

American Speech-Language-Hearing Association (ASHA): The professional, scientific, and credentialing association for audiologists, speech-language pathologists, and speech, language, and hearing scientists.

Audiologists: Professionals that work with people who have hearing, balance, and related ear problems, especially diagnosing and treating hearing loss. Audiology is regulated by licensure or registration in all 50 states.

Baby boomer: Individual born during a period of extreme population increase due to high birth rates. Generally refers to those born in the period following the end of World War II.

Brain drain: The large emigration of individuals with technical skills and knowledge from one (usually developing) country to another (usually developed) country. It generally is due to lack of opportunity, political conflict and instability, and poor working conditions in the home country.

Bureau of Labor Statistics: The principal fact-finding agency for the federal government in the broad field of labor economics and statistics.

Canadian Association of Speech-Language Pathologists and Audiologists (CASLPA): The national body that supports and represents the professional needs of speech-language pathologists, audiologists, and supportive personnel inclusively within one organization. The organization supports and empowers its members to maximize the communication and hearing potential of the people of Canada.

Career mobility: Progress in a chosen profession or during a person's working life.

Certification: A process indicating that an individual or institution has met predetermined standards.

Clinical practice acuity: The complexity of care required to meet patient care needs and goals.

Cohort: Statistically, a group of subjects defined by their common experience of an event in a particular time span.

Commission on Accreditation in Physical Therapy (CAPTE): The accreditation agency recognized by the U.S. Department of Education and the Council for Higher Education Accreditation to accredit entry-level physical therapist and physical therapist assistant education programs.

Council on Academic Accreditation in Audiology and Speech-Language Pathology (CAA): Accreditation board responsible for evaluating and accrediting master's programs in speech-language pathology and clinical doctoral programs in audiology.

Credentials evaluation: An analysis of an individual's qualifications, such as education and licensure, to ensure that they are comparable to U.S. qualifications.

Cultural competence: An ability to interact effectively with people of different cultures, often in the context of health care.

Grandfathering: To exempt a person involved in an activity, business, or profession from new regulations.

Health Care Worker Certificates: Health care worker certification documents indicating that the education, training, licensure, and English language proficiency of foreign health care workers have met U.S. comparability standards.

Internship: The program through which an individual can work as a trainee to gain practical, on-the-job experience for a specified amount of time.

Medical technicians: Medical technicians, or clinical laboratory technicians, perform less complex tests and laboratory procedures than medical technologists, typically have a 2-year specialized education, and are supervised by a medical technologist.

Medical technologists: Health care professionals who perform chemical, hematological, immunological, microscopic, and bacteriological diagnostic analyses on body fluids. Medical technologists, also known as clinical laboratory scientists, have at least a baccalaureate degree and work in clinical laboratories at hospitals, doctors' offices, and biotechnology laboratories.

Mentor: A senior or experienced person in a company or organization who gives guidance and training to a junior colleague; a wise and trusted teacher and counselor.

Mutual Recognition Agreement: An international agreement by which two or more countries agree to recognize one another's education, programs, licensure, and so forth, in an effort to increase mobility between and among the nations that sign the agreement.

National Commission on Certification of Physician Assistants (NCCPA): Credentialing organization for physician assistants in the United States. The credential certifies that the physician assistant meets established standards of knowledge and clinical skills upon entry into practice and throughout his or her career.

North American Free Trade Agreement (NAFTA): A trade agreement that allows for the exchange of products and services in North America, involving the United States, Canada, and Mexico.

Occupational therapists: Occupational therapists use treatments to develop, recover, or maintain the daily living and work skills of their patients. They work with individuals, families, groups, and populations to facilitate health and well-being through engagement or reengagement in an occupation.

Occupational therapy assistant (OTA): An occupational therapist assistant works under the direction of an occupational therapist to provide rehabilitative services to persons with mental, physical, emotional, or developmental impairments.

Physical therapists: Physical therapists provide services that help restore function, improve mobility, relieve pain, and prevent or limit permanent physical disabilities of patients suffering from injuries or disease. They restore, maintain, and promote overall fitness and health.

Physical therapist assistants: Physical therapist assistants and aides help physical therapists to provide treatment that improves patient mobility, relieves pain, and prevents or lessens physical disabilities of patients.

Physical therapy: A health care profession that provides services to clients in order to develop, maintain, and restore maximum movement and functional ability throughout life.

Physician assistants: Individuals formally trained to provide diagnostic, therapeutic, and preventive health care services, as delegated by a physician.

Practice doctorates: Practice-focused doctoral degrees as opposed to a research-focused doctoral degree, such as a PhD.

Preceptor: A specialist in a profession, especially health care, who gives practical training to a student or novice in the profession.

Professional autonomy: Responsible discretionary decision making by a profession or an individual within the profession; the quality or condition of being self-governing.

Professional fluency: The ability to discuss the motivation and reasoning behind research or general research trends in a particular field or profession.

Speech-language pathologists: Individuals with specialized education who assess, diagnose, treat, and help to prevent disorders related to speech, language, cognitive communication, voice, swallowing, and fluency.

U.S. Citizenship and Immigration Services (USCIS): The government agency that oversees lawful immigration to the United States. It establishes immigration services, policies, and priorities, and adjudicates (decides upon) the petitions and applications of potential immigrants.

U.S. Department of Labor (DOL): The government department responsible for improving working conditions and promoting opportunities for profitable employment in the United States.

World Federation of Occupational Therapists (WFOT): The international representative for occupational therapists and occupational therapy around the world and the official international organization for the promotion of occupational therapy.

The U.S. health care industry is rapidly expanding and has added 1.7 million jobs since 2001 (Business Week, September 25, 2006). The United States is facing a continued growth of health care jobs and a concurrent expanding shortage of health care professionals to fill these positions. Driven by a growing aging population (commonly the biggest user of health care services), changing technology, **clinical practice acuity,** *retirements of currently practicing professionals, and changing career choices of younger generations, the health provider shortages are expected to continue and expand.*

U.S. IMMIGRATION PATTERNS

Since its founding the United States has depended on workers from other countries to provide the labor and skills necessary to ensure development of the U.S. agricultural, manufacturing, and export industries. Early immigrant workers ranged from indentured servants and African and Caribbean slaves to Irish, Italian, and Polish mill and mine workers and Chinese railroad builders. Today the face of the immigrant is changing and includes skilled professionals in education, science, and technology from Africa, Asia, and Latin America.

Early Immigration Trends

While immigration has been ongoing since the time of the early U.S. settlers, the United States experienced a major wave of immigration in the 1800s as people began leaving their home countries because of crop failures, land and job shortages, rising taxes, and famine. Many came to the United States because it was seen to be the land of economic opportunity. Others came seeking personal freedom or relief from political and religious persecution. The majority of immigrants during this intense period of immigration arrived from Germany, Ireland, and England.

Migration Trends in the 20th Century

Migration patterns changed considerably in the 1900s. Not only did the number of immigrants increase, but the countries from which they came also changed—with the majority of immigrants coming from non-English-speaking European countries. The principal source of immigrants was now Southern and Eastern Europe, especially Italy, Poland, and Russia, countries quite different in culture and language from the U.S. population of that time, making adaptation to the new country more challenging than for previous immigrants.

Although each ethnic group demonstrated distinctive characteristics, the groups shared one overarching feature: they settled in urban areas and worked in jobs that native-born Americans did not want. In fact, they made up the bulk of the U.S. industrial labor pool, making possible the emergence of such industries as steel, coal, automobile, textile, and garment production, and enabling the United States to move to the front ranks of the world's economic giants.

By the mid-1900s migration patterns changed again. Restriction of immigration occurred sporadically over the course of the late 19th and early 20th centuries, but immediately after World War I (1914–1918) and into the early 1920s, Congress changed the nation's basic policy on immigration (Library of Congress, 2004).

Legislating Immigration

National Origins Act

The National Origins Act (also known as the Reed-Johnson Act) of 1924 not only restricted the number of immigrants who could enter the United States but also assigned slots according to quotas based on national origins. The Act limited the number of immigrants who could be admitted from any country to 2% of the number of persons from that country who were already living in the United States based on the 1890 census.

Approximately 86% of the 165,000 permitted entries were from the British Isles, France, Germany, and other Northern European countries.

The law was aimed at further restricting the Southern and Eastern Europeans who had begun to enter the country in large numbers beginning in the 1890s. However, it set no limits on immigration from the Western hemisphere, thus ushering in a new era in U.S. immigration history. Immigrants could and did move quite freely from Mexico, the Caribbean (including Jamaica, Barbados, and Haiti), and other parts of Central and South America.

Immigration and Nationality Act

The Immigration and Nationality Act (INA) was created in 1952. Before the INA, a variety of rulings governed immigration law but were not organized in one location. The Immigration and Nationality Act collected and codified many existing provisions and reorganized the structure of immigration law. The Act has been amended many times over the years, but is still the basic body of immigration law. The Immigration and Nationality Act of 1952 upheld the national origins quota system established by the Immigration Act of 1924, reinforcing this controversial system of immigrant selection.

The Hart-Celler Act

Immigration policy changed with passage of the Hart-Celler Act, an amendment to the Immigration and Nationality Act in 1965 that was a by-product of the civil rights revolution and a much more liberal immigration law.

This law replaced the quota system with preference categories based on family relationships and job skills, giving particular preference to potential immigrants with relatives in the United States and with occupations deemed critical by the **U.S. Department of Labor.** Immigrants were to be admitted by their skills and professions rather than by their nationality.

Immigration Today

The result of the Hart-Celler Act was that most legal immigrants now come to the United States from Asia and Latin America, rather than Europe. The Act also began the rejuvenation of the Asian American community in the United States by abolishing the strict quotas that had restricted immigration from Asia since 1882. After 1970, following an initial influx from European countries, immigrants began to come to the United States from such countries as Korea, China, India, the Philippines, and Pakistan, as well as countries in Africa, such as Nigeria, Egypt, and Ethiopia. By the beginning of the 21st century immigration to the United States had returned to its 1900 volume, and the United States once again became a nation formed and transformed by immigrants.

LEGISLATING FOREIGN-EDUCATED HEALTH CARE PROFESSIONAL IMMIGRATION

United States immigration policy has evolved over time to respond not just to the country's need for various labor skills but also to health care delivery needs. Foreign-educated health care professionals have been a part of the U.S. workforce for many years. However, their recruitment has ebbed and waned as the health care system has been challenged by demographic and economic changes and changing immigration laws. Today, limited data exist to verify the actual number of foreign-educated health care professionals in the United States.

Because of cyclical and often severe health care professional shortages, several immigration laws and regulations were implemented to facilitate the migration of foreign-educated health care professionals to the United States.

Creation of Schedule A

The Immigration Nursing Relief Act of 1989 created a unique visa category for nurses to address the severe nursing shortage of that time. Also under the Immigrant Nursing Relief Act, the Department of Labor (DOL) established a special category, referred to as Schedule A, in recognition of the continuing shortage not only of registered nurses but also of **physical therapists.**

Schedule A alleviates some of the documentation required of a sponsoring employer by the DOL for its labor **certification** process. Just as immigration can be an expensive process for foreign-educated health care professionals, labor certification is a complicated, labor-intensive, and expensive process for employers. Schedule A's core premise is to precertify those occupations for which there are few qualified, willing, and available U.S. workers. For Schedule A occupations, the Prevailing

Wage Determination request form that employers must complete goes directly to the **U.S. Citizenship and Immigration Services (USCIS)** for processing, bypassing the Department of Labor and streamlining the labor certification process.

Illegal Immigration Reform and Immigrant Responsibility Act

Enactment of the 1996 Illegal Immigration Reform and Immigrant Responsibility Act (IIRIRA) on September 30, 1996, resulted in significant changes to existing U.S. immigration laws. Although IIRIRA was promoted as an illegal immigration bill, its far-reaching provisions have had a serious impact on legal immigration as well. IIRIRA requires that all immigrants and nonimmigrants coming to the United States for the purpose of performing labor as health care workers on either a permanent or temporary basis must submit a Health Care Worker Certificate. This rule includes those seeking a change of nonimmigrant status. The regulations implementing IIRIRA became final in 2003. Health care workers listed under section 343 of IIRIRA include nurses, **occupational therapists, medical technologists, medical technicians,** physical therapists, **physician assistants,** and **speech-language pathologists/audiologists.**

Federal Screening Program

The 1996 Act required that all health care professionals, except physicians, seeking an occupational visa to enter the United States for employment purposes undergo a federal screening program. By law, this screening program requires that foreign health care professionals have their education, licensure, and experience evaluated to ensure comparability to those of an entry-level U.S. health care professional of the same profession. The screening is required for foreign-educated health care professionals seeking an occupational visa to work in the United States. You should be aware that if you were born outside of, but were educated in, the United States, by law you must undergo the federal screening program when applying for an occupational visa.

The occupational visa gives entry into the country. However, to work as a health care professional, you also must meet state requirements for practice. In many states and for most professions, this means having a license to practice that has been granted by the state regulatory body for your profession.

Approved Federal Screening Agencies

CGFNS was named in IIRIRA to conduct the federal screening program for all health care professionals, and developed its VisaScreen® Program to meet the law's requirements. The National Board for Certification in Occupational Therapy (NBCOT®) and the Foreign Credentialing Commission on Physical Therapy (FCCPT) were named in the regulations implementing the 1996 law to conduct the federal screening program for foreign-educated occupational therapists and physical therapists respectively.

The USCIS requires that each of these organizations evaluate the health care worker's education to determine comparability to that required of a U.S. health care entry professional in the same discipline, including specified competencies and clinical or field work experience. Additionally, Section 343 of IIRIRA requires verification of written and spoken English proficiency, through testing by specified examinations, unless the applicant is exempt. Exemptions for the English proficiency requirement include completion of entry professional programs in Australia, Canada (except Quebec), Ireland, New Zealand, the United Kingdom, or the United States when the textbooks and instruction were in English. Finally, the organizations must determine that all of the applicant's current and previously held professional licenses are valid and unencumbered. Please refer to CGFNS (www.cgfns.org), FCCPT (www.fccpt.org), and NBCOT (www.nbcot.org) for detailed requirements and applications. See chapter 3 for a more in-depth discussion of the 1996 law and its requirements.

CGFNS International

CGFNS is an immigration-neutral, nonprofit organization, internationally recognized as an authority on **credentials evaluation** related to the education, registration, and licensure of nurses and other health care professionals worldwide. It protects the public by ensuring that nurses and other health care professionals educated in countries other than the United States are eligible and qualified to meet licensure, immigration, and other practice requirements in the United States. CGFNS not only validates international professional credentials but also supports international regulatory and educational standards for health care professionals.

CGFNS has three programs that are used by foreign-educated health care professionals to meet federal and state requirements for employment in the United States: the VisaScreen Program, the Credentials Evaluation Service, and the New York Credentials Verification Service.

- The VisaScreen Program is a U.S. government-mandated program that ensures that a foreign-educated health care professional's education, licensure, and experience are comparable to those of U.S. graduates; that the individual's license is valid, current, and without penalties; that he or she has proficiency in written and oral English; and that the individual has passed either a test predicting success on the occupation's licensing or certification examination (provided such a test is recognized by a majority of states licensing the occupation for which the certification is issued), or has passed the occupation's licensing or certification examination.
- By law, CGFNS was named to screen all health care professionals, except physicians. Final regulations implementing the 1996 immigration law granted CGFNS approval to issue **Health Care Worker Certificates** to foreign-educated health care professionals coming to the United States to work as **medical technologists** and technicians, nurses, occupational therapists, physical therapists, physician assistants, and speech-language pathologists and audiologists.
- The **Credentials Evaluation Service** (CES) provides a written analysis of a foreign-educated health care professional's education and licensure in terms of U.S. comparability, identifies what the individual's education and licensure give access to in his or her home country and in the United States, and provides an analysis of the individual's coursework based on U.S. standards. The CES provides detailed reports for regulatory bodies, educational programs, and employers. Two levels of report are available: Health Care Profession and Science Course-by-Course Report and Full Education Course-by-Course Report.
- The New York Credentials Verification Service (NYCVS) obtains the academic transcripts and licensure validations of foreign-educated health care professionals directly from the issuing agencies, verifies their authenticity, and provides a report to the New York State Department of Education. The state then evaluates the credentials to determine comparability to U.S. education and licensure. This service is used by nurses, physical therapists,

physical therapist assistants, occupational therapists, and **occupational therapy assistants.**

National Board for Certification in Occupational Therapy

The United States Citizenship and Immigration Services (USCIS) granted the National Board for Certification in Occupational Therapy, Inc. (NBCOT) approval to issue Health Care Worker Certificates to foreign-educated health care professionals coming to the United States to work in the field of occupational therapy. NBCOT's (2008a) Health Care Worker Certificates are known as Visa Credential Verification Certificates (VCVC). For more information on the Visa Credentials Verification program, which meets the federal screening requirements for occupational therapists seeking a visa to enter the United States for employment purposes, you may access the NBCOT Web site at http://www.nbcot.org.

Foreign Credentialing Commission on Physical Therapy

The USCIS granted the Foreign Credentialing Commission on Physical Therapy (FCCPT) approval to issue Health Care Worker Certificates to foreign-educated health care professionals coming to the United States to work in the field of **physical therapy.** FCCPT's (2008a) screening program is known as Visa Credentials Certification (VCC). For more information on the FCCPT Comprehensive Credentials Evaluation (Type I Certificate), which meets the federal screening requirements for physical therapists seeking a visa to enter the United States for employment purposes, access the FCCPT Web site at http://www.fccpt.org.

HISTORY OF FOREIGN-EDUCATED HEALTH CARE PROFESSIONALS IN THE U.S. WORKFORCE

Demographics

The majority of foreign-educated health care professionals seeking a VisaScreen Certificate from CGFNS for visa purposes are in the 29–31 age range. The youngest (29 years) were educated as physical therapists and occupational therapists and the oldest (36 years) were educated as medical technicians.

A review of Health Care Worker Certificates issued by CGFNS, FCCPT, and NBCOT indicates that physical therapists represent the largest number of **allied health professionals** receiving Health Care Worker Certificates, followed by medical technologists, speech-language pathologists, and occupational therapists. Table 1.1 presents the number of certificates (required for the visa process) that were issued by CGFNS (2008), FCCPT (2008b), and NBCOT (2008b) in 2006. Table 1.2 presents the number of certificates issued by the three entities in 2007.

Countries of Education

Data from CGFNS International in 2007, which included nurses in their totals, listed the top five countries of education for VisaScreen applicants as the Philippines, India, United States, Canada, and South Korea. NBCOT's (2008) Visa Credential Verification Certificate Program for

Table 1.1

HEALTH CARE WORKER CERTIFICATES ISSUED BY CGFNS, FCCPT, AND NBCOT IN 2006

	CGFNS	FCCPT	NBCOT	TOTAL
Physical therapist	559	1,049		1,608
Medical technologist (clinical laboratory scientist)	777			777
Speech-language pathologist	135			135
Occupational therapist	39		288	327
Clinical laboratory technician	16			16
Physician assistant	<15			<15
Audiologist	<15			<15

Data compiled from CGFNS VisaScreen® Program data, 2006; FCCPT Summary of Credential Review, 2006; and NBCOT, Visa Credential Verification Year End Review, 2006.

Table 1.2

HEALTH CARE WORKER CERTIFICATES ISSUED BY CGFNS, FCCPT, AND NBCOT IN 2007

	CGFNS	FCCPT	NBCOT	TOTAL
Physical therapist	362	834		1,196
Medical technologist (clinical laboratory scientist)	697			697
Speech-language pathologist	154			154
Occupational therapist	<15		255	255 + less than 15
Clinical laboratory technician	<15			<15
Physician assistant	<15			<15
Audiologist	<15			<15

Data compiled from CGFNS VisaScreen® Program data, 2007; FCCPT Summary of Credential Review, 2007; and NBCOT, Visa Credential Verification Year End Review, 2007.

occupational therapists listed the top five countries of birth for 2007 as the Philippines (153), India (32), Canada (29), Taiwan (10), and Australia (6). These numbers include foreign-born as well as foreign-educated professionals because all foreign-born allied health professionals seeking occupational visas, including those educated in the United States must, by law, obtain a Health Care Worker Certificate.

The United States is one of the top receiving countries for migrating health workers (Association of Academic Health Centers, 2008). Factors attracting immigration include a growing health profession market, higher salaries, better working conditions, and availability of advanced technology. As health care professional shortages continue to grow, many potential U.S. students are investigating other high technological and advanced careers rather than health care–related disciplines. At a time when the United States needs to be actively recruiting foreign health care professionals, changing educational requirements, licensure and regulation requirements, and visa delays are increasingly creating unintended barriers.

EMPLOYMENT TRENDS

Baby Boomers

The **baby boomer** population, the large population **cohort** born from 1946 to 1964, has impacted the United States continually through their large numbers and emerging ideas and expectations. Boomers, as this cohort is known, are enjoying longevity and will be using health care services at unprecedented rates to maximize their functioning as they begin a retirement period that is expected to be more active than that of previous generations. The boomers also are planning retirements in record numbers, which will deplete the health service provider pool.

Health Care Professions

Some health care professions, like nursing, already have documented that their retirements of doctorally prepared professionals are greater than their graduations from doctoral programs in specified regions of the country. Further, study of the emerging generations indicates that many do not view the health professions as a top career choice. Those who do enter the health care professions may desire more part-time opportunities for practice in order to create a more balanced lifestyle. Current employment trends already indicate many health care professionals are choosing part-time employment.

As these trends fueling shortages of qualified health care professionals become more acute, the United States will need to rethink policy and practice to enhance the ease of **career mobility** for all providers (Collier, 2008). Foreign-educated health care professionals offer one strategy for meeting the U.S. and global health care needs of this rapidly growing health services market.

PREDICTED GROWTH IN THE HEALTH CARE PROFESSIONS

The U.S. Department of Labor, **Bureau of Labor Statistics** (BLS, 2008–2009a), documents current employment and predicts employment growth for audiologists, speech-language pathologists, medical technologists, medical technicians, occupational therapists, physician assistants, and physical therapists. Data are updated every 2 years. Although nursing as well as rural and underserved physician markets have large vacancy rates and perhaps represent the largest health care shortage crisis statistics, the shortages in other key health care professions may represent some of the largest needed percentage increases and some of the greatest opportunities for impacting health care delivery as professional roles rebalance to meet market demands.

The use of foreign-educated health care professionals varies by profession and fluctuates as professions grow and evolve with the practice market. Summary occupational data from the Bureau of Labor Statistics (BLS) highlight current market employment and predict significant job market growth by profession.

Demands of an aging population challenge every health profession to expand opportunities and services. Bureau of Labor Statistics data are discussed in the following section for audiologists, speech-language pathologists, medical technologists, medical technicians, occupational therapists, physician assistants, and physical therapists. Table 1.3 summarizes

Table 1.3

HEALTH WORKFORCE EMPLOYMENT 2006–2016

OCCUPATION	EMPLOYMENT NUMBER		CHANGE	
	2006	2016	NUMBER	PERCENT
Physical therapists	173,000	220,000	47,000	27
Medical and clinical laboratory technologists	167,000	188,000	21,000	12
Medical and clinical laboratory technicians	151,000	174,000	23,000	15
Occupational therapists	99,000	122,000	23,000	23
Physician assistants	66,000	83,000	18,000	27
Speech-language pathologists	110,000	121,000	12,000	11
Audiologists	12,000	13,200	1,200	10
Total	**778,000**	**921,200**	**145,200**	

Note: Numbers are rounded.
From U.S. Department of Labor; Bureau of Labor Statistics, 2008–2009a.

the BLS (2008–2009a) current employment data and 10-year employment projection for each of these professions.

Audiology

Audiologists comprise a smaller employment base than many of the other health care professions, approximately 12,000 jobs in 2006. Most audiologists stay employed in their careers until retirement, limiting professional turnover. The BLS (2008–2009b) predicts an average growth of 10% between 2006 and 2016, accounting for an additional 1,200 jobs by 2016.

Certain public health studies look at the immense need for audiologists over the next 10 years. The demand will become great and the supply will have to increase for several reasons. As seniors age and enjoy longevity, the numbers of services needed are expected to grow exponentially to accommodate the expanding population. Approximately 30% of those over 75 years of age will experience hearing loss and require the attention of an audiologist. This is a significant number of people at only one end of the spectrum. The need to look at the universal evaluation of infants is equally important as is evaluation of the adult who experiences hearing loss from extraneous noises, such as iPods®, concerts, and acoustics in public places.

Foreign-Educated Audiologists

Some foreign-educated audiologists are employed in the United States and were employed and licensed prior to the new doctoral preparation standards. However, the new requirement for a doctorate for licensure (effective January, 2009) may slow U.S. production and at least temporarily limit entry of the foreign-educated audiologist into the United States for this profession.

CGFNS (2007) VisaScreen Program data reported that less than 15 foreign-educated audiologists were issued Health Care Worker (VisaScreen) Certificates in 2007. This pattern has held true since 2003 and may be reflective of the U.S. educational requirements for audiologists.

Speech-Language Pathology

Speech-language pathologists held approximately 110,000 jobs in 2006. The profession is projected to grow 11% by 2016, gaining 12,000 additional positions. Growth in employment is expected with the aging population and in school systems with growth in elementary and secondary schools, where about half of all speech-language pathologists are currently employed. The market is expected to be especially favorable for speech-language pathologists who speak a second language to assist with the diversified U.S. population (BLS, 2008–2009c).

Foreign-Educated Speech-Language Pathologists

In reviewing 2004 CGFNS VisaScreen Program Data, Pendergast (2005) found 153 Health Care Worker certificates were issued to speech-language pathologists and audiologists combined. In 2007, 154 Health Care Worker certificates were issued, indicating a stable pattern.

Medical Technology

Medical technology represents a current shortage area in the United States with more vacancies than available professionals. Rapid job growth is anticipated. Together, medical technologists (also referred to as clinical laboratory scientists) and medical technicians (also referred to as clinical laboratory technicians) represented approximately 319,000 jobs in 2006. That total is projected to reach 362,000 by 2016. Foreign-educated health professionals employed as medical laboratory technologists and technicians must meet requirements for practice that vary by state.

For medical technologists, the BLS (2008–2009d) predicts an average growth of 12%, an increase of 21,000 new jobs by 2016. For medical technicians, 15% new job growth is expected, an increase of 23,000 jobs by 2016. As individuals age and develop chronic conditions, primary practitioners routinely monitor laboratory values as part of standard care. This adds to the need for more professionals to manage these tests. Additionally, new testing procedures are evolving as technology grows, not only increasing efficiency but also adding to a greater demand for medical technologists and technicians.

Foreign-Educated Medical Technologists and Technicians

In 2004 CGFNS issued 610 medical technologist (clinical laboratory scientist) VisaScreen certificates. While this number was far below nursing with 15,613 certificates, medical technologists represented the third highest number of Health Care Worker certificates issued.

Medical laboratory technicians were issued only 39 Health Care Worker Certificates. In reviewing CGFNS VisaScreen Program data, 697 VisaScreen Certificates were issued to medical technologists in 2007, showing an increase of 87 certificates over 2004. Medical laboratory technicians in 2007 were recorded as receiving less than 15 certificates, data showing a decrease in certificates issued.

Occupational Therapy

Occupational therapy represents both a shortage market and a rapid growth area for the future. Approximately 99,000 occupational therapists were employed in 2006. The Bureau of Labor Statistics (2008–2009e) predicts the employment of occupational therapists will rise 23% between 2006 and 2016. This will create the need for an additional 23,000 professionals and projected employment of 122,000 occupational therapists. Employment opportunities may be especially abundant with the elderly as a "graying" or aging United States drives the demand for rehabilitation services and assistance with everyday life skills.

Foreign-Educated Occupational Therapists

In 2004, a total of 411 Health Care Worker Certificates were issued to foreign-educated occupational therapists by CGFNS and NBCOT: CGFNS issued 91 of these and NBCOT issued 320. In 2007, occupational therapists were awarded less than 15 certificates from CGFNS and only 131 from NBCOT (2008). The change to a graduate educational requirement (postbaccalaureate) for occupational therapists, the difference in practice areas, and the ability to practice more independently in the United States may have accounted for the change.

Physician Assistants

The physician assistant profession is predicted by BLS (2008–2009f) to be a rapid growth market in the United States, increasing from 66,000 jobs in 2006 to estimates of 83,000 jobs by 2016. This 27% increase is predicted based on the ever-expanding needs of the aging population, coupled with the cost-effective use of physician assistants for routine care and in high physician shortage areas.

Foreign-Educated Physician Assistants

Currently, foreign-educated physician assistants are not employed as physician assistants in the U.S. market as this profession requires graduation from an accredited physician assistant program and these programs have been exclusively in the United States. However, Pendergast (2005) listed four physician assistants as receiving CGFNS VisaScreen Certificates. A foreign-born but U.S-educated health care professional also requires a Health Care Worker Certificate by law and this requirement accounts for the VisaScreen Certificates issued to physician assistants. In the CGFNS data for 2007, physician assistants were recorded as receiving less than 15 certificates.

Physical Therapy

Physical therapy is another rapid-growth health profession market fueled by the aging population and the need for rehabilitation for chronic conditions. The survival of newborns with birth defects and the survival of trauma victims due to enhanced technology and health care practices also will add to the demand for physical therapy services. Most states have a vacancy rate for physical therapists. Physical therapists held approximately 173,000 jobs in 2006 and have a projected employment of 220,000 jobs by 2016, up 47,000 new positions and representing a 27% increase (BLS, 2008–2009g).

Foreign-Educated Physical Therapists

Physical therapy has also been a leader in facilitating the immigration of physical therapists. Physical therapists must meet additional state/jurisdiction requirements to be able to practice in this country. In the Pendergast (2005) analysis of Health Care Worker Certificates issued in 2004, physical therapists received the second-highest number of certificates awarded. Physical therapists received a total of 1,247 Health Care Worker Certificates; CGFNS issued 465 and FCCPT issued 782 certificates.

In 2006, total Health Care Worker Certificates awarded from these two agencies (CGFNS and FCCPT) totaled 1,049, down 198 certificates from the 2004 baseline. However, physical therapists received a total of 1,196 Health Care Worker Certificates in 2007. The CGFNS (2008) reported issuing 362 Health Care Worker Certificates and FCCPT (2008) reported issuing 834 Health Care Worker Certificates in 2007.

While the 2007 number of certificates is still below the 2004 data by 51 certificates, it was higher than 2006. Any downward change represents a disturbing concern since the shortage of physical therapists in the United States is growing rapidly at the same time that the educational level for entry into the profession is increasing rapidly. Refer to Table 1.1 and Table 1.2 for a summary of Health Care Worker Certificates issued across professions during 2006 and 2007.

ISSUES RELATED TO MIGRATION

Cultural Competence

Cultural competence is an area of concern for all health care providers, appearing more and more frequently in articles, research, and educational curriculums across the United States. Cultural competence is the ability to interact effectively with people of different cultures. The concern for health care professionals is one of delivering culturally competent care to patients from very different backgrounds and educational levels.

As the United States rapidly becomes more diverse, educators and providers in all the professions are attempting to recruit students and practitioners from diverse backgrounds to help meet the needs of a diverse population. The foreign-educated health professional has much to contribute to the changing U.S. diversity and also much to learn from that diversity as different cultures mix in the U.S. health care practice environment.

A related but critical issue is English proficiency. In addition to the cultural mix of patients and health care professionals, there also is a mix of languages and accents. Although language proficiency for foreign-educated health care professionals is a required competence prior to coming to the United States, **professional fluency** often may require practice in the country and unique geographic region for full language conversation skill to develop. See chapter 8 for a more in-depth discussion of language issues and challenges.

Ethics of Migration

Globalization of the health care workforce has enabled health care professionals to further their careers through migration. With the increase in global migration, there has been a corresponding increase in the number of international recruiters and recruiting firms, some of which have aggressively pursued health care professionals to work in developed countries. This aggressive recruitment has led, in some instances, to the serious depletion of the health care workforce, particularly in developing countries and countries that could ill afford to lose their health care professionals.

Brain Drain

Since the 1960s, concerns have been raised about the ethical considerations of immigration of highly skilled health care workers from developing countries. The term **brain drain** has been coined and discussed in various arenas, but especially as it relates to the recruitment of foreign-educated health care professionals. Brain drain is the large emigration of individuals with technical skills and knowledge from one (usually developing) country to another (usually developed) country. It generally occurs because of lack of opportunity, political conflict and instability, and poor working conditions in their home country.

Professional Autonomy

Parallel to the concern of brain drain are two issues: the right of the individual to migrate and **professional autonomy.** Professional autonomy is the responsible discretionary decision making by a profession or an individual within the profession—the quality or condition of being self-governing. Proponents of professional choice argue that professionals have the right to select the country and place of practice as well as the right to seek rewarding professional development and career advancement opportunities (Association of Academic Health Centers, 2008). Most health care agencies recognize that quality health care is directly dependent on an adequate supply of health care professionals in the country and also recognize the right of the individual health care professional to migrate.

Interdisciplinary Challenges

Practice in the complex U.S. health market is exciting, sometimes confusing, and often stressful. Professional shortages can contribute to workload strain. Changing educational expectations support expanding roles and often add to interdisciplinary overlap of activities, creating tension and conflict. However, opportunities to provide the highest level of care within a talented interdisciplinary team are equally a part of an evolving everyday practice in the United States.

ENTRY INTO PRACTICE IN THE UNITED STATES

Practice Doctorates

The United States is experiencing a rapid proliferation of expanding educational requirements for health care professionals that is not being paralleled in other countries. Many professions have identified the need for a **practice doctorate** to prepare members for a changing health care environment. Most practice doctorates require approximately 8 years of university education, incorporating varying amounts of clinical supervision. As practice doctorates become established, practice roles probably will change, redefining basic entry and advanced practice requirements throughout the professions.

Within the last 10 years, occupational therapy has changed its requirements for entry into practice from a baccalaureate to a master's degree and is now developing the doctorate. Audiology has moved to a doctorate degree for entry. Physician assistants have elevated education requirements from predominantly baccalaureate preparation to predominantly master's entry preparation. Physical therapy has moved from the bachelor's degree to the master's degree for entry and is rapidly adding practice doctorate programs and approaching the entry doctorate.

Audiology

Audiology now requires the professional doctorate (AuD) as an entry degree in all states. The **Accreditation Commission for Audiology Education (ACAE),** a new accrediting agency, began to award accreditation in 2007. Since January 1, 2007, the **Council on Academic Accreditation in Audiology and Speech-Language Pathology (CAA)** awards candidacy, initial accreditation, or re-accreditation only to doctoral level programs in audiology (CAA, 2008).

The majority of states require audiologists to be licensed or certified. Traditionally, licensure or certification required a master's degree. The **Canadian Association of Speech-Language Pathologists and**

Audiologists (CASLPA) has been actively discussing the professional doctorate since 2002. In a 2007 position paper, CASLPA reported survey results indicating that 51.5% of respondents supported implementing the professional doctorate (AuD) as an entry level to the profession in Canada, while **grandfathering** in practicing master's prepared audiologists.

However, almost two-thirds of the survey's respondents expressed concern regarding the implications that the entry to practice decision will have for the **Mutual Recognition Agreement (MRA)** between CASLPA and the **American Speech-Language-Hearing Association (ASHA).** Both CASLPA and ASHA award professional certification. The MRA mutually recognizes the certification programs of CASLPA and ASHA and expedites the certification review process for individuals to work in the signatory countries. Canada still is exploring the entry issue.

Foreign-Educated Audiologists. The U.S. professional education requirement of a doctorate for audiologists has limited the entry into practice of foreign-educated audiologists. Foreign-educated audiology graduates who do not hold a doctoral degree in the specialty cannot be licensed in the United States at this time because their entry-level degrees do not meet U.S. comparability requirements. Negotiations are under way regarding possibilities for managing this new issue, especially with Canada. Practicing foreign-educated audiologists, who were in the United States and held licensure or certification prior to the doctoral requirement—like U.S.-educated audiologists—may continue to practice but may be limited in movement throughout the 50 states because of state licensure restrictions.

Speech-Language Pathology

Most speech-language pathologists in the United States are educated at the master's level. The American Speech-Language-Hearing Association (ASHA) awards certification to speech-language pathologists, recognizing clinical competence. Speech-language pathologists seeking ASHA certification must possess an earned graduate degree, typically a master's degree.

Foreign-Educated Speech-Language Pathologists. Foreign-educated speech-language pathologists applying for ASHA certification must undergo a credentials evaluation by a recognized credentials review agency. Such an agency provides verification that the individual's degree is comparable to a U.S. master's degree. If degree comparability is confirmed by the evaluating agency, an application for certification may be submitted to ASHA.

Acquisition of the requisite knowledge and skills and the appropriate number of graduate semester credit hours and clinical practicum hours as outlined in the ASHA Certification Standards will be determined. Individuals educated internationally also must complete a clinical fellowship supervised by an individual holding current ASHA certification, must take and pass the Praxis examination offered by the Educational Testing Service (ETS), and must submit appropriate dues/fees.

Mutual Recognition Agreements

A multilateral Mutual Recognition Agreement recognizing the certificate programs in speech-language pathology conducted by six signatories became effective January 1, 2008. The signatories include ASHA, the Canadian Association of Speech-Language Pathologists and Audiologists (CASLPA), the Irish Association of Speech and Language Therapists (IASLT), the New Zealand Speech-Language Therapists' Association (NZSTA), the Royal College of Speech and Language Therapists in the United Kingdom, and the Speech Pathology Association of Australia Limited. This agreement recognizes the degrees earned in these countries as being substantially equivalent to a U.S. master's degree.

The agreement expedites the certification review process for speech-language pathologists wishing to gain certification by the listed countries (ASHA, 2008). It does not, however, guarantee individuals, at least in the United States, that they will be eligible for a state license that will permit them to work.

Medical Technology

The education, certification, and registration of medical technologists and medical technicians are, like other disciplines, changing. Currently, medical technology requires a baccalaureate degree in either medical technology or a related life science. Medical technicians usually hold an associate degree or certificate. Presently 11 states require a technologist to hold the baccalaureate and pass an examination to be licensed or registered, but this varies state to state. Licensure has been proposed in several more states as the profession seeks to enhance regulatory consistency.

Foreign-Educated Medical Technologists and Technicians. A professional doctorate in Clinical Laboratory Science (DCLS) has been proposed by the American Society for Clinical Laboratory Science. The clinical doctorate is not viewed as an entry level for the profession but as an additional level of education to provide new opportunities for the clinical laboratory scientist (medical technologist). The new educational direction should not adversely affect foreign-educated health care professionals seeking employment as medical technologists or medical technicians. Since 697 medical technologists were awarded Health Care Worker Certificates to practice in the United States in 2007, foreign-educated medical technologists are receiving education deemed to be comparable to education in the United States.

Occupational Therapy

A master's degree or higher in occupational therapy, which includes a supervised fieldwork experience, is required for entry into practice. Occupational therapy moved from a baccalaureate requirement as preparation for occupational therapy to a master's requirement for entry into professional practice within the last 10 years. This degree change also reflects higher standards of accepted practice. Currently, occupational therapy has recognized the need for additional education and is developing and opening professional/practice doctorate programs (OTD). These programs are developing as additional education opportunities rather than entry requirements.

Most states require occupational therapists to be licensed. The National Board for Certification in Occupational Therapy (NBCOT) certifies occupational therapists, including foreign-educated occupational therapists. Currently, 47 states, Guam, Puerto Rico, and the District of Columbia require NBCOT certification for the licensing of occupational therapists (NBCOT, 2008).

Foreign-Educated Occupational Therapists. NBCOT and CGFNS issue Health Care Worker Certificates in occupational therapy to foreign-educational occupational therapists. The postbaccalaureate or graduate educational requirement, the difference in practice areas, and the need to practice more independently are at least temporarily restricting some occupational therapists' entry into the United States. The **World Federation of Occupational Therapists (WFOT)** is the official international organization for occupational therapists from around the world.

This organization (www.wfot.org) lists specific educational programs with contact information and the educational requirements of each program from countries around the world (World Federation of Occupational Therapists, 2008).

Physician Assistants

The education of physician assistants (PAs) originated in the United States in the mid-1960s. PAs are academically and clinically prepared to provide medical services under the direction and responsible supervision of a doctor of medicine or osteopathy. The physician/PA team relationship is fundamental to the PA profession and enhances the delivery of high-quality health care.

Although PA programs were originally offered and accredited primarily at the bachelor's level, the vast majority are now offered and accredited at the graduate level and award a master's degree. All jurisdictions require the PA to pass the Physician Assistant National Certifying Examination, which is administered by the **National Commission on Certification of Physician Assistants (NCCPA)** and open only to graduates of nationally accredited physician assistant programs.

All U.S. physician assistant programs are accredited by the **Accreditation Review Commission on Education for Physician Assistants (ARC-PA),** an independent accrediting body authorized to accredit qualified educational programs leading to the professional credential, Physician Assistant (PA). Optional postgraduate (following entry-level education) residencies are available in 15 specialty areas but there is no specialty certification.

Foreign-Educated Physician Assistants. Since no foreign education programs are accredited by the ARC-PA and most foreign programs are just emerging, only graduates of U.S. physician assistant programs currently are eligible to take the examination for entry into practice. Foreign physicians are not eligible to take the exam unless they have attended, and graduated from, an accredited PA program. According to the **American Academy of Physician Assistants (AAPA;** 2008), there are no set standards of education, licensing, credentialing, or reciprocity for PAs to work in other countries. Other countries developing PA practice and education include Canada, the United Kingdom, the Netherlands, and Australia.

Canada has employed U.S.-educated physician assistants for years and has a military Canadian Forces school that was accredited by the

Canadian Medical Association in 2004. In 2007, Canada employed approximately 150 physician assistants, mostly in the military. Canada has recently opened two civilian physician assistant programs at Canadian universities with initial 2-year program graduates expected to emerge in 2010 with different degrees. McMaster University PAs will earn a Bachelor of Health Science degree. The University of Manitoba requires a baccalaureate degree for entry and their graduates will earn a master's degree (Canadian Medical Association, 2008).

The United Kingdom has worked extensively on the development of a PA model and released a competence and curriculum framework for physician assistants. Physician assistants have been working in Scotland as part of a 2-year demonstration since 2006. Australia has launched a South Australia Health PA trial in which U.S. physician assistants are recruited to work one year in surgery, anesthesia, perioperative medicine, and pediatrics (AAPA, 2008).

Physical Therapy

The master's degree and doctoral degree both serve as entry degrees for physical therapists. The profession stopped accrediting baccalaureate programs in physical therapy in 2001. Since 2002, the **Commission on Accreditation in Physical Therapy (CAPTE)** accredits only master's and doctoral programs.

The **American Physical Therapy Association,** or APTA (2008), adopted a vision statement advocating that all physical therapists would have the doctorate (DPT) by 2020 and may have advanced certification. Master's programs are approximately 2 years in length; doctoral programs are approximately three years in length. As of October 2008, more than 92% of programs offered the DPT. A review of the list of CAPTE (2008) accredited programs indicates that most programs no longer offer the master's entry degree as they replace it with the doctorate entry degree. The CAPTE expects that by 2010, 99.5% of all physical therapy programs will offer the doctorate degree. Many programs have added transitional doctorate programs for postprofessional training to licensed physical therapists.

A license is required to practice as a physical therapist in all states. An applicant for the licensure examination must have graduated from an accredited physical therapy program. Specialty certification is available postlicensure in one of seven areas and requires additional hours of practice in the specialty area. It also requires passing a specialty examination, and may require additional education. Residencies are available in five specialty areas and fellowships are available in four areas.

Foreign-Educated Physical Therapists. Three physical therapy programs located outside the United States are listed as being accredited by CAPTE. These are the Robert Gordon University in the United Kingdom offering the master of science in physiotherapy, the University of Toronto in Canada, and the University of Western Ontario, Canada, both offering the master of science in physiology.

IMMIGRATION AND JOB NEEDS IN HEALTH CARE

Immigration is exceedingly complex and time consuming, requiring patience and perseverance. The U.S. Citizenship and Immigration Services (USCIS), a branch of the Department of Homeland Security, requires foreign-educated health care workers to apply for, and receive, authorization to work legally in the United States. Employment visas may be temporary (nonimmigrant) or permanent (immigrant). Temporary visas are valid for a specified time (usually 3 years); a permanent visa continues until it is either revoked or abandoned (Department of Homeland Security, 2003). Temporary visa classifications used by foreign-educated health care professionals include H-1B and the **North American Free Trade Agreement (NAFTA)** or Trade NAFTA (TN) classification.

H-1B Visas

The H-1B visa requires the health care professional to hold the equivalent of a baccalaureate degree—and the position the applicant is seeking must require a baccalaureate degree or higher. Physical therapists, occupational therapists, medical technologists, speech-language pathologists, audiologists, and physician assistants qualify for the H-1B visa. The visa usually is granted for 3 years with an option to renew for another 3 years. There is a 6-year limit. After the 6-year limit, the worker must spend 1 year outside the country to be eligible for another H-1B visa.

Trade NAFTA Status

NAFTA allows for the free movement of trade among the United States, Canada, and Mexico and covers select health professionals known as

"TNs" for "Trade NAFTA." A citizen in a NAFTA country may work in a professional occupation in another NAFTA country provided the profession is identified under NAFTA. Physical therapists, occupational therapists, medical technologists, and registered nurses are on the NAFTA list. Audiologists, speech-language pathologists, physician assistants, and medical technicians are not on the NAFTA list.

Requirements for Canadian citizens and Mexican citizens differ. A TN Canadian physical therapist, occupational therapist, or medical technologist need only show proof of employment, Canadian citizenship, and a Health Care Worker Certificates to enter the United States for employment purposes. The TN status must be renewed every three years but is not limited in the number of times it can be renewed. Mexican citizens must meet additional requirements. The TN health care professional would still be required to meet state licensure requirements before beginning practice in the United States.

Permanent Visas

Permanent residence in the United States is signified by a permanent residence card, often called a green card. Obtaining permanent status is shorter for registered nurses and physical therapists because of the well-established shortages in these disciplines, which allow members of both professions to apply for permanent status as Schedule A workers. For other health care professionals, the process takes longer because it requires that the prospective employer determine if there are any other U.S. workers willing and able to do the job. Once issued, the green card must be renewed every 10 years. For more in-depth information on visas for foreign-educated health care professionals, please see chapter 3.

TRANSITION TO HEALTH CARE PRACTICE IN THE UNITED STATES

Beginning practice in a new country can be both exciting and challenging. You will meet new colleagues and friends, and will be introduced to a new health care system and new technologies. Initially, you may feel intimidated, but over time you will begin to understand the new system and how care is provided within that system.

Navigating immigration, moving to the United States, obtaining state licensure, and becoming comfortable in a health care system different from your own can be a lengthy, sometimes challenging process—a process that balances the needs of migrating health care professionals with protection of the U.S. public. However, meeting the challenges of migration provides unlimited career opportunities.

Orientation to Practice

Because preparation is critical to safe practice, hospitals, long-term care institutions, schools, and other employing facilities want the foreign-educated health care professional to succeed and are willing to create an orientation that truly facilitates your transition to U.S. practice. It is your responsibility to let orientation leaders know how effective the orientation is, answering such questions as: What made sense and what did not? Did you need more information about or assistance with a specific aspect of health care delivery? Did you need more time to process the information? In other words, do not be afraid to speak up so that the orientation is meaningful for you.

Support Systems

Another factor that is crucial to having a smooth transition to practice is having a support system in place. Support systems are vital to a foreign-educated health care professional's ability to adapt to practice in the United States. Be sure to ask if the facility has an **internship** program, or if the facility will provide you with a **preceptor** to assist you through the transition period.

The delivery of health care in the United States can be complex and challenging. A **mentor** or preceptor can guide you through the transition and help you to understand how processes within the health care system relate to each other, thus ensuring safe practice. A mentor is a senior or experienced person in a company or organization who gives guidance and training to a junior colleague. A mentor is considered a wise and trusted teacher and counselor. The mentor relationship is not limited to a specific task or time frame but generally lasts over a period of years. A preceptor is a specialist in a profession, especially health care, who gives practical training to a student or novice in a profession. The relationship may or may not last after completion of the period of preceptorship. The difference between a mentor and a preceptor is that the mentor is chosen by the junior colleague and agrees to serve in that role. Often times the mentoring relationship is lifelong. A preceptor is assigned the role as part of his or her employment responsibilities and the role is time limited.

Variations in Health Care Systems

The more similar your health care system is to that of the United States, the easier your transition and the more comfortable you will be in your chosen clinical setting. You can then focus on specific practice needs rather than the transition process. Since health care systems vary greatly from country to country, it is essential that you have an understanding of how the U.S. system works. This includes a description of the health team, its members, and their roles. Information on health insurance and how the system is accessed by patients also should be included. Although you will not come to understand the system thoroughly until you work within it, preliminary knowledge helps to make the transition to U.S. practice less stressful. See chapter 5 for a more in-depth discussion of the U.S. health care system.

Language Competency

Health care professionals for whom English is a second language have repeatedly indicated to CGFNS that perception of their competence by patients and health care personnel is tied to their ability to speak English. If English is a second language for you, it is best to increase your English language skills as you transition to living and practicing in the United States. Language skills, like practice skills, are primarily obtained through experience. Exercise your language skills by using English as much as possible in your new environment, even if it makes you feel uncomfortable or embarrassed at first. If you don't understand a term, ask for clarification. Look for publications that describe the idioms, abbreviations, and slang terms used in health care practice settings in the United States. If English is your second language, use every opportunity to speak and critically think through clinical scenarios in English. Practice will help make speaking English more natural, thus enhancing your comfort when you enter the United States.

Most of all, do not feel that you have to apologize to your employer or your colleagues for your attempts at using a new language. If you ask for help, most of your colleagues will try to help you to understand the nuances or subtle variations of the language. If one colleague does not take the time to assist you, it does not mean that others will react in the same way. While it may be difficult to say, "I don't understand what you mean," it is the only way to begin understanding the use of words within the context of U.S. health care.

Continuing Professional Development

Our advice to foreign-educated health care professionals would be: Take advantage of the wealth of continuing professional development opportunities while you are in the United States. In-service opportunities with your employer help to enhance skills in your work setting and give you the opportunity to meet others in the organization. Professional workshops with your disciplinary colleagues provide networking opportunities and are focused on knowledge and new developments in your chosen profession. Formal coursework at a university can greatly broaden your skills and knowledge. As you work and take advantage of professional development opportunities, share your perceptions and unique experiences with colleagues. The diversity you bring will tremendously enhance everyone's learning. Attend company or organization social events and social gatherings and talk to your coworkers, neighbors, and people who share interests with you. Make U.S. friends.

Join professional associations in your discipline. Their local, state, and national activities and meetings place you at the heart of professional issues in the United States and often the world. These associations are fertile networking and learning opportunities unique to your profession.

ACCULTURATION

Acculturation—the process of adapting or learning to take on the behaviors and attitudes of another group or culture—is an essential aspect of working in a host country. For health care professionals transitioning to practice in the United States, it generally takes 4 to 6 months to become fully productive, and 12 months to feel fully acclimated to the new setting.

Phases of Acculturation

Acculturation can be divided into four phases: Acquaintance, Indignation, Conflict Resolution, and Integration. Familiarity with the process of acculturation will help you to know what to expect within your first year of practice in a new culture and new work environment.

The *Acquaintance Phase* of acculturation occurs from entry into the culture to 3 months postarrival. It is the stage of initial contact during which time you will be excited about your new life and your new place of employment. This is the time in which you will become oriented not just to the practice environment but also to the community—the time during which you will begin to develop a supportive social network, a network of both colleagues and friends.

The *Indignation Phase* occurs 3 to 6 months postarrival. The feelings of excitement about your new environment give way to feelings of anxiety, which can lead to a sense of isolation and psychological discomfort. Understanding the U.S. health care system and your role in it—what is expected of you and how quickly it is expected—can become overwhelming. It is during this time that a mentor or preceptor will be critical. The support that mentors or preceptors can provide is invaluable because they have knowledge of the system, contacts within and outside of the system, and, most importantly, are willing to work with you so that your experience is a positive one. This also is the time to rely on family, friends, and colleagues for support—and especially those who have been through a similar experience.

It also may be helpful to seek out regional support groups. There are support groups within the United States designed to help immigrants adapt to their new life. These support groups are generally composed of individuals of the same ethnic background who have been through the immigration and transition processes and are willing to share their experiences with those who are new to this country. The Chamber of Commerce in the city or town in which you intend to practice can provide you with a list of support services that are available.

The *Conflict Resolution Phase* generally occurs 6 to 9 months postarrival. This is the time to clarify new roles and development, to gain insight into problem solving, and to make personal and professional decisions about your new workplace and the new community. You may feel that you are a part of two cultures—your native culture and its work values and the culture of the U.S. health care system.

Now is the time to determine what values and beliefs are essential to you. What values and knowledge from your own culture make you comfortable as a health care professional in the United States? Which of the values of the new culture and the new workplace can you incorporate into your practice? What aspects of practice in the

United States do you find difficult to adopt—and why? Again, using a mentor, a preceptor, or someone familiar with the process of adapting to a new culture and work environment to explore these issues will be invaluable.

The *Integration Phase* occurs 9 to 12 months postarrival. It is the phase of renewed enthusiasm for your work and your new country, a time when you have reconciled the differences between your native culture and your host culture, and a time when you feel confident in your ability to practice as a health care professional in the new culture. It is a time when you know you made the right decision to migrate, a time when you will have a sense of belonging to the new culture and, most importantly, a sense of the skills and knowledge that you bring to your profession (Adeniran, Davis, & Nichols, 2005).

ENSURING YOUR U.S. EXPERIENCE IS REWARDING AND GRATIFYING

Planning is the key to a positive experience for the foreign-educated health care professional. Immigration is complex, and moving to the United States to practice a discipline is a complex interaction of immigration and licensure and/or certification requirements. Licensure/certification requirements vary by profession, state, and the nature of practice. For example, some professions require additional education or certifications to work in some specialties.

Make sure that you review all documents carefully and seek answers to questions you might have. Complete your application carefully, because omissions and errors can add months to the process. Apply far in advance of your intended entry date so that delays are minimized.

Prepare carefully for certification examinations, engaging in review courses when available. Many professions offer reviews for certification and licensure examinations and more of these are becoming available online. Being well prepared decreases disappointment and delays in achieving your migration goals.

Choosing a Practice Site

Most professions offer a variety of practice sites including hospitals, outpatient offices, schools, and community agencies. Explore practice in different settings and different states as privileges sometimes vary. Work varies greatly across settings. Check the most recent Bureau of Labor Statistics (BLS) data for average salaries and employment in your profession. This data is updated and published every 2 years and may be accessed at http://www.bls.gov/oco/home.htm. Profession-specific excerpts from the BLS *Occupational Outlook Handbook,* 2008–2009 edition, on audiologists, clinical laboratory scientists and technicians (medical technologists and technicians), occupational therapists, physical therapists, physician assistants, and speech-language pathologists may be found in Appendix A.

Choosing a Place to Live

As you review employment opportunities, research the area where you might decide to live. Consider the culture and lifestyle that would be most appealing to you as a base location as you begin your new adventure. Because of the size and diversity of the United States, you can select almost any climate and geography that you can imagine. The United States abounds with coastlines, mountains, plains, and warmer and colder climates. There are busy cities filled with crowds of different people and bursting with cultural events. There are also rural pastoral communities that surround you with quiet peaceful days for nature enjoyment. Wherever you choose to live, be an avid tourist and visit points of interest near your home location and around the country. Try all the varieties of food and activities and culture that you can imagine. The Internet offers tremendous information regarding communities, conditions, events, and opportunities. Welcome and enjoy.

SUMMARY

The demand for health care professionals in the next decade is expected to increase substantially in the United States. International health care professionals will continue to have a significant impact on the U.S. health care workforce and to contribute to its growth. Since the migration of health care professionals across international borders and their assimilation into the U.S. workforce enables the health care professions to grow, to broaden their perspectives, and to increase their diversity, the successful adaptation of foreign-educated health care professionals to U.S. practice is critical.

REFERENCES

Adeniran, R. K., Davis, C. R., & Nichols, B. L. (2005, May 26). *Empowering internationally educated nurses through collaboration.* Paper presented at the 23rd Quadrennial Congress of the International Council of Nurses, Taipei, Taiwan.

American Academy of Physician Assistants. (2008). *International PA development.* Retrieved December 2, 2008, from http://www.aapa.org/international/practicing.html

American Physical Therapy Association. (2008). Retrieved December 7, 2008, from http://www.apta.org/Vision2020.

American Speech-Language-Hearing Association. (2008). *International frequently asked questions.* Retrieved December 1, 2008, from http://www.asha.org/about/member ship-certification/international/intlfaqs.htm

Association of Academic Health Centers. (2008). *Out of order out of time* (p. 54). Retrieved July 24, 2009, from http://www.aahcdc.org/policy/outofforderoutoftime.php

Bureau of Labor Statistics. (2008–2009a). *Occupational outlook handbook* (2008–2009 ed.). Retrieved April 2, 2009, from http://www.bls.gov/oco/home.htm

Bureau of Labor Statistics. (2008–2009b). *Occupational outlook handbook: Audiologists.* Retrieved November 14, 2008, from http://www.bls.gov/oco/ocos085.htm

Bureau of Labor Statistics. (2008–2009c). *Occupational outlook handbook: Speech-language pathologists.* Retrieved November 14, 2008, from http://www.bls.gov/oco/ocos099.htm

Bureau of Labor Statistics. (2008–2009d). *Occupational outlook handbook: Clinical laboratory technologists and technicians.* Retrieved November 14, 2008, from http://www.bls.gov/oco/ocos096.htm

Bureau of Labor Statistics. (2008–2009e). *Occupational outlook handbook: Occupational therapists.* Retrieved November 14, 2008, from http://www.bls.gov/oco/ocos078.htm

Bureau of Labor Statistics. (2008–2009f). *Occupational outlook handbook: Physician's assistants.* Retrieved November 14, 2008, from http://www.bls.gov/oco/ocos081.htm

Bureau of Labor Statistics. (2008–2009g). *Occupational outlook handbook: Physical therapists.* Retrieved November 14, 2008, from http://www.bls.gov/oco/ocos080.htm

Canadian Association of Speech-Language Pathologists and Audiologists. (2007). *CASLPA position paper on the professional doctorate degree in audiology.* Retrieved December 1, 2008, from http://www.caslpa.ca/english/certification/index.asp

CGFNS International. (2008a). *VisaScreen statistical data.* Retrieved April 2, 2009, from http://www.cgfns.org/sections/tools/stats/vs.shtml

CGFNS International. (2008b). *Credentials evaluation service.* Retrieved December 2, 2008, from http://www.cgfns.org/sections/tools/data/vs/vs_data.shtml

Collier, S. N. (2008). Changes in the health workforce: Trends, issues, and credentialing. In D. E. Holmes (Ed.), *From education to regulation: Dynamic challenges for the health workforce* (pp. 1–19). Washington, DC: Association of Academic Health Centers.

Commission on Accreditation of Physical Therapy Education. (2008). *Directory of programs.* Retrieved December 7, 2008, from http:www.apta.org

Council on Academic Accreditation in Audiology and Speech-Language Pathology. (2008). *Academic program accreditation.* Retrieved December 1, 2008, from http://www.asha.org/about/credentialing/accreditation

Department of Homeland Security. (2003, July 25). Final rules. 8 C.F.R.212.15. *Federal Register, 68*(143).

Foreign Credentialing Commission on Physical Therapy (FCCPT). (2008a). *Services available through the FCCPT.* Retrieved November 25, 2008, from http://www.fccpt. org/forapplicants.html

Foreign Credentialing Commission on Physical Therapy (FCCPT). (2008b). *Summary of credential review results for 2006 and 2007.* Retrieved November 30, 2008, from http://www.fccpt.org/aboutus.html

Illegal Immigration Reform and Immigration Responsibility Act of 1996. Public Law 104–208, Div. C, 110 Stat. 3009-546.

Library of Congress (2004). *American memory timeline: Rise of industrial America, 1876–1900.* Retrieved February 9, 2009, from http://memory.loc.gov/learn/features/ timeline/riseind/immgnts/immgrnts.html

National Board for Certification in Occupational Therapy. (2008a). *Visa Credential Verification Certificate (VCVC) handbook.* Retrieved November 25, 2008, from http:// www.nbcot.org/WebArticles/articlefiles/106-RegulatoryBoardsAndNBCOT_bro chure.pdf

National Board for Certification in Occupational Therapy (2008b). *Report to the profession: Visa credential verification year end review for 2006 & 2007, spring/summer 2007 & 2008.* Retrieved December 7, 2008, from http://www.nbcot.org

Pendergast, J. M. (2005). International health care professional migration. *Journal of Nursing Law, 10*(4), 208–213.

"What's really propping up the economy." (2006, September 25). *Business Week.* Retrieved July 24, 2009, from http://www.businessweek.com/magazine/content/06_39/ b4002001.htm?chan=top+news_top+news+index_businessweek+exclusives

World Federation of Occupational Therapists. (2008). *Recognized occupational therapy programs.* Retrieved December 7, 2008, from http://www.wfot.org

2

Preparing to Leave Your Home Country

CATHERINE R. DAVIS AND DONNA R. RICHARDSON

In This Chapter

Keywords

Acculturation program: A system of procedures or activities that has the specific purpose of training individuals to understand another culture and its practices.

Advocacy: Active support for a cause or position.

Breach of contract: A legal concept in which a binding agreement is *not* honored by one or more of the participants.

Codes of Conduct: A set of rules outlining the responsibilities of, or proper practices for, an individual, a profession, or an organization.

Continuing education: Regular courses or training designed to bring professionals up to date with the latest developments in their particular field.

Department of Homeland Security (DHS): A government agency created in 2003 to handle immigration and other security-related matters. A component of DHS is the U.S. Citizenship and Immigration Services (USCIS), the government agency that oversees lawful immigration to the United States of America.

Garnished: (wages) Monies taken from payroll or royalty checks, or from investment checks, to pay a debt.

Pen pal: Two people, usually in different countries, who become friends through an exchange of letters but who may never meet.

Portfolio: A collection of items or documents outlining one's work experience, achievements, and skills organized in a binder, file, or electronic format.

Remittances: The portions of migrant income that, in the form of either funds or goods, go back into the home country.

Residency programs: The programs through which entry-level professionals work for a specific period of time in a community or a facility to gain experience. In many U.S. facilities such programs are structured learning experiences.

Self-learning modules: Activities designed for participants to do independently when they are unable to attend traditional education sessions.

Migration is the movement of people across borders, usually for the purpose of acquiring a new residence and employment. Migration can occur within countries (internal) or across national borders (external). The annual flow of international migration has continued to increase over the past decades so that in the early 21st century it is estimated that 1 out of every 35 individuals worldwide is an international migrant (Kingma, 2006).

MIGRATION FACTORS

People have many reasons for migrating—usually identified as push factors (reasons for leaving their own country) and pull factors (reasons for choosing a host country). Push factors may include such things as poor wages, poor working conditions, civil war, or other factors that make living and working in a country difficult. Pull factors are those that make a host country desirable and include such things as higher wages, greater professional opportunities, and better work environments.

Push/Pull Factors

The world is seeing a sharp increase in the number of highly skilled workers moving across international borders (Kingma, 2006). Health care professionals make up a significant portion of that increase. In a Commission on Graduates of Foreign Nursing Schools (CGFNS) survey (2007), foreign-educated health care professionals in the United States most frequently cited poor wages and few jobs as the primary reasons for leaving their home countries (push factors). The United States was identified as the destination of choice because of such pull factors as better wages and working conditions, a better way of life, and greater opportunity for advancement. Many health care professionals responding to the survey had family members living in the United States, and this also was cited as a pull factor.

Health care professionals educated outside the United States traditionally have augmented the U.S. workforce during periods of shortage. However, migration patterns and the availability of international health care professionals often change based on environmental, economic, and political considerations. As a result of the aging of its general population and an increased need for health care professionals, the United States is facing a major shortage in a number of health care professions.

BEFORE YOU LEAVE YOUR HOME COUNTRY

Leaving one's home county is a significant event—one that produces many changes in your life. Leaving your home, family, and friends to move to a new land can be daunting, but understanding the migration process, knowing what to expect, and being aware of your rights can smooth the transition and make it a worthwhile experience.

Becoming a health care professional in the United States begins with seeking an occupational visa, which will allow you entry into the country for the purpose of employment. Certain Canadian and Mexican health care professionals, namely, physical therapists, occupational therapists, and clinical laboratory scientists, may obtain trade NAFTA

(North American Free Trade Agreement) status for this purpose. A description of the different types of visas available to health care professionals seeking to come to the United States is outlined in chapter 3 of this publication.

Embracing Life in a New Culture

When you decide to immigrate to the United States, the initial excitement of the decision can fade into a stressful, worrisome time when you realize you have to not only embrace a new life and culture but also say goodbye to family and friends. One of the most important tasks when deciding to move abroad is to get your family and friends involved in the decisions you are making. Often close family feel left out and worried that they do not know what choices you are making. Involving family and friends by discussing with them possible places to live, areas to visit in the United States, and other aspects of your new life can help to allay their concerns. It allows them to see that you are putting plenty of thought into your actions and that their opinions are important to you.

Often the biggest decision when emigrating is the initial one where you decide where you would like to work and when you would like to move. While immigration procedures may affect the timing of your move to the United States, there still are numerous steps you will need to go through in order to have a successful and relatively stress-free move abroad. The best way of ensuring that you have taken care of everything is to prepare a "To Do" list. That way you can take the time to organize the move, identify what needs to be done, check off the completed items, and know what still needs to be accomplished. If nothing else, this should give you a sense of control over the process. Following are some of the steps you will have to take when considering moving to the United States.

Choosing Where You Want to Live

The United States is composed of many geographic regions, each with its own climate, culture, and customs. For example, the Middle Atlantic States of Pennsylvania, New York, and New Jersey enjoy four distinct seasons of the year (summer, fall, winter, and spring). These states were among the original 13 British colonies that founded the United States and are rich in historical tradition. They each include densely populated, major cities with large, ethnically diverse communities and many rural towns and communities. By contrast, California, a Pacific state, contains areas that are considered ideal resort destinations, sunny and dry all year with easy access to the ocean and mountains. California's historical and cultural traditions reflect its origins as part of Mexico prior to gaining U.S. statehood in 1850.

Determining where you want to live is a major decision that may be influenced by the choices of health care professionals who have migrated before you. CGFNS routinely surveys VisaScreen applicants to determine where they intend to work in the United States. Trend data indicate that the most commonly identified states of intended practice were California, New York, Florida, Illinois, and Michigan.

Questions to Ask

Because of the wide geographic diversity in the United States, you should use a library or the Internet to research the different areas of the country and ask yourself such questions as:

- Do I want to live in a climate that is similar to my home country or experience something different?
- Do I want to live in a large city, small city, town, or rural community?
- Do I want to live where I already have friends and family, or do I want to be on my own?
- Do I want to live in a mountainous area, a plains area, or by the ocean?
- Do I want to live close to my employing institution? How do I want to commute? By auto? By public transportation?
- How will I make living arrangements? Who will meet me when I arrive? How will I get to my destination?

Choosing the Type of Employment Facility

Prior to leaving your home country, you should consider the type of U.S. facility in which you would like to work. Foreign-educated health care professionals in all regions of the United States most frequently are employed in hospitals, followed by smaller percentages in long-term care facilities (such as nursing homes), ambulatory care settings, community health, and home health. Those employed in hospital settings work primarily in adult health and critical care.

Questions to Ask

Questions you might consider prior to employment are:

- Do I want to work in a hospital or another type of facility?
- Do I want to work in the community as opposed to a structured facility?
- Do I want to work in a rural or urban area?
- Do I want to work in a small hospital (100 beds) or a large facility (300+ beds)?
- Do I want to work in a public (government-operated) facility, such as a Veterans Administration Hospital, or in a private (nongovernment) facility?
- Do I want to work in a teaching or nonteaching facility? Teaching hospitals serve as training sites for new physicians during their internship and **residency programs.** These hospitals are usually affiliated with a medical school and may be part of an academic health center that includes other health professional schools.
- What specialty areas do I enjoy most (adult health, critical care, maternal infant, pediatrics, etc.)?
- In what areas of practice am I most skilled or proficient?

Selecting a Health Care Facility

Once you have identified potential places of employment, you should carefully research their hiring practices, the units and shifts available, the orientation provided, and the placement of foreign-educated health care professionals.

Questions to Ask

Questions to consider prior to accepting a position in the United States are:

- Do I have to sign a contract? What is the length of the contract? What does the contract require me to do? What is the penalty if I break the contract?
- To what unit, department, or facility will I be assigned? Will I have to move from unit to unit, as needed? How large is the unit? How many patients will I be responsible for at a time?

- To what shift will I be assigned (day, evening, or night shift), and what will be the length of the shift (8 hours, 10 hours, or 12 hours)? How much overtime will I be expected to work? Is overtime mandatory?
- What will my salary be? Is my salary comparable to what other health care professionals are earning?
- Will my health care experience in my home country be considered in my starting salary, my starting position, and in promotion? How often will my performance be evaluated?
- What type of orientation will be provided? How will it be modified to meet my needs? Will I be assigned a preceptor and for how long?
- Is there a **pen pal** or buddy system in place that I can access prior to leaving my home country? Is there a health care professional working in the facility, preferably in my chosen field, with whom I can correspond?

Some of these questions may be addressed by doing an Internet search, while others will have to be asked during the interview process with the specific facility.

Mentors and Preceptors

Most employers considered preceptorship as having the greatest impact on a successful transition to U.S. practice. Employers indicate that, on average, it takes foreign-educated health care professionals 4 to 6 months to feel comfortable with practice in the United States and to exhibit safe practice. For those reasons alone, you should ask if a preceptor will be available to you and for how long.

A preceptor can help you to understand the U.S. health care system, to become acquainted with other staff, to understand the technology used in practice, and to understand how to get things done within the system. A preceptor also can support you when you give or write reports on your patients, show you how to best organize your care, and explain how to get the supplies you need. Most of all, a preceptor can help you to problem solve and can be there when you need some support.

Mastering English

Another critical factor for foreign-educated health care professionals during their first year of practice is good English language skills. If

English is your second language, try to improve your skills prior to leaving your home country, either through classes or **self-learning modules.** When deciding on your U.S. place of employment, ask if the facility offers any English language classes during orientation. A preceptor also may be able to assist you with your language skills, especially with the language of health care practice in the United States (see chapter 8 on communication).

Researching the Environment

Knowing what to expect ahead of time can be critical to your adjustment in the U.S. work setting. Do not hesitate to ask the facility for a brochure or even a video of the facility, the unit or department in which you will work, and the staff with whom you will work. Send pictures or a video of yourself (after you have been offered and accepted employment) so the staff will be familiar with you when you arrive.

Ask for a description of the types and severity of patient conditions that you will encounter as well as the commonly represented cultures of patients and staff members. Ask if the facility would be interested in information on your culture. The more information you and the staff share ahead of time, the more comfortable you will feel when beginning your health care career in the United States.

Preparing for U.S. Licensure

To enter the United States for the purpose of employment, you will need an occupational visa, which allows you entry into the country. However, in order to practice in some of the health care professions in the United States, you must have a license in the state in which you plan to work. Each state sets its own requirements for licensure, so it is important to understand those requirements and to start the process early (see chapter 6 for profession-specific information on entering the U.S. workforce).

Developing Your Portfolio

A **portfolio** is a collection of items or documents outlining work experience, achievements, and skills. It is organized in a binder, file, or electronic format. By collecting this information throughout your health care career, you will become more aware of the skills and abilities you possess, and have an excellent way to market your qualifications to an employer.

A portfolio does two major things: (1) creating it helps you to focus on the milestones of your career, allows you to look back and review your accomplishments, helps you to set goals for your future, and helps to identify what will be needed to achieve those goals; and (2) presenting your portfolio to prospective employers tells the employer that you are serious about your professional career and its advancement, that you are reflective and organized, and that you have identified a career path. The portfolio allows employers to identify your competencies, to design an orientation program that best meets your needs, and to work with you to achieve your identified goals.

A portfolio can be in hard copy, electronic, or both. Electronic portfolios can be designed as Web pages and posted to an Internet location or stored on a CD-ROM, computer wand (flash drive), or DVD to be used as a tool to supplement the hard-copy version of your portfolio. Documents stored electronically should be printed out as needed for employment, academic admission, licensure, and other purposes. Portfolio development consists of a number of steps:

Step 1. Consider your career thus far and determine what you consider to be your most significant achievements.

Step 2. Collect all representative documents that showcase your academic and professional accomplishments and organize them into sections: for example, education, work experience, publications and presentations, memberships, **continuing education,** and awards. You might also provide a separate section for your short-term and long-term goals. Documents can be organized chronologically, from the beginning of your career to the present time.

Step 3. Create a paper file by making copies of original documents. Retain the originals and provide the copies when presenting your portfolio. If you choose to create an electronic portfolio, scan the documents onto a CD-ROM, DVD, or flash drive. Back-up files should be created on your personal computer. Copies of documents collected for portfolios include, but are not limited to:

- academic experiences, for example, transcripts, special reports you developed, presentations you gave, copies of positive faculty evaluations, skills assessments, and summaries of research projects you completed;

- work-related documents, such as letters of recommendation, performance evaluations, special recognitions, and copies of employee newsletters in which you are mentioned;
- community activities that you conducted or in which you participated;
- awards you received, for example, scholarships, academic citations, and newspaper articles noting special honors or activities;
- letters of recommendation;
- a list of your short-term and long-term goals; and
- an updated résumé and cover letter (see Appendix B).

Step 4. Review your completed portfolio to make sure that it is accurate and concise and contains only necessary items. Make sure that it is easy to follow and tells a positive story about you. A portfolio should contain no more than 15–20 pages.

CHOOSING A RECRUITER

Many health care professionals seeking to enter the United States for employment purposes use a recruiter to assist them through the migration process—from obtaining a U.S. work visa to attaining employment in a U.S. facility. The recruiter can be hospital-based (usually a health care professional with experience in recruitment who is an employee of the hospital) or commercial. Commercial recruiters generally charge a fee for their services and work independently or as part of a recruitment firm. Some immigration attorneys also conduct commercial recruitment services. If you plan on using a recruiter, you should choose that recruiter carefully because the health care recruitment industry is largely unregulated.

What to Look for in a Recruiter

Because of the global shortage in various health care professions, there has been a proliferation of commercial recruiters here in the United States and worldwide. There are many recruiters whose policies are transparent (visible and clear) and who use best practices. They often also provide transition and **acculturation program**s to ensure the acceptance and comfort of their recruits in their new employment positions. Several recruitment companies have participated in the development of

Codes of Conduct for recruiters and employers through collaboration with policy makers, unions, professional organizations, and employers (Pittman, Folsom, Bass, & Leonhardy, 2007).

On the other hand, there are some recruiting firms that are poorly funded and often require foreign-educated health care professionals to pay for their own examination review courses and travel expenses. Reportedly, some recruiters have solicited duplicate fees—demanding payment from health care professionals in addition to charging employers fees for each recruited professional. Some recruiters, including health care recruiters, have made unfulfilled promises, misrepresented positions and resources, or charged unwarranted fees. Therefore, you should investigate your recruiter carefully before agreeing to become a client.

Finding a Recruiter

Currently, there is not a public site for reviewing the ethical conduct of recruitment companies, but there are efforts under way for the development of a user-based review system whereby clients can make public comments regarding their experience with health care recruiters. Until such a service is available, you should contact friends and colleagues to determine what recruiters they used and if their experiences with the recruiter were positive. Check Internet postings about the recruiter you are considering, and check to see if the recruiter is a member of the National Association of Healthcare Recruiters (NAHCR) or the American Association of International Healthcare Recruitment.

Rights and Responsibilities of Health Care Recruits

Health care professionals using a recruiting firm to assist with the process of migration have the right to be treated fairly and equitably, to review their contract before signing, to not have their contract modified unless agreed upon by both parties, and to have their interaction with recruiters free from intimidation. Recruiting firms commonly are founded by immigrants themselves, or by individuals who previously lived overseas and are familiar with the language and business opportunities in the source countries (Pittman et al., 2007). Although you may feel more comfortable with a recruiter of the same ethnic background as yours, you should still carefully investigate that recruiter's reputation—just as you would with any recruiter—prior to signing a contract. Ask for the recruiter's references, that is, names of recruited health care professionals and of health care institutions that have hired health care professionals recruited by that firm. Do not rely on spoken promises. Request written documentation of all details.

Knowing Your Rights

Health care professionals have the responsibility of knowing their rights before they leave their home country and of finding out as much as possible about the immigration process of the host country, in this case the United States. Visit the Web site for the U.S. Department of State, which issues visas (www.state.gov). Visit the U.S. Embassy in your country or view its Internet site (which can be located through www.usembassy. gov) to gather information on the United States and its visas. Use the **Department of Homeland Security** (www.dhs.gov) and the U.S. Citizenship and Immigration Services (USCIS; www.uscis.gov) Web sites to gain an understanding of the requirements for immigration.

Signing Contracts

The majority of recruiters have foreign-educated health care professionals sign contracts prior to beginning the immigration process. You must understand that if you sign a contract, you may be legally required to abide by all the terms of the contract. Those contracts may be legally enforceable and can mean significant monetary penalties and even deportation if violated or broken. Therefore, you should read everything carefully before signing, and you should not sign anything without taking sufficient time to review it. If you do not understand the terms of the contract, ask to have them explained until you thoroughly understand what you are signing. It may be best to have an outside attorney (an attorney not employed by the recruiter) or a trusted family member or friend read the contract before you sign it. Do not sign a contract that you cannot explain to others or that you do not understand.

Reviewing Your Contract

You have the right to receive a copy of the contract prior to signing so that you can review it. You also have the right to a signed copy of the contract for your records. Contracts should:

- Be in writing and should describe the roles and responsibilities of the recruiter as well as those of the recruited health care professional

- Outline which fees are to be paid by the recruiter and which, if any, are to be paid by the health care professional
- Identify the health care professional's proposed geographic work location, place of employment, and housing, if provided
- Identify the length of the contract and fees charged, if any, for **breach of contract**

Recruitment Costs

The financial costs of immigration can be high. The typical fees include visa filing fees for the visa applicant(s); medical examination fees; certification fees charged by organizations that conduct credentials evaluation, such as CGFNS, NBCOT, and FCCPT; English proficiency examination fees; travel fees; and licensure fees, if applicable (varies by state and profession). Unless your recruiter or the employer who is sponsoring your visa agrees to cover those costs and travel expenses, you will be required to pay for them directly or have them deducted from your future salary. It is important to receive a detailed account of all charges for which you will be responsible.

Breach of Contract

Generally, recruitment contracts involve a 2- to 3-year commitment and identify a buy-out or breach fee that can range from $8,000 to $50,000 if the recruit does not fulfill the contract. Breach fees are usually proportionate to the investment made by the recruiter in bringing the health care professional to the United States and for facilitating visa, immigration, licensure, and placement processes (Pittman et al., 2007). Before signing a contract make sure that the breach fee, if any, is reasonable and will be prorated for the amount of work you have provided. Also ensure that if you breach your contract, you will not be required to pay the fee in one lump sum, but rather in installments. In focus groups conducted jointly by CGFNS and AcademyHealth in 2007, one Filipino health care professional reported,

> I talked to my agent last Friday (who is Filipino) because I wanted to buy out my contract. My agent told me that buying out my contract would ruin his relationship with the mother company, which is one of his biggest clients. He also told me that my buying out my contract might result in revocation of my immigrant visa since it was [that company] who petitioned it. Also, if I opted to buy out, I will need to pay the whole amount in a one-time

payment only, which is $13,650. For now, I can only pay them one-fourth of the buy-out price. (CGFNS/AcademyHealth Focus Group, 2007)

Be aware of fees for which you may have to reimburse your recruiter both during the contract and for early termination. Find out if your wages will be **garnished** (held by your employing facility and given directly to the recruiter) to reimburse the recruiter for unpaid fees, how much will be deducted from each paycheck (will your entire pay be garnished until the fees are paid, or will there be a certain percentage taken out of each paycheck), and for what length of time will the garnishment extend.

Pitfalls and How to Avoid Them

Immigrating health care professionals commonly report several types of contract violations by some recruiters and employing institutions. These violations typically include: forced changes in the place or location of employment; changes from being direct hires of the facility (which is preferred by most foreign-educated health care professionals) to employees of staffing agencies; lower salaries than anticipated, or being paid less than U.S. health care professionals, which is illegal; and restricted or lacking benefits, including health insurance, vacation time, or sick leave (Pittman et al., 2007). Immigrant health care professionals have reported being threatened with deportation for not adhering to contracts—as well as having their VisaScreen Certificates and green cards withheld by recruiters.

Recognizing Unethical Recruitment Practices

Because the shortage of certain health care professionals is of such global proportion, your refusal to sign on with one recruiter will not end your chances to immigrate. The more information you have, the less chance that you will be intimidated or taken advantage of by recruiters or those who profess to be immigration agents or facilitators. Self-described "immigration agents" will falsely claim to be able to make immigration move faster for the right amount of money.

Health care professionals who plan to migrate to the United States can go to the U.S. Department of Labor (DOL) Web site (www.dol. gov) to access information about employment, rights of women, unions, wages, and civil rights. The DOL fosters and promotes the welfare of job seekers, wage earners, and retirees of the United States by improving their working conditions, advancing their opportunities for profitable employment, protecting their retirement and health care benefits, helping employers find workers, strengthening free collective bargaining, and tracking changes in employment, prices, and other national economic measurements. In carrying out this mission, the DOL administers a variety of federal labor laws, including those that guarantee workers' rights to safe and healthful working conditions, a minimum hourly wage and overtime pay, freedom from employment discrimination, unemployment insurance, and other income support.

There also are immigration **advocacy** groups that can provide you with reliable and correct information on U.S. immigration laws and referrals to immigration law firms. You should be aware that not every attorney is knowledgeable about immigration. Immigration law is very complicated. There are specialists in immigration law who focus on health care workers. You may want to ask the attorney about his/her experience in immigration law and about the type of clients he/she serves.

Third Party Authorizations

Another factor to be aware of is the use of third-party authorizations. These authorizations can give someone else the right to receive and open your correspondence—the right to receive your test scores, your CGFNS VisaScreen Certificate, and even your green card—rather than the correspondence and documents going directly to you. Read everything carefully before signing any documents to ensure that you are not giving up rights that should be retained by you. In most cases, your signature on such a document makes it legally binding. If you believe that you have been wronged during the immigration process, seek an independent immigration attorney or civil rights attorney who can review your case with you, determine if your rights have been violated, and assist you in seeking recourse.

Ethical Recruitment of Health Care Professionals

The globalization of the health care workforce has enabled health care professionals to further their careers through migration. With the increase in global migration, there has been a corresponding increase in the number of international recruiters and recruiting firms, some of whom have aggressively pursued health care professionals to work in developed countries. This aggressive recruitment has led, in some instances, to the serious depletion of the health care professional workforce, particularly in developing countries and in countries that could ill afford to lose their health care professionals. While health care professionals have the right to migrate to countries for employment purposes, large-scale migration can have a devastating impact on the health systems of the source country. Widespread concerns also have been raised about unethical and unfair recruitment practices.

World Health Organization

In response to this evolving global health challenge, member states of the World Health Organization (WHO) mandated that the WHO Director-General develop a code of practice on the international recruitment of health personnel in consultation with WHO member states and all relevant partners. Web-based hearings were held on the draft code through September 2008, providing an opportunity for member states, health workers, recruiters, employers, health professional organizations, and various other regional and international organizations to comment on the code.

Voluntary Code of Ethical Conduct

The Code of Practice will be a nonbinding, international instrument designed to be a first step in developing an effective framework for national and international cooperation. It will address the benefits and potential negative impact of international health care worker migration and the need to safeguard the rights of migrant health care workers. The proposed Code balances the collective interests of many in emphasizing guidelines that effectively plan for sustaining the global health workforce and retaining health workers.

The draft Code sets out guiding principles and voluntary international standards for the recruitment of health workers. Its goal is to increase the consistency of national policies and discourage unethical practices, while promoting an equitable balance of interests among health workers, source countries, and destination countries. Consistent with contemporary international legal practice, the initial draft of the Code also aims to establish an international procedural structure to foster national dialogue, commitments, and action on health worker migration (Dayrit et al., 2008). Information on the proposed code may be accessed at http://www.who.int/bulletin/volumes/86/10/08-058578/en/print.html.

World Federation of Public Health Associations

In 2005 the General Assembly of the World Federation of Public Health Associations also acknowledged that health professionals from less prosperous countries were moving across international boundaries and into the more developed countries to the detriment of health care delivery in the less prosperous nations. Their General Assembly recommended that health worker employers in developed countries voluntarily adopt a code of ethics to judiciously manage the employment of health professionals from abroad. Their report and recommendations may be accessed at http://www.wfpha.org/Archives/05_policy_Recruitment.pdf.

REMITTANCES

One of the lessons learned from migration is that source countries need to benefit as well. Foreign-educated health care professionals traditionally have sent **remittances** back to their home countries. Remittance refers to the portion of migrant income that, in the form of either funds or goods, goes back into the home country, primarily to support families back home, to cut poverty, and to improve education and health within the family (Focus Migration, 2006). The World Bank estimates that in 2001, remittances sent back to developing countries reached a level of $70 billion. This is 40% more than the development assistance the countries in question received (Carballo & Mboup, 2005). However, it should be noted that although remittances provide some compensation for sending countries, those sent by health workers (even if they can be identified) are not directly reinvested in human capital for the health system. This means that those countries sending more health professionals than they are either receiving or producing will end up with a net loss of human capital in the health system. Even though the capacity of the country may ultimately be strengthened in the long term, the short-term loss of health professionals could have serious implications for coverage of and access to services in developing countries (Stilwell et al., 2003).

Sending Remittances to Your Home Country

If you plan on sending money back to your family or friends, you should discuss this before you depart from your home country so that you know the best way to send money and goods. Look into fees for the transfer of money (what it will cost you to send money and what it will cost the recipient in your home country to receive it). Fees that money-sending services such as Western Union charge are usually higher than bank fees. You also should consider the security of the transfer of funds, especially if the funds are sent through more informal channels. It might be helpful to talk to someone who has migrated from your home country to the United States and is sending remittances back home. This will give you a good idea of the cost and the processes involved.

SUMMARY

Migrating to a new country can be challenging and time consuming, but the more research you do on immigration requirements while still in your home country, the smoother the process will be. Be cautious if you are using a recruiter, and gather as much information as possible on the recruitment process prior to entering the United States. This way you can reduce your risk of mistreatment and intimidation and increase the likelihood of achieving your professional goals.

RESOURCES

Anticipating Your Move to the United States

Twelve Months to Go

With a year still to go before a move, many people think they have plenty of time to arrange things, so they just put it off or forget about it. It is best to start the process as early as possible so that you have adequate time to put your affairs in order and to prepare for migration.

At this point in time, you should be ensuring that your passport has plenty of time left on it (usually 2 years) and checking that you have original copies of all your birth/marriage/divorce paperwork. This also should be done for anyone who may be traveling with you. If you have any outstanding debts, try to get those in order and start educating yourself on the job market of the place to which you would like to move. Check on visa policies and procedures at the U.S. Department of State Web site at http://www.travel.state.gov/visa/visa_1750.html.

Six Months to Go

At this point, time generally starts to move very quickly. It is a good idea to obtain quotes from shipping companies and to check flight prices so that you can get the best deals, especially if you are paying for the flight yourself. If you can, open a bank account in the United States. Because official paperwork can often take a while, you should at this point ask your bank for credit references. Also, ask your dentist and doctor for your records so that you can take these with you when you sign up with new health care professionals in the United States. Check on immunizations that you will need before entering the United States, and develop a timetable for receiving them. Make sure that you have a copy of your immunizations to take with you. For a list of immunizations for U.S. immigration, check the Department of State Web site at http://travel.state. gov/visa/immigrants/info/info_1331.html.

Two Months to Go

At this stage, you will find that most of your time is spent thinking about moving or organizing the move. If you are responsible for making living arrangements in the United States, they should be in progress now. If you will be traveling with children, see if you can register them for their new schools and make sure they have all their friends' contact information to take with them. Start saying goodbye to friends now as time will run out quickly.

One Month to Go

With only 1 month left to go, you need to ensure that you have informed all the official agencies (such as the postal service) and service providers (such as telephone companies) of your move. You should start packing any nonessential items and ensure that you have all your important paperwork in a small travel file. This will make your life much easier when you are searching for things on arrival. Also, start transferring money to your foreign bank account so it is there when you arrive.

One Week to Go

At this stage, everything should be finalized, and you should be getting excited about your new venture in life. Cancel any newspaper subscriptions or milk deliveries, and if you have sold your car, cancel the insurance on it. Make sure that your goods are already shipped, and get rid of anything else that you don't need. Set aside some time to spend with friends and family, as you will miss them when you are gone. If you want to have local currency when you arrive in the United States, buy some of that. Make sure that you have copies of your travelers' check numbers, insurance policy numbers, passport, and visa documents in a separate and safe place in case they are lost or stolen. As an added precaution, leave copies with family or friends.

Saying Goodbye

Make sure you leave plenty of time to say goodbye to people, and plan how you will keep in contact with them. Remember that in the first few weeks you will be very busy settling in. Therefore, be realistic about how often you will make contact so that your friends and family will not worry about you. It is helpful to obtain contact information for all those people close to you. There will be times when you cannot find your address book or the paper on which you wrote the information. Put all the information on your computer, if you have one, on a computer disc or wand that you can take with you, or in a file with the rest of your important paperwork.

REFERENCES

Carballo, M., & Mboup, M. (2005). *International migration and health.* Retrieved May 1, 2009, from http://www.gcim.org/attachements/TP13.pdf

Commission on Graduates of Foreign Nursing Schools. (2007). *Trends in international health care migration.* Unpublished research study.

Commission on Graduates of Foreign Nursing Schools & AcademyHealth. (2007). *Focus group report on international health care recruitment.* Unpublished report.

Dayrit, M., Taylor, A., Yan, J., Braichet, J., Zurn, P., & Shainblum, E. (2008). *WHO code of practice on the international recruitment of health personnel.* Retrieved April 14, 2009, at http://www.who.int/bulletin/volumes/86/10/08-058578/en/print.html

Focus Migration. (2006). *Remittances—A bridge between migration and development.* Retrieved February 10, 2009, from http://www.focusmigration.de/uploads/tx_wilpubdb/PB05_Remit.pdf

Kingma, M. (2006). *Nurses on the move.* Ithaca, NY: Cornell University Press.

Pittman, P., Folsom, A., Bass, E., & Leonhardy, K. (2007). *U.S. based international nurse recruitment: Structure and practices of a burgeoning industry.* Washington, DC: AcademyHealth.

Stilwell, B., Diallo, K., Zurn, P., Dal Poz, M., Adams, O., & Buchan, J. (2003). *Developing evidence-based ethical policies on the migration of health workers: Conceptual and practical challenges.* Retrieved April 14, 2009, at http://www.pubmedcentral.nih.gov/articlerender.fcgi?artid=272935

3 Entry Into the United States

DONNA R. RICHARDSON AND CATHERINE R. DAVIS

In This Chapter

Keywords

Affidavit: A sworn statement or a written declaration made in the presence of someone authorized to administer pledges.

Associate degree: A degree earned on completion of a 2-year program of study at a community college, junior college, technical school, or other institution of higher education.

Asylum status: Protection and immunity from extradition granted by a government to a foreign political refugee.

Attestation: A statement that something is true, especially in a formal written document.

Backlog: A quantity of unfinished business or work that has built up over a period of time and must be dealt with before progress can be made.

Compliance: A state in which someone or something is in accordance with established guidelines, specifications, or legislation. The adjective form is **compliant** and indicates readiness to conform or agree to do something.

Consular: Term pertaining to an official appointed by the government to reside in a foreign country to represent the commercial interests of foreign citizens who come from the official's home country.

Petition: An appeal to or a request for something from a higher authority.

Refugee status: Protection granted by a government to someone who has fled another country, often because of political oppression or persecution.

Retribution: Something given or demanded in repayment, especially punishment.

Retrogression: The procedural delay in issuing an immigrant visa when there are more people applying for immigrant visas in a given year than the total number of visas available.

Third-party authorization: Occurs when the individual for whose benefit a contract is created gives another person the right to act on that individual's behalf.

Unencumbered: Not held back or delayed because of difficulties or problems, for example, a professional license that is not revoked, suspended, or made probationary or conditional by a licensing or regulatory authority as a result of disciplinary action.

U.S. Department of State: The U.S. government department that sets and maintains foreign policies, runs consular offices abroad, and makes decisions about nonimmigrant visas and immigrant visas that are processed through U.S. consulates.

Health care professionals who plan to enter the United States to practice their professions will have to satisfy requirements set both by immigration and licensing agencies. These include requirements that have been established for entry into the United States and for practicing the profession in states within the United States. This chapter will discuss the various immigration processes required of foreign-educated health care professionals who wish to enter the United States to practice.

IMMIGRATION: ENTERING THE UNITED STATES

Immigration requirements establish the conditions that noncitizens must meet in order to enter the United States. A health care professional who wishes to enter the United States to work will encounter three main U.S. federal agencies involved in the immigration process. The U.S. Citizenship and Immigration Services (USCIS) is an agency within the U.S. Department of Homeland Security (DHS) that is responsible for processing immigrant visa applications and **petitions** for occupational visas. The U.S. Department of Labor (DOL) is responsible for processing labor certifications. A labor certification is a document filed by a U.S. employer that demonstrates a lack of American workers available to fill vacant health care professional positions. Finally, the **U.S. Department of State (DOS)** is responsible for granting the visa upon receipt of all required documents, fingerprints, and medical and background checks.

A listing of common visa terms and their meanings as well as frequently asked questions about admission to the United States are included in Appendix C.

Selecting a Visa Type

The type of visa for which you will apply depends on whether you are attempting to enter the United States to work, study, visit, or join family. Requirements will differ based on your desired length of stay and your country of origin. There are several types of visas that provide health care professionals entry into the United States. The majority of health care workers enter the United States on occupational or work visas. Others arrive as spouses or family members of immigrants who are now residents of the United States. Some have married U.S. citizens. Table 3.1 outlines the most common types of U.S. visas available to foreign-educated health care professionals.

Table 3.1

OCCUPATIONAL VISAS AND IMMIGRATION OPTIONS FOR NURSES AND ALLIED HEALTH CARE WORKERS

VISA TYPE/ CLASSIFICATION	CATEGORY	WHO QUALIFIES	DESCRIPTION
Green Card	Permanent	RNs, LPNs, Physical Therapists, Occupational Therapists, Medical Technologists, Medical Technicians, Speech-Language Pathologists, Audiologists, and Physician Assistants	Foreign health care workers may qualify for a permanent visa through various processes. Registered nurses and physical therapists may qualify under a process known as Schedule A designation, while others will need to go through the labor certification.
H-1B Visa	Temporary	Physical Therapists, Occupational Therapists, Medical Technologists, Speech-Language Pathologists, Audiologists, Physician Assistants, and RNs with a bachelor's degree working in a nursing job that requires a bachelor or higher degree	Allows a foreign national to work in a position that requires at least a bachelor's degree. There are two criteria for an H-1B visa: (1) the position must require at least a bachelor's degree; and (2) the foreign worker must have at least a bachelor's degree.
H-1C Visa	Temporary	RNs	Created in 1999 when Congress passed the Nursing Relief for Disadvantaged Areas Act. It applies only to health care facilities in medically disadvantaged areas. The Act was renewed in 2006.
TN Status	Temporary (Renewable)	Canadian or Mexican: RNs, Physical Therapists, Occupational Therapists, and Medical Technologists	The North American Free Trade Agreement (NAFTA) allows employers to hire Canadian or Mexican citizens to work in the United States under a streamlined process.
F-1 Visa	Temporary (Renewable)	Students such as those attending RN-to-BSN programs	Eligible to adjust to H-1B or permanent status after completion of education.

Visa Issues

An issue to be aware of as you consider applying for a visa is that requests for visas from some countries (e.g., the Philippines, China, and India), always exceed the yearly quota. It may therefore take up to 14 years for that applicant's visa number to be called. Similar delays also occur for family visas, for example, when the visa holder has parents or siblings who will come later or when the spouse and minor children do not accompany the immigrant.

There are quotas for visas. Each country is allowed so many visas per year. Each visa category also has a limited number of visas. Once the country quota is reached, no more visas can be processed until the next year. Until 2005, approximately 20,000 visas remained each year, because of a USCIS **backlog.** Since 2005 USCIS has streamlined its procedures and is able to process visa applications more efficiently.

Retrogression

Retrogression is the procedural delay in issuing visas when more visa applications have been received than visa slots exist. The Department of State determines when it is necessary to impose limits on the allocation of immigrant visa numbers. They also determine to which countries retrogression will apply. In 2004 when retrogression was ordered, it only applied to China, India, and the Philippines.

Under retrogression, visa applications are not processed until the backlog is completed. Retrogression may be limited to immigrants from select countries or from all countries. Retrogression was declared in November 2006 for all countries and continues to the present, effectively causing a major decrease in the recruitment and certification of foreign-educated health care professionals.

OCCUPATIONAL VISAS

Occupational visas require an employer sponsor and **compliance** with the labor certification process. Occupational visas can be permanent or temporary.

A permanent visa allows an immigrant to stay in the United States indefinitely. A permanent visa recipient is granted a permanent resident card, commonly called a *green card.* Although it has not actually been green since 1964, the permanent resident card is still universally referred to as a green card. You can retain legal permanent resident status as long as you do not leave the United States for longer than a year without a re-entry permit. The green card must be renewed every 10 years. Foreign-educated health care professionals are eligible for a permanent visa or green card.

A temporary visa limits the amount of time a health care professional can stay in the United States. Those who enter the country on temporary visas are considered nonimmigrants. Temporary occupational visas are not available to everyone. Most foreign-educated health care professionals are eligible for the H-1B temporary (nonimmigrant) visa. They also may qualify for student or training visas, which allow a limited number of hours that an allied health care professional may work. Certain professions also are eligible for Trade NAFTA (North American Free Trade Agreement), or TN, status.

Trade NAFTA Status

Trade NAFTA (TN) status is available to clinical laboratory scientists, also known as medical technologists, physical therapists, and occupational therapists from Canada or Mexico. The North American Free Trade Agreement (NAFTA) eased restrictions on the immigration of workers and importation of products among the United States, Canada, and Mexico.

Physical therapists, occupational therapists, and clinical laboratory scientists are among those professionals who can enter the United States with TN status. They must be citizens of either Canada or Mexico, must have a written job offer from a U.S. employer, and must hold a license in the U.S. state of intended practice/employment (if applicable). Further, clinical laboratory scientists must have a VisaScreen® Certificate from CGFNS; physical therapists must have either a VisaScreen Certificate from CGFNS or a Health Care Worker Certificate from the Foreign Credentialing Commission for Physical Therapy (FCCPT); and occupational therapists must have either a VisaScreen Certificate from CGFNS or a Health Care Worker Certificate from the National Board for Certification in Occupational Therapy (NBCOT®).

Foreign-educated health care professionals who immigrated to either Canada or Mexico and became citizens of those countries are eligible for TN status if they meet the qualifications listed above. For example, many health care professionals from Canada who are in the United States on TN status were born in India, Jamaica, the Philippines, or the United Kingdom.

Duration of Trade NAFTA Status

Initially, TN status duration was for a 1-year period and required annual renewal. However, on October 16, 2008, the Department of Homeland Security announced that TN status would be extended for up to three years.

The number of renewals for which a foreign-educated health care professional may apply is currently unlimited, although some immigration opponents believe that renewal of TN status should be limited, and should not be used as a permanent form of temporary status. A benefit of TN status is that it is not affected by external factors such as retrogression.

Canadian Health Care Professionals

The majority of health care professionals holding TN status are from Canada, and are not required to have a visa to enter the United States. Many TN workers commute between Canada and the states of Michigan, Maine, and Minnesota on a daily basis.

The Canadian health care professional applies for TN status to work in the United States and needs only to show proof of citizenship, a letter of intended employment, the required licenses and the VisaScreen or Health Care Worker Certificate at the Canadian port of entry, which can be at a border crossing or an airport. The process can be completed in less than one day.

Mexican Health Care Professionals

The TN process for Mexican health care professionals is more complex. It requires a visa and **consular** processing. The employer must file a labor certification and an I-129 petition for nonimmigrant workers. The process can take a day or up to a week. The Mexican health care professional must present a VisaScreen Certificate from CGFNS or a Health Care Worker Certificate from FCCPT or NBCOT as needed for his/her profession.

The H-1B Nonimmigrant Visa

The H-1B is a temporary or nonimmigrant visa, which is given for a 3-year term, after which it can be extended for an additional 3 years. H-1B visas require that the individual hold a baccalaureate degree and are available only for individuals who have been recruited for employment in the United States that requires a minimum of a baccalaureate degree. A clinical laboratory technician does not qualify for an H-1B visa because the entry-level education in the United States for the technician is 2 years or less and is comparable to an **associate degree.**

The H-1B visa is most frequently used by foreign-educated health care professionals for an entry-level position. Nonimmigrants from Free Trade countries such as Chile, Singapore, and Australia are eligible for additional H-1B slots. Although H-1B visas are limited to 65,000 per year, many health care employers may be exempt from the quota because they are nonprofit organizations and/or research institutions.

The H-1B status is available to those foreign-educated health care professionals who qualify as meeting the definition of a specialty occupation. A specialty occupation is defined as a field of employment that requires theoretical and practical application of a body of specialized knowledge, and a bachelor's or higher degree in the specific specialty (or its foreign degree equivalent), which is a minimum for entry into the United States.

Physical therapists, occupational therapists, clinical laboratory scientists, speech-language pathologists, and audiologists meet the specialty occupation requirements. Currently, PTs, OTs, speech-language pathologists (SLPs), and audiologists are educated at the master's level in the United States. Medical technologists or clinical laboratory scientists and physician assistants are graduates of baccalaureate programs. Medical technicians are typically graduates of 2-year programs and do not meet the specialty occupation requirements.

Specialty Occupation Requirements

In order to meet specialty occupation requirements, the foreign-educated health care professional must meet certain criteria. They must (a) have full state licensure to practice in the occupation, if such licensure is required to practice in the occupation, (b) have completed the degree required for the occupation, or (c) have experience in the specialty equivalent to the completion of such degree (in other words, have a combination of education, training, and work experience in the specialty occupation comparable to a U.S. bachelor's degree or higher); and (d) recognition of expertise in the specialty through progressively more responsible positions relating to the specialty.

Licensure Requirements

Physical therapists entering the United States under an H-1B visa must pass the National Physical Therapy Examination (NPTE) to meet the licensing requirement of a specialty occupation. Currently, the foreign-educated physical therapist must enter the United States to take this examination. Many physical therapists will do this on a visitor's visa and then return home to wait for the H-1B visa. Others may be in the United States on an F-1 student visa. Holders of student visas must meet specific deadlines regarding filing for adjustment of status from a student to an occupational visa.

The licensing requirements also are applicable to clinical laboratory scientists, speech-language pathologists, occupational therapists, and audiologists. All states require occupational therapists and audiologists to be licensed. However, only 12 states license clinical laboratory scientists and 47 states license speech-language pathologists.

Labor Certification Process

Foreign-educated health care professionals also must comply with the Department of Labor's labor certification process before the U.S. Citizenship and Immigration Services (USCIS) can act on an immigration petition (I-140). The employer sponsor must provide written documentation to the Department of Labor of how all labor certification requirements were met, including posting of intent to hire foreign-educated workers, job descriptions, prevailing wages, copies of advertisements, employer's financial status, and **attestation** regarding absence of union or organizing activity, to name a few.

Visa Caps

H-1B visas currently are limited to 65,000 per year. Furthermore, health care professionals must compete with other professionals, including engineers and computer specialists, for those limited visa slots. In the last 2 years when the visa process opened on April 1, the quota was filled within 3 days. Those eligible were chosen by lottery. All excess applications over the quota were returned to the applicants. However, in 2009, visa slots were not filled as quickly, probably due to the worldwide economic downturn.

An exemption from the visa cap is available for employers who employ health care professionals in higher education institutions, nonprofit entities affiliated to institutions of higher education, or nonprofit or governmental research organizations. An additional 20,000 visas are available for those who hold master's or doctoral degrees and who are to be employed in positions that require the higher degrees. There also are additional visas for those covered by the Chile and Singapore Agreement and for foreign-educated professionals from Australia.

Student Visas

Those who are in the United States on student or training visas must apply to adjust to another status if they wish to stay in the United States either temporarily or permanently upon completion of the program. Because those actions must be done within a limited time period, it is important for the health care worker to consult his/her immigration attorney or the academic institution's Office of International Students for advice regarding the adjustment process.

APPLYING FOR A VISA

The petition for immigration, an I-140 form (visa application), must be filed. Members of the health care professions are considered "skilled workers"—based on 2 years of postsecondary education—as well as professionals, which makes them eligible for employment-based (EB), Third Preference visas. Third Preference generally refers to a category used in employment-based immigration to identify skilled workers capable of performing a job requiring at least 2 years of training or experience; professionals with a baccalaureate degree, or members of a profession with at least a university bachelor's degree; and other workers, capable of filling positions requiring less than 2 years of training or experience.

Visa Application Documents

In addition to submitting an I-140 form and the required fees, the employer and/or employee also must submit the following necessary documents:

- A statement of valid prevailing wage
- Copies of all in-house media, printed, and electronic job advertisements

- A VisaScreen Certificate from CGFNS International (all professions) or a Health Care Worker Certificate from FCCPT (PTs only) or NBCOT (OTs only); or a U.S. license; or a letter confirming eligibility to work
- A diploma or degree
- School transcripts
- A marriage certificate, if married
- Divorce decrees, if divorced

Schedule A

Physical therapists are included under the designation *Schedule A,* which precertifies only three categories of employees. This precertification documents that there is a shortage of U.S. workers available in that occupation. Because Schedule A bypasses the Department of Labor's certification process, the physical therapist is not subject to all the requirements that other H-1B nonimmigrants must meet. The physical therapist is required only to show a letter of eligibility from the state of intended employment.

Physical therapists and registered nurses (RNs) are the only professions that historically have been listed under Schedule A because of a continual manpower shortage in the United States. Occupations listed under Schedule A have a streamlined labor certification process. Schedule A occupations are determined by the Secretary of the Department of Labor not to have a sufficient supply of qualified, willing, and available U.S. workers. The DOL also has established that similarly employed U.S. workers will not have their wages and working conditions adversely affected by the employment of immigrants. Because of retrogression, there have been no available Schedule A visas beginning October 2006 and continuing to the present. Immigration advocates have proposed expanding the quotas under Schedule A or removing them totally.

Labor Certification

The labor certification process is a mandatory requirement of employers, such as hospitals, who wish to hire foreign-educated health care professionals. The process was designed to assure the public that U.S. jobs would not be given to foreign workers without well-documented proof of a shortage of U.S. workers in a particular field. Employers must submit a labor certification for each worker they recruit from abroad.

The Department of Labor requires that a notice regarding the job for which the health care worker is being recruited be posted at the site of intended employment for at least 10 business days. The posting must list the prevailing wage and the job requirements. A wage survey must be completed and the employer must also show proof of the ability to pay the wages (20 CFR 656.10Ld).

Visa Process

The time to complete the immigration process is not predictable. It varies from country to country and is affected by your ability to obtain all required documents. Another factor that influences the process is the time it takes you to successfully complete any required certification and/or licensure examinations and obtain the required scores on the English language proficiency exams. All of these documents are needed to support your application for the VisaScreen Certificate or the Health Care Worker Certificate, which must be submitted at your visa interview.

Employee Sponsor

An applicant for a permanent occupational visa needs an employer sponsor. The sponsor must file the Form I-140, Petition for Alien Worker. Different forms are required for other visa categories. The form must be filed at the United States Citizenship and Immigration Services (USCIS) Service Center.

In order to file an I-140 form the employer must have certain documents. You must submit your health care profession diploma, health care profession school transcripts, health care profession license from your country of education, proof of passing the required certification and/or licensure examinations, and a copy of your passport.

Visa Petition

The employer and/or immigration attorney will request the required documentation for the labor certification required by the Department of Labor (DOL). That information must document the employer's intent to hire foreign-educated health care professionals and its financial status. The DOL grants the labor certification application (LCA).

Once the labor certification has been granted, the visa petition is filed. USCIS will approve the petition and send it to the National Visa Center (NVC) at Portsmouth, New Hampshire. The NVC will assign you a case number. Then fees will be requested and must be submitted to NVC.

Visa Interview

Depending on the country in which you are located, you may be able to submit copies of your documents but, generally, the NVC requires originals. You will receive an Interview Notice from the U.S. Embassy in which you applied.

You must submit all required forms at the visa interview, including the medical examination report. Embassy staff will conduct the interview and will inform you if your visa is approved. If you lack required documents, then the petition will be denied and you will be given a Request for Evidence (RFE) and a time frame in which the required documents must be submitted to USCIS.

If approved, you will receive your passport with immigrant visa stamps. The visa must be used within six months. The passport and other documents from the embassy must be provided to U.S. immigration at the airport or border. You must carry your green card with you at all times.

Adjustment of Visa Status

When health care professionals seek to change their visa from temporary to permanent, they must request an adjustment of status. If the time limit on a foreign-educated worker's temporary occupational visa expires, then the worker must return home, or adjust his or her visa status to permanent.

A health care worker who came to the United States on a temporary visa in order to take the licensing examination may decide to request an H-1B or permanent visa in a different category. TN workers may wish to adjust to H-1B or permanent status. Canadians may do so without losing their Canadian citizenship.

When contemplating such changes, you should consult with an immigration attorney. If filing for an adjustment is not timely or is procedurally in error, you might lose your visa and/or have to return home.

IMMIGRATION REQUIREMENTS FOR FOREIGN-EDUCATED HEALTH CARE PROFESSIONALS

Section 343 of the 1996 Illegal Immigration Reform and Immigrant Responsibility Act (IIRIRA) mandated that health care professionals not born or educated in the United States must undergo a federal screening program in order to receive an occupational visa. Section 343 authorized CGFNS, through its division the International Commission on Healthcare Professions (ICHP), to conduct such a program by verifying and evaluating the educational and licensure credentials of seven allied health professions, including physical therapists, occupational therapists, audiologists, speech-language pathologists, medical technologists and technicians (also known as clinical laboratory scientists and technicians), and physician assistants. The law also authorized CGFNS to screen registered nurses and practical nurses. CGFNS designated this process as VisaScreen: Visa Credentials Assessment. Regulations implementing the 1996 law authorized two other organizations to conduct the screening program for their respective professions: the Foreign Credentialing Commission on Physical Therapy (FCCPT) for physical therapists only and the National Board for Certification in Occupational Therapy (NBCOT) for occupational therapists only.

Section 343 Screening

Section 343 screening of the seven allied health care professions named above includes an assessment of the individual's education to ensure that it is comparable to that of a U.S. graduate in the same profession; verification that licenses are valid and **unencumbered;** demonstration of written and oral English language proficiency; and passage of a test predicting success on the occupation's licensing or certification examination, provided such a test is recognized by a majority of states licensing the occupation for which the certification is issued, or passing the occupation's licensing or certification examination.

Medical Technologists

The medical technologist category has been used as an umbrella term for a variety of allied health professions. The Department of Homeland Security has defined a medical technologist as a clinical laboratory scientist. Medical technologists are not the same professional as all other disciplines with *technologist* in their title. There are differences in education, clinical experience, licensure/certification requirements, and functions.

The medical technologist works in five major areas of the laboratory: blood banking, chemistry, hematology, immunology, and microbiology. The medical technologist performs a full range of analytical laboratory tests on blood, tissues, and body fluids to provide laboratory information for the detection, diagnosis, and treatment of human diseases. The educational requirement is a Bachelor of Science (BS) degree.

Professions Restricted From Designation Medical Technologist. Based on the requirements and description of medical technologists cited above, the molecular diagnostic categorical technologist, nuclear medical technologists, medical ophthalmic technologist, ultrasound technologist, and the medical sonographic technologist, to name a few, are not clinical laboratory scientists. Likewise, specialists in clinical laboratory sciences such as cytotechnologists or genetic technologists are not subject to the VisaScreen requirement. These specialists do not have the range of courses and clinical experiences that a generalist clinical laboratory scientist has.

You must be aware of the job and functions that your employer or recruiter describes on your visa application. The medical technologist category is often chosen because these workers are eligible for entry under H-1B and more importantly Trade NAFTA (TN) status. Remember, TN health care workers are not subject to retrogression and their immigration process is less burdensome.

Feldchers. Foreign-educated health care professionals must be able to verify that their education was designed to produce the specific health care professional who can perform the job that the U.S worker performs. Often feldchers, who are health care workers educated in Eastern Europe, will attempt to apply for an occupational visa as a physician assistant or a nurse. A review of their education has demonstrated that the feldcher's education is not comparable to either profession.

Physicians. Similarly some foreign-educated physicians have sought to apply for VisaScreen as allied health professionals. Although they are educated in the same sciences, their education in their profession's philosophy, science, professional autonomy, responsibility, and skills differs from allied health education. Therefore, a foreign-educated physician is not eligible to receive a VisaScreen Certificate or Health Care Worker Certificate as a physical therapist, occupational therapist, physician assistant, or a nurse.

However, many employers have recruited foreign-educated physicians to work in various laboratory positions and have filed petitions designating them as medical technologists. Although foreign-educated physicians have laboratory exposure, it lacks the variety and the quantity required for a clinical laboratory scientist in the United States. The difference in quantity and variety of lab experiences raises questions regarding the comparability of foreign-educated physicians' education for that position.

English Language Proficiency Examinations

The English language proficiency examinations and their required scores are mandated in the 2003 final regulations implementing Section 343 of IIRIRA. Health care professionals must demonstrate competency in oral and written English on English tests approved by the U.S. Departments of Education and Health and Human Services, as recommended to the Department of Homeland Security (DHS).

Physical therapists and occupational therapists must take either the (a) Test of English as a Foreign Language (TOEFL), plus the Test of Written English (TWE) and Test of Spoken English (TSE); or (b) TOEFL iBT (Internet-based TOEFL). Clinical laboratory scientists, speech-language pathologists, audiologists, and physician assistants must take one of the following English language assessments:

1. Test of English as a Foreign Language (TOEFL), plus the Test of Written English (TWE) and Test of Spoken English (TSE);
2. TOEFL iBT (Internet-based TOEFL);
3. Test of English for International Communication (TOEIC), plus TWE and TSE; *or* the
4. International English Language Testing System (IELTS).

English test scores are valid for 2 years so they must be current when all other required visa screening documentation has been received. Scores from the ETS tests (TOEFL, TWE, TSE, iBT, and TOEIC) and the IELTS examinations cannot be interchanged. See Table 3.2 for the required English scores by profession. Those educated in designated English-speaking countries are exempt from this requirement. Take note

Table 3.2

SECTION 343 ENGLISH LANGUAGE SCORE REQUIREMENTS BY PROFESSION

Health Care Profession	ETS OPTION 1[a]			ETS OPTION 2[a]			ETS OPTION 3[a]		IELTS OPTION 4	
	TOEFL Test of English as a Foreign Language[b]	TWE Test of Written English	TSE Test of Spoken English	TOEIC Test of English for International Communication	TWE Test of Written English	TSE Test of Spoken English	TOEFL iBT Test of English as a Foreign Language Internet-Based Test (total)	TOEFL iBT Test of English as a Foreign Language Internet-Based Test (speaking section)	IELTS International English Language Testing System (overall)	IELTS International English Language Testing System (spoken band)
Registered Nurse	207 (540)	4.0	50	725	4.0	50	83	26	6.5 (Academic)	7
Practical/ Vocational Nurse	197 (530)	4.0	50	700	4.0	50	79	26	6.0 (General) or 6.0 (Academic)	7
Physical Therapist	220 (560)	4.5	50	—	—	—	89	26	—	—
Occupational Therapist	220 (560)	4.5	50	—	—	—	89	26	—	—
Speech-Language Pathologist	207 (540)	4.0	50	725	4.0	50	83	26	6.5 (Academic)	7

(Continued)

Table 3.2

SECTION 343 ENGLISH LANGUAGE SCORE REQUIREMENTS BY PROFESSION (*CONTINUED*)

Health Care Profession	ETS OPTION 1[a] TOEFL Test of English as a Foreign Language[b]	TWE Test of Written English	TSE Test of Spoken English	ETS OPTION 2[a] TOEIC Test of English for International Communication (listening and reading test)	TWE Test of Written English	TSE Test of Spoken English	ETS OPTION 3[a] TOEFL iBT Test of English as a Foreign Language Internet-Based Test (total)	TOEFL iBT Test of English as a Foreign Language Internet-Based Test (speaking section)	IELTS OPTION 4 IELTS International English Language Testing System (overall)	IELTS International English Language Testing System (spoken band)
Audiologist	207 (540)	4.0	50	725	4.0	50	83	26	6.5 (Academic)	7
Clinical Laboratory Scientist (Medical Technologist)	207 (540)	4.0	50	725	4.0	50	83	26	6.5 (Academic)	7
Clinical Laboratory Technician (Medical Technician)	197 (530)	4.0	50	700	4.0	50	79	26	6.0 (General) or 6.0 (Academic)	7
Physician Assistant	207 (540)	4.0	50	725	4.0	50	83	26	6.5 (Academic)	7

[a]ETS (Educational Testing Service) administers the tests shown in Options 1, 2, and 3.

[b]Numbers in parentheses indicate required score on pencil and paper version of TOEFL.

Note: Combining passing test scores from both IELTS and ETS administered tests is not acceptable.

that state licensure boards also may have English proficiency requirements that may differ regarding score requirements and exempt criteria.

THE VISASCREEN® PROGRAM

The CGFNS VisaScreen Program is composed of three elements: educational analysis (including analysis of clinical experiences), licensure validation, and English language proficiency assessment. The VisaScreen Program is administered by the International Commission on Health Care Professions (ICHP), a division of CGFNS.

Educational Analysis

The educational analysis ensures that the applicant's professional education meets all applicable statutory and regulatory requirements for the profession, and is comparable to the education of a U.S. graduate seeking licensure. Transcripts of professional education must come directly to CGFNS from the academic institution. For physical therapists, occupational therapists, clinical laboratory scientists and technicians, speech-language pathologists, and audiologists, more comprehensive details are required regarding their clinical experience with patients. For specific requirements by profession, please access http://www.cgfns.org/files/pdf/req/vs-requirements.pdf.

Request for Academic Records

Applicants submit a Request for Academic Records form to each school listed in the Professional Education section of the VisaScreen application. Physical therapists must submit a self-report of their clinical experience during their education. The report requires more than just hours completed. It must describe not only patient contacts but also a description of the clinical facilities to ensure educational comparability.

Occupational therapists must have a similar report of patient contacts and clinical supervision submitted by their professional school. Clinical laboratory scientists and technicians must contact their professional school and have them send directly to CGFNS/ICHP details of their clinical laboratory practice hours in the following areas: clinical chemistry, hematology, hemostasis, urine and body fluid analysis, specimen collection and handling, parasitology, mycology, microbiology, virology,

and immunohematology and immunology. Speech-language pathologists and audiologists must contact their professional school and have
them send directly to CGFNS/ICHP details of their clinical observation
and clinical practicum hours for the evaluation and treatment of speech
disorders in both children and adults, and the evaluation and treatment
of language disorders in both children and adults.

Licensure Review

The licensure review evaluates all professional licenses to ensure that
they are valid and unencumbered. Applicants submit a Request for Validation of Registration/Licensure form to the licensing/registration authorities in their country of education and in all other jurisdictions in
which they have ever been licensed, whether current or expired. When
the country does not have a licensure system, the individual's diploma
grants the right to practice in that country and is validated as such for
VisaScreen purposes. CGFNS validates all licenses, past and present, to
ensure that they have not been revoked or suspended. If such action occurred, the resolution must be documented by the licensing authority.

English Language Proficiency

The English language proficiency assessment confirms that the applicant has demonstrated the required competency in oral and written
English by submitting scores on tests approved by the U.S. Department
of Education and the U.S. Department of Health and Human Services
as described above.

VisaScreen Certification

Once the applicant has successfully completed all elements of the
VisaScreen Program, the applicant is awarded a VisaScreen Certificate,
which must be presented to a consular office or, in the case of adjustment of status, to the attorney general as part of the visa application.
Trade NAFTA applicants must present their VisaScreen Certificate at
the port of entry into the United States or to border agents.

VisaScreen Documents

Documents and test scores required for VisaScreen also may be required
by state licensure boards as well as by the Department of Homeland

Security for immigration. Because CGFNS must receive these documents directly from the school and licensing authority in the applicant's country of education, processing times may vary; processing cannot occur until all required documents have been received.

CGFNS is mindful of deadlines for immigration and licensing application purposes. It works with applicants to facilitate the necessary VisaScreen processing to meet applicant deadlines. Most countries and schools assess fees for licensure validation and transcripts. These fees vary from a few dollars to more than US$100. They also may charge mailing and stamp fees.

THE VISASCREEN PROCESS

In addition to all the documents that must be submitted to support the employee's petition with the employer's labor certification, there are extensive documentation requirements that must be met in order to obtain your VisaScreen Certificate. This certificate will be required by the USCIS in order to set up your visa appointment at the consulate or U.S. embassy.

Beginning the Process

The VisaScreen process should be started as soon as the health care professional begins to consider coming to the United States. The applicant should contact CGFNS International, preferably via the Web, at www. cgfns.org. Written correspondence can be mailed to 3600 Market Street, Suite 400, Philadelphia, PA 19104. Telephone assistance is available from 8:00 A.M. to 12:00 P.M. Eastern Time (ET) at (215) 349–8767. The application process and credentials review do not begin until a complete application and fee are received and accepted by CGFNS.

Application Form and Handbook

The VisaScreen application and handbook are available on line. To avoid confusion and mistakes in the application process, you should read all instructions and the handbook before filling out any forms. Inconsistent information will result in processing delays. All inconsistencies require written confirmation by the issuing agency as well as written clarification by the applicant.

Source Documents

Since all transcripts and licensure validations must come directly to CGFNS from the professional schools and licensing authorities, you must submit a request to those agencies authorizing them to release your information to CGFNS. You are responsible for paying any processing fees, taxes, or postage fees related to the application. You should request all necessary documents as soon as possible when applying for VisaScreen, since the submitting agency's response can be affected by its staffing, computerization, and budget capabilities.

The submitting agencies also should be advised that you might be required to have the same documents sent to several different places, as the state licensure boards, employers, and USCIS usually do not share documents. Confidentiality and privacy laws may prohibit information from being exchanged between agencies or with nongovernmental bodies.

International Mail

To ensure timely delivery of documents to CGFNS, you should provide a prepaid, preaddressed envelope to the submitting agencies for the documents to be sent to CGFNS. Remember the documents must come directly from the agency to CGFNS. Documents that are sent by a third party, such as you (the applicant) or a recruiter, will *not* be accepted.

Always be sure to use a mail or courier service that provides a tracking number, such as Federal Express (FedEx) or United Parcel Service (UPS), when submitting important documents to CGFNS. Traceable mail alleviates the stress of locating mail that cannot be matched to applications, and confirms for the sender, applicant, and recipient that the documents have been sent and received.

Preventing Processing Delays

Common reasons for delays in processing include incomplete information, missing signatures, inconsistent information between the documents and the application, and expired documents. Licenses must be validated by the issuing agency if more than 3 years old. This is required even when licenses are deemed lifetime to ensure that no adverse incidents have affected the applicant's right to provide care to patients. All English scores must have been achieved within 2 years of the receipt of all required VisaScreen documents.

One way that you can decrease the processing time for your VisaScreen application is by making sure that you identify all the names you have ever used, including unmarried (maiden) names and names from previous marriages, if any, when completing the application form. All name changes should be accompanied by verifying documents, such as birth certificates, marriage licenses, and divorce decrees.

Completing the Application Correctly. Dates are critical. Double-check dates of school attendance, graduation, and date of birth. Remember to write out the name of the months. The European and U.S. styles of using numerical dates are different, which can cause confusion. If you are aware of date conflicts in any of your documents, provide a written explanation (**affidavit**).

When providing information on your education, give the name of all schools attended, dates when you attended, and degrees and diplomas or certificates you received. Provide the exact full name of all schools. Do not use abbreviations or initials. If your school has closed or merged with another, check with the Ministry of Health or Education—or the licensing authority in your country—to find out where the school's records are now kept and request them to be sent to CGFNS.

Using Your CGFNS Identification Number. It is helpful to include your CGFNS identification number on all documents and correspondence so that when CGFNS receives them they can be matched with your file. CGFNS has files on over 500,000 nurses and allied health professionals. In many countries there are birth and surnames that are very common. For example, there are over 11,000 files with the name Maria Lopez in the CGFNS database. Without middle names, dates of birth, and other vital data, appropriate and timely matching of documents is difficult.

All documents are scanned by CGFNS and an electronic file is created. This allows examination of all your documents by those at CGFNS when inquiries are received. No information about you will be shared with anyone, including spouses and employers, without a release (**third-party authorization** form) signed and submitted by you. Your CGFNS file is permanent, which means that the same file and ID number is used if you subsequently apply for any additional CGFNS services.

Maintaining Document Integrity. It is important to treat all documents with the same care and integrity that you would a patient's record and documentation. Under no circumstances should you alter any information on any document.

If a mistake is made, do not cover it up, but instead draw a strike through the mistake and initial it. Altering a document in any way may result in the sealing of your CGFNS file and may prevent CGFNS from providing services to you in the future.

Document Review

CGFNS procedures require that CGFNS international credentials evaluators verify all documents. The evaluators compare dates of educational attendance, names, and dates of birth. They verify all seals, signatures, and watermarks, and also may confirm documents with the agencies. Table 3.3 lists select terms related to VisaScreen processing, document review, and certificate renewal.

Academic Transcripts

Schools are asked to provide full transcripts and a breakdown of your clinical and theory hours to determine the comparability of your education to that of a health care professional educated in the United States.

Table 3.3

COMMON TERMS USED IN THE VISASCREEN PROCESS

Educational Requirements Deficient: Status given to an applicant file when the applicant's education has a deficiency that makes him or her ineligible for a VisaScreen Certificate.

Expired Application Order: Applicant orders expire when the requirements of the VisaScreen Program are not met and completed within 12 months of application. A *Reprocess an Expired Order* must be submitted within 12 months of expiration if an applicant wants to continue the service.

Renewal Certificate: VisaScreen Certificates expire after 5 years from the date of issue. A Renewal VisaScreen application order may be placed for a VisaScreen Renewal Certificate.

Restrictions on Credential: Status given to an applicant file when an international credentials evaluator has reviewed a credential (license) and identified a restriction (the license was restricted, disciplined, or suspended by the regulatory body).

Sealed File: Action taken because of misrepresentation or fraud related to submitted VisaScreen documents.

When asked to provide your professional title, use the exact terminology used in your country of education. If your country of education requires completion of military or community service, you may have to verify that service in order to receive your transcripts. Transcripts may be denied or held by the professional school if you did not complete your military or community service.

Licenses

All foreign and U.S. licenses are reviewed to ensure that they are valid and have not been revoked or suspended. Health care professionals should be mindful of the licensure requirements in their country of education to ensure efficient responses to their requests for licensure validations. Some countries require payment of registration fees, even retroactively (e.g., Egypt and the Philippines), before they will provide licensure validation to CGFNS and state licensure boards.

CGFNS is aware that some countries may have additional requirements for health care professionals who are not citizens or residents. The Philippines requires a reciprocal process with the health care professional's home country. In some countries, there may be language proficiency requirements in order for a foreign-educated health care professional to be eligible for licensure.

VisaScreen Attestation

It is critical to answer all application form questions thoughtfully and truthfully. A VisaScreen application can be slowed, suspended, or sealed because of altered, misrepresented, or fraudulent information. Applicants must take the attestation required on the application seriously. The VisaScreen process is relied upon by the Department of Homeland Security for immigration. It also is valued by state licensure boards and employers as it ensures that the recruitment and migration of qualified health care professionals protects the health and safety of patients in the United States.

Refugee Status

Special procedures have been established for applicants who have official **refugee status** or **asylum status.** These are individuals who have left their country to avoid persecution or requested to stay in the United

States because of fear of persecution or **retribution** if they return home.

CGFNS recognizes that these professionals may not be able to request or obtain educational or licensure documents because of political restrictions and loss or destruction of documents and/or infrastructure, such as the closing of agencies and the loss of knowledge of how policies and procedures were implemented.

Streamlined Certification Process

A Streamlined Certification Process is in place for U.S.-educated health care professionals who were born outside the United States. Such health care professionals are exempt from the educational comparability review and English language proficiency testing generally required to obtain an occupational visa. The Streamlined Process applies to the following health care professionals:

1. An occupational therapist who has graduated from a program accredited by the Accreditation Council for Occupational Therapy Education (ACOTE) of the American Occupational Therapy Association (AOTA)
2. A physical therapist who has graduated from a program accredited by the Commission on Accreditation in Physical Therapy Education (CAPTE) of the American Physical Therapy Association (APTA)
3. A speech-language pathologist and/or audiologist who has graduated from a program accredited by the Council on Academic Accreditation in Audiology and Speech-Language Pathology (CAA) of the American Speech-Language-Hearing Association (ASHA)

The school/program must provide a statement verifying graduation. All licenses have to be verified as unencumbered by the issuing agency.

Appeals Process

CGFNS has an appeals process in place through which a health care professional who has applied for VisaScreen Certification or who holds a VisaScreen Certificate is entitled to appeal a decision or an action taken against him or her to the ICHP Appeals Committee. A copy of the Appeals Procedure is mailed to any applicant whose file is sealed due to falsification of documents or any other fraudulent practices, to an applicant who wishes to appeal a certification decision, and to certificate holders whose certificate is revoked.

SUMMARY

Foreign-educated health care professionals must meet state licensure and immigration requirements to practice in the United States. The foreign-educated health care professional's stay in the United States is determined by the type of visa for which he/she qualifies. Most foreign-educated health care professionals use occupational visas, which can be temporary or permanent. Special procedures have been established under Trade NAFTA for designated Canadian and Mexican health care workers.

The VisaScreen process has been mandated by the Department of Homeland Security to ensure the foreign-educated health care professional's educational comparability, licensure validity, and English language proficiency, and to certify the individual's capability to provide safe patient care in the United States. The process can be navigated more easily by accessing the CGFNS Web site (www.cgfns.org) and customer service materials.

4 Employment in the United States

MICHAEL D. WARD

In This Chapter

Keywords

Acculturation program: A system of procedures or activities that has the specific purpose of training individuals to understand another culture and its practices.

Collective bargaining: Negotiations between management and a union about pay and conditions of employment on behalf of all the workers in the union.

Entitlement: Guarantee of access to benefits because of right or by agreement through law. Also refers to one's belief that he or she is deserving of some particular reward or benefit.

Mandatory overtime: Term for overtime that is *required* by an employer rather than being optional for the employee.

National Labor Relations Board: An independent federal agency created by Congress in 1935 to administer the National Labor Relations Act, the primary law governing relations between unions and employers in the private sector. The statute guarantees the right of employees to organize and to bargain collectively with their employers, to engage in other protected concerted activity with or without a union, or to refrain from all such activity.

Networking: Making connections among people or groups of a like kind.

Union: A trade union or labor union is an organization run by and for workers who have banded together to achieve common goals in key areas and working conditions.

Videoconference: Live audio and visual transmission of meeting activities that enables people at different sites to interact remotely in real time.

This chapter will provide information on the characteristics of a supportive work environment and review your employee rights and obligations. While you may have selected a geographical area of the country in which to live based on personal preferences—such as the presence of family or friends, the climate, or the cost of living—there are still many important factors to consider when selecting a workplace. We hope you find this chapter helpful in finding and obtaining employment in an organization that meets your expectations and gives you a long, fulfilling career.

ALLIED HEALTH PROFESSIONALS

When allied health professionals are looking for a job in the United States, there are important factors to consider. However, one must first have an understanding about the usage of the term *allied health*. Allied health (or health-related professions) is a term used to identify a cluster of health professions that encompasses over 200 health careers. In general, the allied health professions are clinical health care professions distinct from medicine, nursing, and dentistry.

Roles of Allied Health Professionals

Allied health providers, the largest and most diverse constituency within the health care workforce, have tremendous potential for addressing questions of cost, quality, and access in our health care system. They work in a variety of disciplines to make up the majority of the health care workforce and thus, form a vital part of the primary, secondary, and tertiary health care infrastructure. Working in a multitude of settings, allied health professionals also are diverse in terms of the work they perform, their educational backgrounds, and the regulatory control over their activities.

Patient Care

When you work in allied health professions, you are involved both directly and indirectly with the well-being and overall health of the patient, and should be regarded as an expert in your field. Some allied health professionals practice independently; others work as part of a health care team, providing continual evaluation and assessment of patient needs. They also play a major role in informing the attending clinician of the patient's progress and response to treatment.

More than twice the size of nursing, the over 200 allied health professions together represent the other core of the health care workforce that not only runs the machines of the high-tech health care system, but also provides much of the face-to-face care and specialized services that make the health system work. These health professionals range from those in entry-level positions to doctorally prepared professionals who can generate practice incomes that rival physicians.

EMPLOYMENT IN THE UNITED STATES

What to Look for in a Work Environment

As you approach your decision to work for a particular employer, you must consider that there are two aspects to the work environment, the physical and the mental. No matter where you work, you want to be in a setting that is supportive and provides you what you need to lead to high job satisfaction.

According to Drafke (1994), the physical work environment consists of the equipment and surroundings in which employees must function.

The mental work environment is the psychological atmosphere in which employees must operate. Both of these affect the employees' work and satisfaction. It is at the intersection of the physical environment and the mental environment that you will find the employee.

Characteristics of a Supportive Work Environment

Physical Work Environment

Unless it is overwhelmingly good or bad, potential employees often overlook the *physical work environment* when applying for a job. Usually the real assessment of the environment doesn't take place until the employee has been on the job for some time. Many times a poor physical work environment results in inefficiency, unnecessary fatigue, low morale, increased turnover and absenteeism, lost time, and low productivity, according to Alexander and Pulat (1985).

Properly identifying the source of a physical work environment problem is the first step toward resolving it. Some examples of factors of the physical environment that affect people are such things as temperature and humidity, ventilation, light, noise, location, layout, equipment, color and decor, and security.

Mental Work Environment

Alexander and Pulat (1985) indicate that the *mental work environment* (also called the psychological work environment) could impact a potential employee's level of satisfaction in the job. The mental work environment is the environment that the employee perceives; it reflects the work itself, the managerial atmosphere, coworkers' attitudes, and the employee's own attitude.

Work Pace. The work itself has a major impact on the mental environment. For example, the *pace* of the work, that is, the time required to perform a job task and the time between each task, can pose a strain on the employee and should be considered when deciding to accept a position. Some jobs are fast-paced. They have a very short interval between the end of one task and the beginning of the next, or a task that can (or must) be completed quickly. Others are slow-paced, perhaps because the diagnostic agents involved are slow-acting or because the patient is just beginning therapy and cannot move fast. Generally, according to O'Reilly (1990), as the pace of the work increases, stress increases.

Some employees enjoy jobs that are fast-paced and could not imagine themselves working in an environment that is slower. In health care, patient flow is often the prime determinant of the variability of the work pace. For example, radiologic technologists who work with magnetic resonance imaging (MRI) scanners and computed tomography (CT) scanners often have lower variability of pace. The equipment takes a certain known amount of time, and the throughput (production over a period of time) is fairly stable. At the other extreme of the pace scale is the rapid pace of the emergency room. The volume of work is never really predictable, and the time to tend each patient is highly variable. According to Herzberg (1966), as the variability of the pace increases, stress increases.

Managerial Atmosphere. The managerial atmosphere has a major impact on the mental work environment. The key influences on the management atmosphere include the overall philosophy of the organization, the tasks the employee performs, and the supervisor's style, level of management training, and experience on the job. Each of these components could affect your decision to choose a particular work place.

Some supervisors are very supportive of their employees and seek ways to make the workplace satisfying by focusing on meeting the needs of the employees and their personal development. On the other hand, some supervisors are task oriented and merely focus on how to obtain the most productivity out of each staff member without regard for their overall satisfaction.

Attitude of Coworkers. The attitude of coworkers can play an important factor in the overall job satisfaction of you, the employee. There are many people who feel that the employees in a work group should, at the very least, be on civil, speaking terms with one another. These people recognize the social aspects of work. Some managers may come from a philosophy where they believe that employees are being paid to work— they are not being paid to like each other.

How your coworkers feel and how you feel about this issue will affect the way that you are treated and will impact the informal organization (the social aspects) of work. It is important to find a good match between how you feel coworkers should act and how the others in a department feel. If social interactions on the job are not important to you, then you may be more comfortable working alone in a small clinic or hospital or on late shifts.

Your Attitude and the Work Environment. Finally, your own attitude has a major impact on a satisfying work environment. No matter what shift you work on, the supervisor's management style, or the level of interaction with your co-workers, it is important to realize that how *you* act or react to the work environment leads to your job satisfaction. Eventually you will come into contact with other workers. Many people would never think to include themselves as part of the mental work environment. According to Drafke (1994), some people's view may be that the world acts upon them—it is an external force that intrudes on them.

It must be noted that how you act can make things better or worse for you. Possibly the two most important factors in coworker relations are not to take other people too seriously and to remember that everyone is human. Today's work environment stresses the importance of working together in teams and the need to assist one another. Understanding that everyone on the team is a professional and is an expert in his or her field will go a long way to make the workplace more supportive and enriching.

Getting Information About Job Opportunities

There are some common methods for locating leads on jobs in the United States. They are advertisements in professional journals, newspapers, trade (equipment and supply) magazines, and the Internet.

Use of the Internet

According to Pappas and Claborn (2006), electronic job searches have replaced newspapers and other methods that were effective in the past. By going directly to the Web site of the hospital where you may potentially seek employment, you can search for position openings and read the job qualifications and job descriptions. These Web sites can also provide information about benefits, tuition reimbursement programs, and health care benefits. Many employers now offer the ability to apply for positions online and allow for submission of your résumé and references electronically.

Word of Mouth

Besides using the Internet to get information about possible positions or about a prospective employer, word of mouth (or informal conversations about the employer with current employees) is often beneficial. However, you never know if you are talking to the *right* person to get an unbiased impression.

Professional **networking** is also helpful in order to obtain answers to questions that you may need to help you with your decision to select a specific employer. In this case, you may get a better feel about an organization if you are seeking the input or advice from someone that you know and, most importantly, that you trust.

Use of Employment Agencies

Finally, some allied health professionals rely on the assistance of an employment agency for finding employment. These agencies may be able to do a much better job of finding openings because of their broad resources and wide networking capabilities.

Obtaining a Job

After you have decided the part of the country in which you like to live and the type of workplace in which you feel most comfortable, and you have picked the place that offers the type of compensation and benefits necessary for you to be comfortable, it is time to actually concentrate on getting the job.

Preparing a Résumé

Drafke (1994) describes the first function of the résumé as a record that is actually more for you than for the prospective employers. It lists your education, work experience, and other items in an organized fashion. Résumés serve an important purpose since they are the initial contact between you and the prospective employer. Along with a cover letter, your résumé introduces you, notifies employers that you are interested in seeking employment with them, and can save time.

Sending résumés is faster than visiting a number of places in person, especially if you are looking to relocate out of state or to another country. According to Pappas and Claborn (2006), the résumé can be submitted on paper by regular mail or it can be submitted electronically. Both paper and electronic versions include the same general format and the same important information: demographic data, professional objective, education, professional experience, licensure, professional organizations, honors and awards, and references (see Appendix B for a sample résumé).

Demographic Data. According to Pappas and Claborn (2006), the demographic data describes who you are to the prospective employer. This includes your name, address, e-mail address, and telephone number. You should not include personal information such as social security number, marital status, height, weight, age, number of children, or a photograph of yourself.

Professional Objective. Your professional objective should describe your short-term and long-term goals. After carefully assessing the information listed about the job, you should have a good understanding about the position and the necessary qualifications needed to get the job. Your professional objective (sometimes called the "career objective") should show that you have given serious consideration to your professional career and the direction you would like to see it take. Your short-term goal might be a listing of specific qualities that make you best suited for the job. A long-term goal would be what you ultimately hope to achieve in your career, such as obtaining a position in administration, or higher degrees or certifications that you hope to achieve (Pappas & Claborn, 2006).

Educational Background. The résumé should include a section listing your educational background, which identifies each degree earned in chronological order, beginning with the most recent education and continuing through all education you have had. High school or secondary school typically is not listed unless it happened to be the highest level of schooling completed.

This section should include all degrees, naming the institution, type of studies, and dates of attendance. This section also includes certifications or special training, where you received them, and the date you completed them.

Licensure. The section on licensure should answer the question, "What can you do and where can you do it?" If you already have licensure in the United States, you need to include the list of states in which you are licensed to practice. If you are seeking licensure in the state in which you are applying for a job, it is recommended that you place special emphasis on that in your résumé (Pappas & Claborn, 2006).

Because it may take several weeks or even several months to make your way through the process of seeking a license in some states, it is advisable to do your search for licensure requirements well in advance of the job search in that particular state. Not all allied health professions in the United States require licensure, so check with the licensure board in your intended state of practice to make sure that you are familiar with the licensure requirements in that state.

Professional Organizations, Honors, and Awards. Finally, you should list any professional, civic, or volunteer organizations to which you belong, and any honors and awards you have received in the past. Membership in organizations indicates your ability to work with others, possibly in a leadership position, and that you have broad and diverse interests. Honors and awards speak to your dedication to your career and the ability to exceed what is expected of you on the job.

References. The final section, references, may be completed by simply stating, "References will be provided upon request." Providing the names and contact information for references usually comes later in the job search process. However, it is advisable to have at least three references ready, two of which should be former employers or people with whom you have worked in the past, and one personal reference. Always be sure to ask if you can use someone's name as a reference, so that you have that individual's permission to do so. For suggested formats or examples of résumés, you can check http://resume.monster.com (Pappas & Claborn, 2006).

Cover Letter

Your résumé and its cover letter have only one purpose: to get you an interview. In three minutes' reading time or less, the two of them together should project a positive image of you and your qualifications to a potential employer. The cover letter acts as an introduction that is written in a way that causes the employer to want to meet with you for an interview.

Your cover letter should give the employer the reason why you are applying for the position and why you fit the organization or position. The letter also should demonstrate that you know something about the organization and how you would be a good fit with their culture (see Appendix B for a sample cover letter).

According to Drafke (1994), if copies of your cover letter and résumé are being sent to other areas within one institution, you may indicate this as the last line on the letter. For example, if the letter is being sent to a department manager with a copy to the human resources department, you may indicate this with "cc: Human Resources." The "cc" stands for "carbon copy," a term that dates back to the time before computers and photocopies were commonplace.

Proofreading Your Résumé

It is recommended that you find someone that you trust to proofread your résumé for typographical errors, spelling errors, or grammatical errors. Write the résumé in the third person, avoiding "I" or "me" statements. The résumé is a distillation. Don't try to tell your whole story; save the details for the interview or the application form. Prioritize, and only include the most powerful information. Given 10 candidates with relatively equal qualifications, the employer is always going to hire the person he or she likes the most or sees fitting into the organization the best.

Recruiters and Staffing Agencies

Recruitment is a proactive, positive mechanism. There are many recruitment agencies that assist and represent health care professionals around the world to find jobs in other countries, including the United States. Recruiters and staffing agencies are able to assist outside of the United States, can assess your chances of being successful in an international job search, and can guide you through the necessary procedures for obtaining your licensure in the state(s) where you would be seeking employment, if it is required. These agencies also are helpful with assessing English language proficiency, issues related to culture, career experience factors, and any required educational preparation that is necessary for the job.

Role of Recruiters and Staffing Agencies

Health care professionals outside of the United States should select recruiters who can assist them in dealing with social and cultural isolation after moving to the United States. Many of the hospital systems have departments, especially in larger medical centers, that have strong **acculturation programs** in place to make the transition a lot smoother. These programs will assist with establishing housing, help a new employee find a bank, and even help with opening an account.

The employer will pay the staffing agency and the agency pays the health care professional for his or her work in the hospital or clinical setting. The majority of the staffing agencies are local and provide temporary staffing in a small, defined geographical area such as a city or a general metropolitan area (Brewer & Rosenthal, 2008). For a more in-depth discussion of recruiters and how to select a recruiter, please see chapter 2.

Interviewing

As a health care professional seeking a job in the United States, your interview may be arranged by a recruitment agency that represents you, or it may be an interview that you have arranged yourself through presenting you résumé and cover letter to prospective employers. This interview could be set up for you in the country in which you live or with the prospective employer traveling there to interview you.

In many cases the interview will be held by having you travel to the United States to be interviewed in person with the employer. In order to reduce the expense of traveling overseas for an interview, another common way to conduct an interview is by telephone or through **videoconferencing,** with you and the interviewer in your separate locations, each seated before a camera and monitor. This will enable both of you to see and hear each other just as you would in person.

Purpose of the Interview. According to Metzger (2004), the interview has been described as a conversation with a purpose. It is intended to match people with jobs, elicit from the application the data relevant to making a sound employment decision, provide the applicant with necessary information about the job, and, not the least, serve as a means of creating good feelings toward the institution. The in-depth interview with the employer determines specifically whether the candidate meets the detailed requirements of the job and whether his or her work habits, attitudes, and personality are compatible with working in the institution.

Your Role During the Interview. It is vital that you be prepared prior to going into the interview. Find out as much as you can about the hospital or the institution beforehand. Anticipate what the prospective employer might want to know about you and be ready to respond clearly and in a manner that reflects confidence. You should be a good communicator, that is, be easy to talk with. Help carry the conversation and avoid a simple yes or no answer unless that is the only answer that is being sought. Answer all questions as clearly and concisely as possible. It is important to always be honest. If you don't know the answer, say so.

Be yourself during the interview. Make sure the impressions you make during the interview are the same ones the organization will have of you if you should work for them. Active listening is the most important part of the interview. It means more than just hearing what is said. Within the bounds of honesty and being yourself, make sure the interviewer learns how capable you are and how you would contribute to the organization.

Be alert, be curious, and show drive and initiative. In general, don't *react to* your interviewers; instead, *interact with* them. The interviewer is trying to learn enough about you to safely predict your character and behavior in the position. Always keep in mind that the interviewer is handling the interview in such a way as to allow him or her to make some sort of estimate of your aspirations, motivations, attitudes, and general traits.

Dressing for the Interview. According to Pappas and Claborn (2006), one of the most important strategies for successful interviewing is to dress for success. Consider a suit or jacket with coordinated slacks, shirt, and tie for men. Women also should be conservative in their dress, wearing a women's business suit with a skirt or a pantsuit, and being conservative in makeup and hairdo. Both men and women should wear minimal jewelry—you do not want to jingle or rattle with every move.

Conducting Yourself During the Interview. Arriving early may give you a chance to look over additional information about the institution or possibly give you more time for the interview. Be aware of your body language; that is, establish eye contact with the interviewer and maintain reasonable eye contact during the interview. It may be difficult, but try to avoid or minimize distracting nervous mannerisms. Keep your hands positioned in your lap or in some other comfortable position. Do not chew gum or have anything in your mouth during the interview.

Smile when you are introduced and offer to shake hands. Women sometimes have a problem with shaking hands and practicing this prior to the interview will make a woman more comfortable when meeting the interviewer. If you want to take notes during the interview, ask the interviewer if he or she minds. Taking notes is generally quite acceptable.

Before the end of the interview, be sure you thank the interviewer for his or her time and consideration. It is also a good idea to obtain his or her contact information (usually by requesting a business card) for questions you may think of later and for the purpose of writing the interviewer a thank-you letter (see Appendix B for a sample thank-you letter following an interview).

Hiring Process

The job offer may come at the close of the interview or it may occur sometime later. It is appropriate at this time to have a clear understanding of the salary and benefits that accompany the position. Should you already have a salary expectation in mind, be ready to allow room for negotiation.

If you are offered the position, according to Pappas and Claborn (2006), there are three possible reactions that you may face. One is that you may not be ready to accept the position; this is true especially if you are interviewing with other places of employment. A second is that you may want the position and decide to accept the job offer. Or, in a third scenario, you may not want the position and decide to decline the offer.

Declining the Job Offer

Whether you decide to take the position or not, it is always in your best interest to be polite and honest. If you know that the offer does not interest you, decline it graciously and express appreciation for the interest that the employer had in you. You should not feel pressured to say yes to a job offer if you are not ready to commit to the job or feel that the position doesn't meet your particular needs (Pappas & Claborn, 2006).

Not Being Offered a Job

Despite your interest and preparation, should you not be offered the position, it is helpful to ask why. Knowing what may not have gotten you the job for one employer may provide you a way to make corrections for the next interview process. If you do not find out about the rejection until sometime later and receive the rejection by correspondence in the mail, consider making a personal call to the employer for more information if the reason for the rejection was not made clear in the letter.

Accepting a Job Offer

Once you have accepted the position, now it is time to establish the date you will begin working and going through the orientation process. If you are moving to the United States, you will also need to make sure that you understand housing arrangements, transportation arrangements, and whether the employer has acculturation benefits or other means to make your transition from your country of origin to the United States easier for you. So that there is no misunderstanding, it is important to have all of your salary and benefits information provided to you in writing.

Contracts

Depending on where you may be employed, some recruitment agencies or employers may offer you a contract as a part of the hiring process. Contracts are legally binding lists of rights and responsibilities of both the employer and the employee. An employment contract most often will include your orientation schedule, salary, benefits, and other agreements that make up the compensation package.

Before you sign your employment contract, make sure that you read everything carefully and do not feel compelled to sign the contract until your questions have been answered and clarifications have been made. You will find, however, that most employment in the United States is not contractual, unless there is a contract covering **collective bargaining,** a topic that will be covered later in this chapter.

Networking

Networking involves developing personal contacts that can assist you in a job search and in your career in general. It is important that you begin networking, or developing a pool of people who can give you moral support and help make the transition into the job much easier. Networks typically begin with the people you know—friends, relatives, and professional colleagues. An excellent place to begin networking is through your local, state, and national professional associations. Virtually every health profession has associations where you can begin to make beneficial and sometimes lifelong contacts (Drafke, 1994).

Select activities and events to participate in that will bring you into contact with new people. Contacts outside of the professional arena also can provide opportunities. Religious organizations and community organizations, like volunteer groups, have members throughout the job world. Becoming a member of various clubs also may be of help.

Whether you choose a club or professional association to begin your networking journey, the greatest success will come from joining early and participating. According to Drafke (1994), the real power of networking does not come from people that you personally contacted helping you. Rather, the real power of networking is that all of the people that you have contact with also have contacts of their own and can help spread the word about your qualifications and abilities.

WORKPLACE RIGHTS AND OBLIGATIONS

Working in the United States has its rights and obligations. As you prepare for your new position, it is important to know that you have the obligation to work according to the policies shared with you by your new employer, both during the interview process as well as the selection and orientation process. Now that you are an employee within the United States, you have certain rights that are guaranteed to you by law.

Collective Bargaining

The working relationship between employees and their supervisor greatly affects employee morale and performance. This in turn can have an impact on the operations of the institution. According to Boone and Kurtz (1999), collective bargaining is "a process of negotiation between management and **union** representatives for the purpose of arriving at mutually acceptable wages and working conditions for employees." Furthermore, collective bargaining is the performance of the mutual obligation of the employer and representatives of the employees to meet at reasonable times and confer in good faith with respect to fair wages, hours, and other terms and conditions of employment or the negotiation of any agreement or any questions arising from those terms and conditions (Evans & Hicks, 2007).

Collective Bargaining Process

The collective bargaining process begins when the majority of employees of an organization vote to be represented by a specific union. The **National Labor Relations Board** then certifies the union. At this point, the management of the organization must recognize the union as the collective bargaining agent (representative) for all employees of that organization. Once this part of the process is completed, collective bargaining can begin.

Bargaining Models

Many different negotiation styles can be used when union and labor representatives sit down at the bargaining table. The two basic models of bargaining are traditional bargaining and partnership bargaining.

Traditional Bargaining. The traditional style of collective bargaining often is adversarial and pits one side against the other with little or no understanding of, or education about, the other on the part of either party. Each side places its demands and proposals on the table, and the other side responds to them with counterproposals. The process is often negative and involves a struggle of give-and-take on most issues.

Partnership Bargaining. The partnership style of bargaining is the more modern approach to negotiations. It strives for mutual understanding and common education on the part of both labor and management, and it focuses on the goals and concerns common to both parties. Partnership-style bargaining is also known as interest-based bargaining because of its emphasis on each side's being aware of the issues concerning the other side. In this process, labor and management each list and explain their needs, and the ensuing discussion revolves around ways to meet those needs that will be not only acceptable but also beneficial to both parties. This style of bargaining is very positive and imparts a much more congenial atmosphere to the negotiating process (Boone & Kurtz, 1999).

Membership in the Union

It may be important for you to inquire whether the allied health staff in the organization where you are accepting employment is unionized or not. For some professionals in health care, collective bargaining is not considered appropriate or desirable. On the other hand, some health care professionals support collective bargaining in the workplace as a way to control their practice and have input into the direction of the health care organization itself. Often, your membership in the union is voluntary, but you may still be required to pay union dues. These issues raise questions you will want to ask as you make your decision to accept the position.

Civil Rights

Citizens of the United States and those who are legal immigrants are extended rights referred to as *civil rights*. According to Pozgar (1990), there are several significant pieces of legislation that govern the civil rights of employees in the United States.

Civil Rights Act

Title VII of the Civil Rights Act of 1964, as amended, is one of the most significant pieces of legislation affecting equal employment opportunities. This act prohibits employers from discriminating against individuals on the basis of race, sex, religion, color, or national origin. The law's coverage extends to all phases of the employment relationship, which include hiring, firing, compensation, promotion, and so forth. In 1991, the Act was further broadened to include the issue of sexual harassment in the workplace (Pozgar, 1990).

Age Discrimination in Employment Act

The Age Discrimination in Employment Act of 1967, as amended, prohibits age-based employment discrimination against individuals between 40 and 70 years of age. The purpose of this law is to promote employment of older persons on the basis of their ability, without regard to their age. Later, this Act was extended to remove mandatory retirement at a certain age from employment practices in the United States (Pozgar, 1990).

Americans With Disabilities Act

Title I of the Americans with Disabilities Act (ADA) of 1990 prohibits private employers, state and local governments, employment agencies, and labor unions from discriminating against qualified individuals with disabilities in job application procedures, hiring, firing, advancement, compensation, job training, and other terms, conditions, and privileges of employment. This legislation requires an employer to make a reasonable accommodation to the known disability of a qualified applicant or employee, if it would not impose an "undue hardship" on the operation of the employer's business. This particular Act effectively makes it unlawful to discriminate against disabled persons unless they are not qualified or otherwise are unable to perform the job (Pozgar, 1990).

Labor Standards

Within the United States there are certain areas of labor policy that you need to be aware of as a part of the hiring and employment process. It is important that you have an understanding of these policies and you should feel comfortable with asking your employer about them should you need clarification.

Mandatory Overtime

Overtime is usually considered by law as work in excess of 8 hours a day, or 40 hours of work in a given workweek. Requiring staff members to stay on duty after the shift ends in order to fill staffing vacancies or to complete a task is called **mandatory overtime.** At this time there is no federal law limiting overtime hours or preventing mandatory overtime; however, legislation has been passed in some states, and is being considered in others, to prohibit mandatory overtime.

To solve the problem of inadequate health care professional staffing, employers have used mandatory overtime to staff facilities. Concerns for the long-term effects of overtime include its impact on the caregiver's health, the potential for errors or near misses caused by fatigue, and the diminished quality of care provided. Research indicates that risk of making an error increases significantly when work shifts were longer than 12 hours, when staff worked overtime, and when staff worked more than 40 hours per week (Rogers, Hwang, Scott, Aiken, & Dinges, 2004).

Wage and Hour Requirements

The Fair Labor Standards Act (FLSA) is a federal law that establishes standards for minimum wages, equal pay, overtime, and child labor in the United States. Federal law requires that workers who are paid hourly are paid the agreed wage for the hours they work. Generally speaking, any hours in excess of 40 hours per week are required to be paid at one and one-half times the regular hourly rate of pay.

State legislation establishing minimum wage rates is of lesser importance because the 1966 amendment to the federal FLSA provides hospital personnel with coverage under the Act. However, where state minimum wage standards are higher than federal standards, the state's standards are applicable to hospital employees (Pozgar, 1990).

Workers' Compensation

A comprehensive compensation program that is equitable, competitive, and cost-effective should be a primary objective for every health care institution. A fair and equitable classification and salary plan, coordinated with a competitive benefits program, is directly related to an institution's ability to attract, retain, and reward competent health care workers and other hospital staff.

There is federal legislation governing equal pay in the United States. The Equal Pay Act of 1963 is essentially an amendment to the Fair Labor Standards Act and was passed to address wage disparities based on gender. The law applies everywhere that the minimum wage law is applicable. The Equal Pay Act, simply stated, requires that employees who perform equal work receive equal pay (Pozgar, 1990).

Benefits

Benefits are an important part of the total compensation program, in addition to the salary, that you will receive from the employer. The benefit packages made available to employees are now recognized as employee **entitlement**s and in many instances are negotiable. However, in some cases, especially among state institutions, they may be determined by law. Some employers provide benefits only to employees who are considered full-time workers and are regularly scheduled to work 40 hours per week.

Health Insurance

Hospitalization and major medical care are typically covered in the health insurance plan that the employer provides. The hospitalization plans normally provide benefits for inpatients, semiprivate accommodations, such as room and board, special diets, general nursing services, use of the operating room, and drugs and medicines. Payments usually are based on fee schedules, which are fixed, or (in the wording of many health insurance contracts), "reasonable and customary."

These plans either provide for payment of claims directly to the hospital or doctor, or reimburse the insured for payments that they made directly to the doctor or hospital. Major medical plans are designed to meet the costs of catastrophic or extraordinary medical expenses. Normally, such plans carry large benefit amounts per family member, and reimburse a high percentage of covered expenses exceeding a deductible amount or an amount not reimbursed by a base plan.

Your Cost for Health Insurance. Most employer-provided health plans require the employee to pay some of the cost of their medical care. In addition, most plans require the employee to pay part of their health insurance premium (the fee that is paid to the health insurance company). Generally, this amount is deducted from the employee's paycheck. Some employers may require employees to pay only a small amount each month toward the cost of health insurance premiums; other employers may require more significant payments.

In most workplaces, your health insurance plan also can cover your spouse and dependent children. Most employers require you to pay an additional amount for family coverage. However, this benefit may be very useful if your spouse is not working, or is working in a job that either does not provide health insurance or provides health insurance benefits that are not as good or comprehensive as the benefits provided by your employer.

Life Insurance

Life insurance programs available from most employers in the United States provide a certain amount of money to your family or those you designate if you should die while employed by the hospital or health care institution. Accidental death and dismemberment coverage provides a certain amount of money to your survivors if you should die while actually on the job or if you are seriously injured through dismemberment, such as loss of sight, or loss of limbs or other body injury as a result of an accident on the job.

Sick Leave

Sick pay or sick leave is traditionally provided to employees as a means to protect against loss of pay because of illness or injury that does not occur on the job. Sick pay provides payment, usually at your regular rate of pay, when you are ill for a brief period of time (e.g., one day or a few days). Employers differ in terms of how much sick leave they will offer an employee and the conditions under which it can be used.

Vacation Pay

Vacation pay is a benefit that provides paid days off so that you can find time to enjoy travel or to simply rest and relax. Vacations generally are not given in advance, that is, employees typically earn vacation days by working a specified period of time before being eligible to use the vacation benefit.

Bereavement Leave

Funeral leave with pay is provided by most employers for one to three days following the death of a member of your immediate family.

Holiday Pay

Holiday pay is offered by employers and is typically given for federally recognized holidays and other days established by the employer. Most employers provide employees with paid days off for specified holidays. Employers may differ in terms of which holidays they recognize for the purpose of holiday pay. Since hospitals in particular must function every day of the year, health care professionals employed by hospitals often have to work on holidays.

Many employers provide additional pay for working on a holiday. Some provide another paid day off when an employee works on a holiday and still others offer both additional pay and another day off. In hospitals in which health care professionals are represented by a union, the union contract will include details on holiday pay. Table 4.1 lists the federal holidays observed in the United States.

The Uniform Holidays Bill of 1968 (taking effect in 1971) declared that official holidays are to be observed on a Monday, except for New Year's Day, Independence Day, Veterans' Day, Thanksgiving, and Christmas. In the United States, most retail businesses close on Thanksgiving and Christmas, but remain open on all other holidays. Private businesses often observe only the major holidays (New Year's Day, Memorial Day, Independence Day, Labor Day, Thanksgiving, and Christmas). Some also add the Friday after Thanksgiving, or one or more of the other federal holidays.

Table 4.1

TRADITIONAL HOLIDAYS IN THE UNITED STATES

DATE	OFFICIAL NAME	REMARKS
January 1	New Year's Day	First day of the calendar year.
Third Monday in January	Martin Luther King Day	Honors Dr. Martin Luther King, Jr., civil rights leader. A day devoted to volunteering in the community.
Third Monday in February	Washington's Birthday or President's Day	Traditionally honors the first president of the United States, George Washington. In recent years has been known as Presidents' Day to honor all U.S. presidents.
Last Monday in May	Memorial Day	Honors the nation's war dead from the Civil War forward; marks the unofficial beginning of the summer season.
July 4	Independence Day or the Fourth of July	Celebrates the signing of the U.S. Declaration of Independence in 1776.
First Monday in September	Labor Day	Celebrates the achievements of workers and the labor movement; marks the unofficial end of the summer season.
Second Monday in October	Columbus Day	Honors Christopher Columbus, traditional discoverer of the Americas. In some areas this day also is a celebration of Native American culture.
November 11	Veterans Day	Honors all veterans of the U.S. Armed Forces.
Fourth Thursday in November	Thanksgiving Day	Traditionally celebrates the giving of thanks for the autumn harvest; also the giving of thanks for one's family and possessions.

Retirement Plan

A retirement plan is a benefit that allows you to save money for your retirement. The money that you save for retirement is usually matched at a certain percentage by the employer. Retirement benefits provide employees with income when they retire from employment. Most employees who retire qualify for Social Security benefits from the federal government (see section on Social Security later in this chapter), but these benefits are generally modest (the maximum benefit amount in 2009 is $2,323 per month). However, retirement plans provide an important additional source of income for retirees.

Traditionally, in the United States, retirement plans provided a specific amount of income to an employee after retirement. This retirement income was calculated either as a specific dollar amount or as a percentage of the employee's preretirement salary. Today, many employers have moved away from offering such plans, instead offering employees the opportunity to put a percentage of their salary into a fund on which they can draw following retirement. Many employers, as part of their benefits package, pay a specified amount of money into the employee's retirement fund as well. These retirement funds are commonly referred to as 401(k) plans or 503(b) plans.

While you may be many years away from retirement, you should start contributing to the plan your employer offers as soon as you are eligible to do so, especially if the employer's contribution is dependent on the percentage you contribute.

Dental and Vision Insurance

Dental and vision insurance plans are typically provided by employers so that you and your family can have basic dental procedures and cleaning done, as well as vision testing provided on an annual basis.

Other Benefits

Other benefits extended to employees include tuition reimbursement programs, which pay you a certain amount per year to seek additional education and training. Provision of free or reduced cost for parking your vehicle also is considered a benefit of employment. An increased focus on health and wellness has spurred many employers to provide some sort of incentive for staff to exercise and manage a healthier diet. Some hospitals even provide access to gyms or other exercise facilities (Pappas & Claborn, 2006).

Social Security

The Social Security Administration oversees the nation's social insurance program, which is funded by contributions from both employers and employees. The funds are pooled into special trusts so that when the earnings of an employee are reduced or discontinued due to death or disability, Social Security benefits are paid to assist the employee and his or her family. A portion of the Social Security contributions are placed into a separate hospital insurance trust fund. These funds are designated for hospital benefits for senior citizens (persons over 65 years of age) and their dependents.

Social Security benefits are considered an integral part of retirement planning and funding. As a legal United States immigrant, you will have taxes automatically deducted from your paycheck by your employer to pay into the Social Security Administration system. Workers who have been United States residents for a specified number of years and have paid into the Social Security system are eligible for Medicare coverage upon reaching a certain age. Substantial reimbursement for health care expenses for a covered individual is provided by Medicare. Medicare Part A covers inpatient hospital stays while Medicare Part B covers physician and outpatient services (Hunt & Knickman, 2008). The details related to these specific benefits may be a bit confusing at times, so it is recommended that you discuss questions related to Social Security and Medicare benefits with the human resources department of your employer. For a more in-depth discussion of Medicare, please see chapter 5.

Family Medical Leave

The Family and Medical Leave Act (FMLA) of 1993 was passed due to the large numbers of single-parent and two-parent households in the United States in which the single parent or both parents are employed full-time, placing job security and parenting at odds. This Act was written in an attempt to balance the demands of the workplace with the demands of the family, allowing employed individuals to take leave for medical reasons, including the birth or adoption of children and the care of a spouse, child, or parent who has serious health problems. These benefits are sometimes provided all at one time or intermittently as needed and are carefully tracked by your employer following strict guidelines.

To be eligible under the Act, the employee must have worked for at least 12 months and worked at least 1,250 hours during the preceding 12-month period. The employee may take up to 12 weeks of unpaid leave, and the Act allows the employer to require the employee to use all or part of any paid time off that has been accrued as part of the 12-week leave. Employees are required to give their employer 30 days' notice, or such notice as is practical in emergency cases, before using the medical leave (Guido, 2007).

WORKPLACE HAZARDS

Generally speaking, the workplace should be a safe environment that is free from hazards. Of course, in the health care environment there are any numbers of situations in which employees will potentially be exposed to workplace hazards. Protective equipment, including protective equipment for eyes, face, head, and extremities, protective gowns or clothing, respiratory devices, and protective shields and barriers, shall be provided, used, and maintained in a reliable condition wherever it is necessary by reason of hazards to protect yourself while carrying out your job duties.

Occupational Safety and Health Act

The Occupational Safety and Health Act (OSHA) of 1970 affects almost every employer in the United States, including hospitals and health care institutions. In essence, OSHA authorized the Department of Labor to enforce health and safety regulations and provided for the regulations' enforcement. The law requires isolation procedures, radiation safety, proper grounding of electrical equipment, protective storage of flammable and combustible liquids, and the gloving of all personnel when handling body fluids (Guido, 2007).

Musculoskeletal Injuries

OSHA standards were issued in 2000 addressing musculoskeletal disorders that are caused when the worker and the actual physical demands of the work itself are not appropriately matched. Both work-related and non–work-related conditions can individually, or by interacting with each other, give rise to musculoskeletal disorders. There are several approaches that may be used to determine whether conditions in the workplace might be contributing to employees developing these disorders. Employers will sometimes have an analysis of the job or work tasks themselves to identify potential problems before employees injuries occur. Common injuries in the hospital environment include back injuries caused by lifting patients or moving equipment improperly. It is important to use proper body mechanics when lifting, moving, or transporting patients or other heavy objects (United States Department of Labor, 2008).

PROFESSIONAL WORKPLACE PRACTICE

The workplace practice of allied health professionals varies greatly depending on which profession may be discussed. However, general concepts, such as the level of responsibility and authority, the level of autonomy, the division of labor, and motivation on the job, are common concerns among the vast array of health care professions.

Responsibility and Authority

According to Drafke (1994), responsibility and authority should act in concert with each other. Responsibility means that you are held accountable for certain results, while authority means you have been given the ability to fulfill your responsibilities. Problems, and stress, increase when someone has the responsibility for a task but management has not delegated that person the authority to carry it out. For example, you will not be successful if you are given the responsibility for revising the procedures manual in your department without being given the authority to make changes in the procedures. Health care professionals are sometimes placed in a position where they have responsibility for something without the necessary authority. This not only causes stress on the job, but it increases frustration and decreases overall productivity.

Level of Autonomy

Many health care professionals desire a certain level of autonomy in their jobs. As the level of autonomy required of workers increases, stress increases. However, this typically is not a problem unless the workers have not been adequately trained or oriented to their job or have not been given adequate direction on how to perform a task or their job in general.

Removing individual actions and decisions from work can be detrimental as doing so increases boredom and decreases productivity. Therefore, if a job requires that people work autonomously, they must be trained to work independently, and they must be given the authority to do so. As professionals, they should then be held responsible for their actions. Autonomy is a necessary part of every job and leads to a higher level of job satisfaction when properly implemented (Drafke, 1994).

Division of Labor

Management principles have been developed to address ways to improve the operation of organizations in the United States. It is helpful to understand certain principles as a means to improve your understanding of how organizations function and why organizations are the way they are.

The division of labor principle is actually a very old concept. It states that great efficiency is obtained when large jobs are divided into their individual component tasks. Each task is typically performed by one person. For example, the job of removing a patient's gallbladder begins with admitting department personnel processing the patient and the paperwork. A transporter would assist the patient to a hospital room. Nurses would provide care before and after surgery. Medical technologists would perform laboratory exams. Radiology personnel would obtain medical images of the gallbladder and surrounding structures. Pharmacists, dietitians, surgeons, anesthesiologists, housekeepers, and others would all perform their tasks.

Of course, although unlikely, it would be possible for one person to perform all of these tasks. It would not be very efficient, however. One person attempting to perform all of these tasks would have to have had extraordinary training, and even then the job would take much longer. It would also be difficult for one person to perform all of these tasks adequately. This is true for a simple operation like a gallbladder removal. Larger jobs, like open heart surgery, are virtually impossible for one person to perform. The division of labor principle applies to these, and concerns about efficiency. When discussing professional workplace practice, it is actually the division of labor principle that has created the various health professions and the specialties within each profession (Drafke, 1994).

Motivation on the Job

Among several prominent theories of motivation in the workplace, Victor Vroom's Expectancy Theory is helpful to gather a sense of what motivates health care professionals on the job. Essentially, Vroom says that in order for anything to be motivational, the person who is to be motivated must want what is being offered and the person must believe he or she has the chance to earn what is being offered. Note that the second part of the theory doesn't matter if the person actually has a chance at earning the reward—only what the person believes is important.

According to Vroom's theory, the manager can be perfectly fair and equitable in these matters, but if the employee believes he or she is not capable of earning the reward, then it will not be motivational. Only if the reward is something you want and something you believe you have a chance of receiving will it motivate you (Drafke, 1994).

Choosing the Best Workplace Environment

When you are in the interview phase of seeking a job with a potential employer in the United States, you should inquire about the type of professional workplace environment you will be working in. How does the work get done? What is the motivation level of employees? How much autonomy is afforded to health care professionals? How are decisions made? Knowing such things in advance can help you to choose an employer who fits your particular needs and workplace environment.

INTERNATIONAL RIGHTS

The General Assembly of the United Nations, on December 10, 1948, adopted and proclaimed the Universal Declaration of Human Rights. The purpose of the Universal Declaration was to establish a common standard of achievement for all people and all nations, to the end that every individual and every aspect of society shall strive to promote respect for the rights and freedoms of all people in their respective territories under their jurisdiction. As you review the 30 articles of the Declaration, several stand out.

Article 2 of the declaration states, "Everyone is entitled to all the rights and freedoms set forth in this Declaration, without distinction of any kind, such as race, color, sex, language, religion, political or other opinion, national or social origin, property, birth or other status. Furthermore, no distinction shall be made on the basis of the political, jurisdictional, or international status of the country or territory to which a person belongs, whether it be independent, trust, non-self-governing or under any other limitation of sovereignty." This article is congruent with the Civil Rights laws and nondiscrimination laws that are in effect in the United States, which state that everyone should be afforded certain rights and freedoms without discrimination or bias based upon their personal characteristics or place of origin.

Article 6 of the declaration states, "Everyone has the right to recognition everywhere as a person for the law." This article attempts to express that every person has certain basic rights no matter where they are in the world.

Article 7 of the declaration states that, "All are equal before the law and are entitled without any discrimination to equal protection of the law. All are entitled to equal protection against any discrimination in violation of this Declaration and against any incitement to such discrimination." This article attempts to express that every person should have the right of equal treatment throughout the world despite his or her background or nation of origin.

Article 8 of the declaration states that, "Everyone has the right to an effective remedy by the competent national tribunals for acts violating the fundamental rights granted him by the constitution or by law." This article makes it clear that there should be the expectation that a third-party judge or tribunal would review infractions or violations of people's rights.

Article 18 states that, "Everyone has the right to freedom of thought, conscience and religion; this right includes freedom to change his religion or belief, and freedom, either alone or in community with others and in public or private, to manifest his religion or belief in teaching, practice, worship and observance." This article secures the right to worship as one pleases without fear of reprisal.

Article 23 of the declaration states that, "(1) Everyone has the right to work, to free choice of employment, to just and favorable conditions of work and to protection against unemployment. (2) Everyone, without any discrimination, has the right to equal pay for equal work. (3) Everyone who works has the right to just and favorable remuneration, ensuring for himself and his family an existence worthy of human dignity, and supplemented, if necessary, by other means of social protection. (4) Everyone has the right to form and to join trade unions for the protection of his interests."

Article 25 states, "(1) Everyone has the right to a standard of living adequate for the health and well-being of himself and of his family, including food, clothing, housing and medical care and necessary social services, and the right to security in the event of unemployment, sickness, disability, widowhood, old age or other lack of livelihood in circumstances beyond his control. (2) Motherhood and childhood are entitled to special care and assistance. All children, whether born in or out of wedlock, shall enjoy the same social protection." This article speaks directly to social services that should be made available to benefit the well-being of adults and children across the world.

Article 26 of the declaration states, "(1) Everyone has the right to education. Education shall be free, at least in the elementary and fundamental stages. Elementary education shall be compulsory. Technical and professional education shall be made generally available and higher education shall be equally accessible to all on the basis of merit. (2) Education shall be directed to the full development of the human personality and to the strengthening of respect for human rights and fundamental freedoms. It shall promote understanding, tolerance and friendship among all nations, racial or religious groups, and shall further the activities of the United Nations for the maintenance of peace. (3) Parents have a prior right to choose the kind of education that shall be given to their children." This article clearly states the value of education and the basic rights that should be afforded to everyone to inquire and learn (United Nations, 2008).

Protection of Rights

After reviewing the Universal Declaration of Human Rights that has been established by the United Nations, it should be observed that they are congruent with the basic tenets of the labor laws of the United States. Those who are United States citizens or legal immigrants are protected under these rights and should be welcome as a citizen of the world. The history of this country will demonstrate that most of its inhabitants are from other parts of the world, either in the current or past generations. International rights for health professionals who are legal immigrants from anywhere in the world are protected by the laws and regulations of the United States.

SUMMARY

Employment as a health care professional in the United States can be a rich and rewarding experience when you select employment that meets your needs and matches your skills and qualifications. The United States is a nation of immigrants—people who came to the country from other parts of the world, either in the current generation or in past genera-tions. Laws that protect the U.S. worker provide protection for U.S. citi-zens and legal immigrants from all over the world. International rights for health care professionals who are legal immigrants from any country in the world are protected by U.S. law.

REFERENCES

Alexander, D. C., & Pulat, B. M. (1985). *Industrial ergonomics.* Norcross, GA: Industrial Engineering and Management Press.

Boone, L. E., & Kurtz, D. L. (1999). *Contemporary business.* Fort Worth, TX: Dryden Press.

Brewer, C. S., & Rosenthal, T. C. (2008). The health care workforce. In A. R. Kovner & J. R. Knickman (Eds.), *Jonas & Kovner's health care delivery in the United States* (9th ed., pp. 320–355). New York: Springer Publishing.

Drafke, M. W. (1994). *Working in health care: What you need to know to succeed.* Phila-delphia: F. A. Davis Company.

Evans, M. L., & Hicks, F. (2007). Collective action. In P. S. Yoder-Wise (Ed.), *Leading and managing in nursing* (4th ed., pp. 151–167). St. Louis: Mosby.

Guido, G. W. (2007). Legal and ethical issues. In P. S. Yoder-Wise (Ed.), *Leading and managing in nursing* (4th ed., pp. 35–57). St. Louis: Mosby.

Herzberg, F. (1966). *Work and the nature of man.* Cleveland: World.

Hunt, K. A., & Knickman, J. R. (2008). Financing health care. In A. R. Kovner & J. R. Knickman (Eds.), *Jonas & Kovner's health care delivery in the United States* (9th ed., pp. 56–83). New York: Springer Publishing.

Metzger, N. (2004). Human resources management. In L. F. Wolper (Ed.), *Health care administration: Planning, implementing, and managing organized delivery systems* (4th ed., pp. 249–294). Sudbury, MA: Jones and Bartlett.

O'Reilly, B. (1990, March 12). Is your company asking too much? *Fortune,* 38–46.

Pappas, A. B., & Claborn, J. C. (2006). Employment considerations: Opportunities, re-sumes, and interviewing. In J. Zerwekh & J. C. Claborn (Eds.), *Nursing today: Tran-sition and trends* (5th ed.). St. Louis: Saunders.

Pozgar, G. D. (1990). *Legal aspects of health care administration* (4th ed.). Rockville, MD: Aspen.

Rogers, A., Hwang, W., Scott, L. D., Aiken, L. H., & Dinges, D. F. (2004). The working hours of hospital staff nurses and patient safety. *Health Affairs, 23*(4), 202–212.

United Nations. (2008). *Universal declaration of human rights.* Retrieved December 24, 2008, from http://www.un.org/Overview/rights.html

United States Department of Labor. (2008). *Ergonomics—contributing conditions.* Re-trieved December 24, 2008, from http://www.osha.gov/SLTC/ergonomics/contributing_conditions.html

5 The U.S. Health Care System

NANCY C. SHARTS-HOPKO

In This Chapter

Keywords

Alternative therapies: A variety of therapeutic or preventive health care practices, such as homeopathy, naturopathy, chiropractic, and herbal medicine, that complement generally accepted medical methods.

Biomedical research: Medical research and evaluation of new treatments for both safety and efficacy, in what are termed clinical trials, and all other research that contributes to the development of new treatments.

Botanicals: Drugs or products made directly from plants.

Centers for Medicare and Medicaid Services (CMS): The federal agency responsible for administering the Medicare, Medicaid, SCHIP (State Children's Health Insurance), HIPAA (Health Insurance Portability and Accountability Act), CLIA (Clinical Laboratory Improvement Amendments), and several other health-related programs. Formerly known as the Health Care Financing Administration (HCFA).

Community-based care: Services provided in one's own home or other community settings. This system supplies a variety of health care options that allow people to stay in their homes, while still providing important health care support.

Coordinated care: Strategies to make health care systems more cost-effective and responsive to the needs of people with complex chronic illnesses.

Curative care: Refers to treatment and therapies provided to a patient with intent to improve symptoms and cure the patient's medical problem.

Disaster preparedness: Process of ensuring that an organization is prepared in the event of a forecasted disaster to minimize loss of life, injury, and damage to property; and can provide rescue, relief, rehabilitation, and other services after the disaster.

Hospice: A usually small residential institution for terminally ill patients where treatment focuses on the patient's well-being rather than a cure. It includes drugs for pain management and often spiritual counseling.

Meals on Wheels: Provides home-delivered meals to people in need, usually the elderly or the disabled.

Municipal hospitals: Hospitals controlled by the city government.

Palliative care: A specialized form of care focused on the pain, symptoms, and stress of serious illness.

Whether you are considering coming to the United States for employment or you already have begun the visa and licensure processes, understanding the scope and structure of the U.S. health care system can be a daunting task for foreign-educated health care professionals. Those who have basic knowledge of the way health services are organized in the

*United States will be better able to function competently and to help pa-
tients and families navigate the system's many channels. The purpose of
this chapter is to provide you with an understanding of how health care
decisions are made, both economically and organizationally, by physicians, other health care providers, patients, and their families.*

ORGANIZATION OF THE HEALTH CARE SYSTEM

In the United States, individuals access health care services through a
complex array of public or private clinics, private practices, commercial
walk-in settings, employee or school health services, urgent care settings, and hospital systems. The system is large, with over 7,500 hospitals, 2.4 million registered nurses, and 560,000 physicians (Bureau of
Labor Statistics, 2008).

Public Versus Private Health Care

The U.S. health care system includes large numbers of both public and
private health care providers. *Public* sources of health care are directly
managed and funded by a government agency. They include federal,
state, county, and **municipal hospitals** and clinics. Examples of services
provided by the federal government include those of the Veterans Health
Administration, which cares for former active duty military personnel,
and the Indian Health Service, which provides care to those who live on
Native American tribal lands. Other examples include city and county
hospitals such as Bellevue Hospital Center and other hospitals in the
New York City Health and Hospitals Corporation, San Francisco General Hospital, Los Angeles County–University of Southern California
(USC) Medical Center, and Cook County Stroger Hospital in Chicago.

Public clinics and hospitals provide care primarily for lower-income
individuals and families. The system of publicly provided care has diminished over the past 30 years as many governments shifted away from
direct provision of services to contracting with insurance companies
to provide services through private hospitals. While public clinics and
hospitals can and do charge for their services, they usually are heavily
funded by tax dollars.

Private sources of health care include not-for-profit and for-profit
clinics, practices, and hospitals. Not-for-profit hospitals and clinics
charge for services and receive insurance reimbursement for care but

they do not expect to make a profit. All revenue beyond their expenses is to be used for the benefit of the organization. For-profit entities, on the other hand, are operated to generate profits for private owners or shareholders.

Primary, Secondary, and Tertiary Care

In the United States, the level of health care is designated as primary, secondary, or tertiary. These terms refer both to the acuity of care that is provided as well as the nature and location of that care.

Primary Care

The Institute of Medicine (IOM, 1994) defines primary care as "care that is accessible, comprehensive, coordinated, continuous, and accountable." Primary care providers include physicians, nurse practitioners, and physician assistants. Ideally they provide care for people over time that includes health promotion and prevention, the management of acute illnesses or injuries, and the management of chronic conditions. The primary care provider is the point of referral for in-patient or specialty services.

Secondary Care

Primary care providers refer people with complex problems to specialists, or secondary care providers, for their greater, more specific expertise. Common examples include medical specialties such as ophthalmology or dermatology, or nonroutine services such as physical therapy.

Tertiary Care

Tertiary care is advanced or complex care that is provided by medical specialists in referral centers—often academic medical centers that have strong programs of research and the facilities designed for specialized diagnostic and treatment procedures.

Managed Care

Managed care refers to a system of care that became widespread in the United States beginning in 1973 with passage of the Health Maintenance

Organization Act, which is federal legislation that was intended to help reduce health care costs. Originally, managed care referred to the enrollment of people in health maintenance organizations (HMOs), a system or network of health care providers and services that encompassed all levels of care. These HMOs sought to contain costs by ordering bulk purchases of goods and services; limiting diagnostic tests, prescriptions, and referrals to specialty service providers; and using incentives for people to reduce their illness risks by incorporating healthy lifestyle changes and using early screening and other preventive services.

Role of Insurance Providers

Today, most health insurance companies operate using managed care approaches, in which insurers contract with health care providers, such as physicians and nurse practitioners, who agree to operate within the insurer's financial parameters. Most managed care organizations require patients to select their primary care provider from a list approved by the insurance company. This listing of approved providers is called the insurer's *network*.

In many managed care plans, primary care providers function as *gatekeepers,* meaning that a patient is required to get a referral from his or her primary care provider (and, in many cases, approval from the managed care plan) before seeing a specialist. While these requirements were intended to reduce unnecessary use of specialist services, many people feel that they result in additional time and expense as well as in reduced access to services. In recent years, many managed care plans have loosened or eliminated some of their requirements for referrals or prior approval for specialist visits.

When using a managed care plan for in-patient hospital care, the patient is restricted to using only hospitals and providers within the insurer's network. If the patient selects a provider or hospital that is not in-network, the patient pays additional costs. This occurs because the insurance companies contract with certain providers and hospitals that agree to accept reimbursement at a lower, negotiated rate.

Public Health

Public health services are directed at communities and populations for the prevention, management, or elimination of disease and for health promotion. Disease surveillance and vaccination programs, health education for risk reduction, food safety oversight, and the operation of sexually transmitted disease clinics are examples of common public health strategies in the United States.

Centers for Disease Control and Prevention

Since the World Trade Center attacks in 2001 and Hurricane Katrina in 2005, local and state health departments have increasingly focused on planning and preparedness for natural or man-made disasters. Nationally, the Centers for Disease Control and Prevention (CDC), an agency within the U.S. Department of Health and Human Services (HHS), plays a leading role in coordinating and funding public health activities, including **disaster preparedness** efforts.

The CDC monitors the health, illness, and injury of the U.S. population; advocates for national health policies focused on health promotion and disease prevention; and promotes health education. The program units within CDC address workplace health and safety, infectious disease management, terrorism and emergency preparedness, environmental health, health promotion, health information, and global health (CDC, 2008a).

Environmental Health

Within the field of public health, the practice of environmental health has grown significantly in the past several years. Health care providers and health care institutions are increasingly attentive to their impact on the environment. Whether to use disposable versus recyclable equipment is now more than a cost concern; it has become an environmental consideration. How toxic or infectious substances, including medications, are disposed of is a concern because of their potential for contaminating the food and water supply or for spreading infection.

The international coalition *Health Care Without Harm* has been formed to sensitize health care workers to the need to address pollution by the health care industry. One example of the coalition's work is its agenda of eradicating the use, and safely disposing, of mercury thermometers (Health Care Without Harm, 2008).

Ambulatory Care

Ambulatory care is health care delivered outside of an inpatient or residential setting. Ambulatory care settings include physician, nurse practitioner, and dental practices, hospital outpatient clinics, community clinics, school and employee health centers, and urgent care centers.

Urgent Care Centers

Urgent care centers are walk-in (or ambulatory care) facilities usually operating for extended hours where people can be treated for acute illnesses and injuries that are beyond the scope of a primary care provider. There are over 8,000 urgent care facilities in the United States, and their appeal is the accessibility of care as well as the favorable cost compared to hospital emergency department visits (Urgent Care Association of America, 2008). The CDC estimates that over 80% of emergency department visits do not require that level of care; urgent care is filling a gap in the health care system.

Walk-In Clinics

A more recent trend is the emergence of walk-in clinics in commercial venues, such as discount stores or pharmacies. Also referred to as convenient care clinics, retail clinics, and minute clinics, they offer a limited range of primary care services that are more convenient, and typically less expensive, than a visit to a primary care provider's office or an emergency department. They are usually staffed by nurse practitioners, although physician assistants and physicians also work in these sites.

Ambulatory or Day Surgery

Ambulatory surgery can be defined as any surgical procedure that does not require an overnight stay in the hospital. At this time, about 65% of all surgical procedures performed in the United States are performed on a same-day basis.

While the original impetus for this trend was cost savings, there are additional benefits. The risk of hospital-acquired infection is reduced when people return quickly to their homes from a hospital environment, and people tend to recover more quickly in a familiar environment. The technology that has enabled procedures to be performed as same-day procedures is less invasive, so the healing that is required is lessened. Patients are monitored for a few hours after their procedure—typically until they are awake, have stable vital signs, are able to tolerate oral fluids, and can urinate. Day surgery requires that patients and their family members receive clear instructions for postoperative care and symptoms that require immediate attention. It is common for a nurse or surgeon to call patients within a few hours or days of discharge to monitor their status.

Home Care and Community-Based Care

Home care is care provided in the home by health care workers. Most commonly health care professionals, such as nurses, physical therapists, or occupational therapists monitor and manage care on a daily to weekly basis. Nurses may perform procedures such as changing intravenous lines, physical therapists and occupational therapists may attend to the patient's physical and occupational abilities, and routine daily care may be provided by home health aides or by family members. The rise in home care has accompanied the reduction in hospital admissions and hospital lengths of stay. Health care agencies that provide home care are eligible for certification by The Joint Commission, the same agency that certifies hospitals (Joint Commission, 2008), or by the Community Health Accreditation Program (http://www.chapinc.org). Another term that is used when health care services are provided in the patient's home is **community-based care.** Community-based care provides a variety of health care options that allow people to stay in their homes, while still providing important health care support.

Hospice Care

Hospice care is professional support for individuals and their families who face a life-threatening illness, usually terminal or end-stage (Hospicenet, 2008). Hospice care may be provided in hospital settings, but it is more commonly provided in the patient's home or in a home-like setting. Hospice care is based on the principle that death is a normal part of life, and quality of life while a person is dying is a paramount value. Moreover, people who are dying and their family members should be treated compassionately and with dignity.

Hospice care is authorized when the provider indicates that death is imminent or expected within a certain time frame. Care is provided by a team including a physician, a nurse, a chaplain or other spiritual advisor, if desired, and other team members as needed. The management of symptoms such as pain, dyspnea, and anxiety is a primary concern, and spiritual care is often a significant part of hospice care. Care is planned in accordance with the patient's wishes and the family's needs.

Family members are likely to be the primary day-to-day caregivers, while health professionals ensure that they have the knowledge and resources they need to allow their family member to die as comfortably and as peacefully as possible. The hospice team can refer family members to resources for bereavement support following the patient's death.

Long-Term Care

Long-term care refers to a variety of medical and nonmedical services to people with a chronic illness or disability (Medicare, 2008). Most long-term care is provided to assist people with activities of daily living such as eating, dressing, bathing, or going to the bathroom. Long-term care is not age-specific or place-specific. People with temporary or permanent disabilities at any age may require long-term care. Most of the time, the term is used in association with care for elderly persons.

In 2007, 9 million individuals required long-term care; by 2010, it is estimated that 12 million older adults will require this service. The U.S. Department of Health and Human Services, which administers Medicare, estimates that among adults who reach the age of 65, 40% will enter a nursing home, and 10% will be there for 5 or more years. As noted previously, this is a dauntingly expensive proposition. As Medicare describes long-term care, the options range from community-based services to home health, including senior or disabled housing, assisted living, continuing or life-care communities, and nursing homes, to name a few.

Community-Based Services

Community-based services include free or low-cost services that help older adults remain safely and healthily in their homes. These can include adult day care, senior centers, **Meals on Wheels,** financial guidance and assistance with filing taxes, case management, and daily telephone reassurance.

Some older adults may move in with a family member, or conversely, rent space in their homes to an individual who will in return provide some daily assistance. Senior or disabled housing is available, and these facilities are often publicly subsidized so that the resident pays only a portion of the monthly cost. Residents live in their own apartments and typically have services such as laundry, shopping, or housekeeping available.

Assisted Living

Assisted living is a costlier approach to long-term care than community-based services. Residents typically live in their own apartment within a complex and have available such options as assistance with activities of daily living and group meals. Social and recreational activities are commonly provided. On-site health care services also may be available. The cost of assisted living can range widely—up to many thousands of dollars a month for a large apartment in an expensive part of the country. Neither long-term care nor Medicare contributes to the costs of assisted care.

Continuing Care Retirement Communities

Continuing care retirement communities, or life-care communities, offer levels of care as the resident needs them. A healthy older person or a couple might move into an apartment or cottage and live totally independently. Later, the person or couple might require assisted living. Finally, the person will move into the nursing home associated with the community. This is an expensive option. Medicare reports that in 2004 entry fees ranged from $38,000 to $400,000 and the monthly fee ranged from $650 to $3,500 (Medicare, 2008). Long-term care and Medicare will not contribute to costs associated with continuing care retirement communities. Residents often sign over their homes and other assets to fund their residency at such facilities.

Nursing Homes

Nursing homes provide a wide range of personal care and health services, such as activities of daily living for people with a variety of physical, emotional, or cognitive problems. Individuals must fund this care privately or with special insurance because Medicare does not cover this aspect of nursing home care.

Medicare does pay for time-limited skilled nursing care after an illness or injury, and, depending on the facility, Medicaid will cover nursing home costs after an individual's personal assets are spent. In general, it is more likely that individuals will be able to use Medicaid to remain in the setting after their funds are exhausted if it is a nonprofit entity.

Continuing care retirement communities, as well as nursing homes, can be operated as voluntary, nonprofit, or for-profit organizations. Many nonprofit facilities are affiliated with religious groups.

HEALTH CARE FINANCING

In many countries, both private and public sources of health insurance are used. That is the case in the United States, but what is unique in this country is that private insurance is dominant (Chua, 2006). In 2003, 62% of nonelderly Americans had private employer-sponsored insurance, 5% purchased private insurance individually, 15% were insured by public programs such as Medicaid, and 18% were uninsured. Nearly all people age 65 and older are insured through the public program Medicare.

Private Employer-Sponsored Insurance

Private employer-sponsored insurance has been a mainstay of employee benefits since World War II. Employers contract with insurance companies to offer a specific coverage package in which employees can either participate or not. Employees pay some portion of the insurance costs, particularly as they enroll other family members in the plan. The benefits that are covered vary across employers; for instance, some employers provide dental or vision coverage while others do not.

Individual Insurance

Individuals can purchase health insurance directly from insurance companies—the cost is completely borne by the individual subscriber in this case. The cost of health insurance varies widely depending on the insurance company; the scope of benefits the individual seeks; and the person's age, health status, and presence of known health risk factors or preexisting conditions (diagnoses that existed in the past or exist at the time the person seeks health insurance).

Medicare

Medicare is a federal insurance program that covers the health care costs of people age 65 and older as well as some people with disabilities. Medicare is financed through taxes as well as individual premiums for certain benefits. Medicare Part A covers hospitalization costs and requires no premium copay. People may enroll in additional coverage, for which they pay premiums. Medicare Part B covers physician services; Medicare Part C is administered through health management organizations (HMOs) and is referred to as Medicare Advantage; and Medicare Part D is the recently implemented drug plan.

While Medicare has been successful in ensuring access to care for older and disabled Americans, there are gaps in coverage, including incomplete nursing home and health prevention coverage. On average, older individuals spend about 22% of their income on health-related costs despite having Medicare.

Medicaid

Medicaid is a joint federal and state program that provides insurance to many lower-income individuals. Although the federal government provides much of the funding and sets basic criteria for services and coverage, each state administers its own Medicaid program, and thus both covered services and eligibility criteria vary from state to state.

The State Children's Health Insurance Program

The State Children's Health Insurance Program (S-CHIP) was initiated in 1997 to extend coverage to children in low-income families who do not qualify for Medicaid. Like Medicaid, it is jointly funded by federal and state governments and is administered by each state.

Veterans Health Administration

The Veterans Health Administration (VHA) provides health care to veterans of the U.S. armed forces. In general, care is supposed to be provided free or at low cost for conditions directly related to individuals' military service. In reality, many veterans rely on the VHA system for all or most of their care, generally in hospitals and clinics operated directly by the VHA.

Health Care Reform

Numerous solutions have been proposed to address the major issues facing the U.S. health system—providing access to care for all Americans, controlling health care costs, and ensuring quality. Some proposals focus on market-based approaches, such as providing financial incentives to encourage more uninsured Americans to purchase health insurance. Other proposals emphasize greater direct government involvement to ensure universal coverage.

A comprehensive proposal for health reform was proposed to the U.S. Congress by President Bill Clinton in 1993, but after contentious national debate, Congress failed to pass any reform proposals. In the years since then, different approaches have been suggested by political leaders and by organizations representing physicians, nurses, hospitals, insurers, and others. With the election of President Obama, health reform again has been deemed a national political priority.

RECENT TRENDS IN HEALTH CARE

Health care in the United States is provided in a variety of settings by a team of professionals. Depending on the patient's needs, the team may include nurses, advanced practice nurses, physicians, medical social workers, speech therapists, physical therapists, occupational therapists, nutritionists, chaplains, and other specialized professionals. Traditionally the physician was in charge of a patient's care; now, particularly with the advent of managed care, the team works collaboratively, and it may be a case manager working in the health care institution or the patient's health insurance company who oversees the patient's progress through the system or through the illness episode.

While it is impossible to anticipate the future of health care in a rapidly changing environment, several trends in the United States are worth noting: the demographic shift leading to large numbers of older individuals needing health care; the impact of chronic illness and the obesity epidemic on health care delivery; the growing sensitivity to the need for **palliative care** (symptom management), particularly at the end of life; a resurgence in direct provision of health care by employers; and the emergence of concierge care.

Demographic Shift

First and foremost, worldwide there is a demographic shift as life spans increase. In wealthy, industrialized nations, we are faced with the retirement of the baby boom generation, the individuals who were born between approximately 1946 and 1965, after World War II. In the United States, this is the largest group in our nation's history and nearly double the size of the next generation to follow. Because of the size of the baby boom generation, the United States will experience an increasing demand for health care services by older adults—along with a shortage in the labor force available to provide care for them.

Increase in Chronic Illness and Obesity

Chronic illnesses, such as heart disease, stroke, cancer, and diabetes, are among the most prevalent, costly, and preventable of all health problems in the United States—and their incidence is expected to grow (CDC, 2008b). The prolonged course of illness and disability from such chronic diseases can result in a decreased quality of life and an increased use of health care resources. The impact of HIV/AIDS on the minority community and women also will tax the system.

In addition, the U.S. obesity epidemic has many health care implications ranging from anticipated financial demands on the system to physical demands on providers working with larger numbers of obese patients. As of 2006, over one-third of U.S. men and women are obese, and the prevalence of obesity in children is increasing (CDC, 2008c). This will not only exacerbate the incidence of chronic disease, but in the case of childhood obesity, it will also decrease the age of onset of these diseases. It will be an enormous challenge not only to provide services that are needed, but also to control health care costs as this likely scenario unfolds.

Increase in Palliative Care

There is growing sensitivity to the need to shift from **curative care** to palliative care (symptom management) at the end of life. The emergence of intensive care units in the United States in the 1960s led to an explosion of technology—and to its pervasiveness and daily use in health care settings. However, research in recent years has confirmed that patients and families desire compassionate and peaceful deaths without many technological interventions.

A number of organizations have formed to advocate on behalf of people who are dying and their families; one example is a coalition of health care systems, the Supportive Care Coalition (2008). This organization seeks to foster holistic, **coordinated care** for terminally ill people, to enable those who want to die in their homes, and to diminish the number of elders dying in intensive care settings. Fortunately, there seems to be a trend toward promoting palliative care.

Employer-Provided Care

Employer-provided, on-site health care was commonplace before the emergence of managed care and the growth in litigation of the 1970s and 1980s. On-site employee health services are once again emerging as a convenient, low-cost strategy for improving employee health and curtailing overhead costs associated with health care. Moreover, this strategy addresses the needs—which may affect productivity—of employees who decline the company health insurance plan because they cannot afford their portion of the premiums. Companies that have successfully provided on-site care include Coca Cola, Goldman Sachs, Toyota, and Novartis among others (Corporate Research Group, 2008).

Concierge Health Care

Concierge health care, also referred to as boutique care, is controversial because it targets affluent individuals. It is the payment of an annual retainer to a primary care physician, ranging from $50 to $20,000 per family member per year, in return for which he or she will be available to the client at all times. Wait times are reduced, visits are longer, care is more individualized, house calls are available, and some practitioners will accompany their patients to specialists.

The concept emerged out of physician dissatisfaction with managed care and the extreme limitation on their time with each patient—an average per visit of as few as 7 minutes. Hospital attitudes toward concierge care have ranged from regarding it as ethically unacceptable to seizing it as economic opportunity. While many people in the health care industry have ethical concerns with the concept of concierge care, in essence, it does not differ from the already existing opportunity for people to buy expensive and inclusive health care insurance or to pay cash for luxury care—both of which are fully accepted in the U.S. health care system. Data on health outcomes associated with concierge care is not yet available.

QUALITY AND SAFETY IN HEALTH CARE

In 1999, the Institute of Medicine (IOM), composed of respected national leaders in health care, launched an initiative to highlight concerns about safety and quality of health care in the United States. This initiative captured the nation's attention when it reported that as many as 98,000 people die in U.S. hospitals each year due to health care error (IOM, 1999). Other researchers have estimated that U.S. hospital deaths due to error could be as much as five times higher than the IOM's estimate (see, e.g., Zhan & Miller, 2003). Needless to say, these reports and others like them have received attention from consumers, government entities, and the health care industry.

Agency for Healthcare Research and Quality

The Agency for Healthcare Research and Quality (AHRQ, 2008) is the governmental entity within the Department of Health and Human Services charged specifically with promoting health care quality, safety, and effectiveness. AHRQ's efforts have included funding research on improving patient safety and quality, promoting the use of health information technology, and advancing evidence-based practice.

Institute for Healthcare Improvement

To hasten the movement to improve health care quality, the Institute for Healthcare Improvement (IHI) launched the 100,000 Lives Campaign in December 2004 (Berwick, Calkins, McCannon, & Hackbarth, 2006). The nation's hospitals were invited to enroll with a goal that each hospital implement six highly feasible interventions based on published evidence. The six interventions included:

- Deploying rapid response teams with critical care expertise to respond to all codes
- Following published guidelines from the American College of Cardiology and the American Heart Association in caring for people with acute myocardial infarctions
- Reconciling medications at each and every transition in a given patient's site of care
- Following the CDC guidelines for prevention of central line infection
- Following the CDC guidelines for prevention of surgical site infections
- Following the CDC guidelines for prevention of ventilator-associated pneumonia

None of these strategies represent care that is technologically challenging. By July 2006, 50% more hospitals had enrolled than anticipated, and over 123,000 lives had been saved. As a result of the initial success, IHI then launched a campaign to save 5 million lives in the 2006–2008 biennium (Institute for Healthcare Improvement, 2008).

The Centers for Medicare and Medicaid Services

In July 2008, the **Centers for Medicare and Medicaid Services (CMS)** announced that Medicare and Medicaid would no longer cover costs associated with several types of preventable harmful events, including stage III and IV pressure ulcers, falls and trauma involving nursing home or hospital patients, surgical site infections after certain procedures, vascular catheter infections, catheter-associated urinary tract infections, administration of incompatible blood, air embolism, or unintended retention of a foreign object after surgery (CMS, 2008). The intent behind this policy is that avoiding the costs associated with these events will motivate health care systems to institute measures to reduce their occurrence.

Corporate Quality and Safety

One initiative for improving quality and safety has come from the corporate, non–health-care sector. The Leapfrog Group is an organization of large companies that purchase employee health insurance. These companies came together in 1998 in order to use their purchasing power on behalf of patient safety and health care quality. The Leapfrog Group specifically advocates four practices to improve quality and cost-efficiency of care: use of electronic health records, use of evidence-based hospital referrals, staffing intensive care units with physicians specializing in intensive care, and evaluating hospital performance on 30 patient safety indicators endorsed by the National Quality Forum (The Leapfrog Group, 2008).

Electronic Health Records

One of the great hopes for reducing health care errors is the widespread implementation of information technology. For example, many patient safety experts have advocated the use of computerized physician order entry to reduce medication errors, including errors associated with reading handwritten physician orders.

In addition, there are many benefits anticipated to result from the use of electronic health (or medical) records (EHRs). One benefit is that EHRs will be accessible across providers and health systems, thus ensuring clear and complete communication on behalf of patients as they use various services. Online health records would have been helpful in the aftermath of Hurricane Katrina, for example, when large numbers of people were displaced with no records and no identification. In some cases, health records and vital statistics data were permanently lost.

One concern with EHRs is that information must be backed up regularly in the event of a system failure. Ensuring privacy of information remains another concern.

To date, fewer than 20% of hospitals or physician practices in the United States use EHRs. Purchasing and implementing the needed technology is costly, and many systems are reluctant to spend large amounts of money on implementing EHRs until consensus is reached about the standardization and interface of records across systems.

Disaster Preparedness

Disaster preparedness has been a part of health care protocols for many years, but it has taken a more prominent role in health care delivery since the World Trade Center events of September 11, 2001, and Hurricane Katrina in 2005. Disasters, always a part of everyday life, have been increasing due to the global instability, economic downturns, political upheavals and collapse of government structures, violence, civil conflicts, famine, and mass population displacements seen in the late 20th and early 21st centuries. The escalating nature and scope of disasters and their growing complexity provide challenges to health care institutions and health care workers responsible for disaster planning. Disasters are sudden, catastrophic events that can result in great damage, loss, injury, and death. They can be grouped into two types: unintentional and intentional.

Unintentional Disasters

Unintentional disasters are those that occur predominantly as a result of natural events. Natural disasters usually occur suddenly and are often uncontrollable; however, they frequently cluster in a certain time period or geographic location and, therefore, are somewhat predictable. In the

United States and other developed countries, most natural disasters tend to cause extensive damage and social disruption with comparatively little loss of life. Unintentional disasters include such events as tsunamis, floods, typhoons, earthquakes, and epidemics. The response to unintentional disasters may be local or worldwide depending on the magnitude of the event. The most frequent natural or unintentional disasters experienced in the United States are floods, earthquakes, hurricanes, tornados, and fires.

Intentional Disasters

Intentional disasters are those that occur as the result of human purpose; that is, they are man-made or the result of human intervention and include such events as terrorism, bioterrorism, chemical releases, nuclear accidents, and explosions directly associated with human action. They can be caused by deliberate malicious activities or when industrial facilities are disrupted by natural disasters. Intentional disasters share many of the characteristics of natural ones but are typically less predictable.

Role of Health Care Professionals

Health care workers are on the front lines when a disaster occurs; therefore, all health care personnel need to have a basic understanding of disaster preparedness. All health care professionals need to know how to keep themselves and their patients and families safe during any disaster event.

Disaster care differs from emergency care in several ways. Emergency care usually involves care for patients with acute injuries or life-threatening illnesses and is usually administered in an emergency department or on a trauma unit. Disaster care involves providing care in response to natural and man-made events that affect entire communities.

The widespread injury and disruption associated with disasters can pose difficult problems for health care providers, including the triage of mass casualties, disruption of infrastructure (e.g., loss of power and fresh water), and the need to deal with the mental anguish associated with uncertainty and the loss of loved ones. The outcome of a disaster is influenced by many factors, including population location and density, timing of the event, and community preparedness (e.g., emergency response infrastructure).

Similarly, recovery after a disaster is influenced by resources (e.g., savings, insurance, and relief aid), preexisting conditions (e.g., season of the year, local infrastructure, etc.), experience, and access to information. In almost all cases, disasters are associated with mental and physical stress (both during and after the event) that can increase morbidity and mortality over and above that caused directly by the event itself (Veenema, 2007).

Disaster Plans

Most hospitals and other health care facilities have disaster plans in place. These plans should address four phases: preparedness, identification, response, and recovery. All health care providers should be aware of the plans drawn up by their institution and know their role should a disaster occur. States and cities have implemented disaster preparedness procedures to coordinate government and health system effectiveness.

Preparedness. Developing, testing, and maintaining a plan for handling unexpected events will yield a fast and effective response should a disaster occur. Preparedness includes identifying key emergency personnel (e.g., law enforcement, health care and fire personnel, and school administrators), identifying areas of vulnerability (e.g., events/facilities that have a large number of people present, food and water systems, etc.), developing a comprehensive security plan and disaster response plan, and conducting and maintaining the training of responders. In this stage, the community's and the health care institution's ability to respond is assessed.

Identification. A basic element for minimizing loss during a disaster is rapid identification that an event has occurred. That translates into knowing when something unusual is occurring within the local community, recognizing it, and reporting it to the appropriate authorities.

Response. While a disaster is unfolding and until control of the event has been established, the two-way communication of information becomes paramount. Questions, concerns, and facts should be collected and channeled to appropriate agencies while information from those agencies is disseminated to responders and to the public. Volunteers and first responders, such as police, fire, and health care personnel, are mobilized to assess the extent of the disaster and to respond.

Recovery. Recovery from a disaster will be a long process and will require local personnel and agencies that know and understand the community and how it functions. Impacted areas will require follow-up interaction, education, and assistance to minimize short-term and long-term consequences. Because this is a long-term process, the approach will require an evaluation of the disaster response team and the development of a new or revised plan of work for recovery.

ACCESS TO HEALTH CARE INFORMATION

Access to information on health care providers and health conditions is increasingly available to consumers through a variety of sources. For example, Medicare provides public access to information related to quality of care in hospitals, skilled nursing facilities, and home health agencies via the Internet. Many states are creating publicly accessible databases that enable health care consumers to examine quality outcome data about providers and hospitals. The Agency for Healthcare Research and Quality (AHRQ) offers consumers an extensive Web site with information about safety in general and standards of care for specific conditions (2008).

The Internet has generated an explosion of information that consumers can and do access. Hospitals, particularly academic medical centers, often have extensive Web sites that offer information to patients about specific conditions and how they are managed. U.S. organizations that advocate on behalf of the prevention and treatment of specific diseases and conditions, such as the American Cancer Society and the American Heart Association, offer extensive information about these conditions. It is increasingly common for patients to approach health care providers with information about their condition. Information shared by patients should be regarded with respect and patients need to be viewed as collaborators in their own care. That does not mean that all health information is of high quality; therefore, all health care professionals need to help patients understand which information is useful and why.

Access to information on health care providers and health conditions is increasingly available to consumers through a variety of sources. For example, Medicare provides public access to information related to quality of care in hospitals, skilled nursing facilities, and home health agencies via the Internet. Many states are creating publicly accessible databases that enable health care consumers to examine quality outcome data about providers and hospitals. The AHRQ offers consumers an extensive Web site with information about safety in general and standards of care for specific conditions (2008).

The Internet has generated an explosion of information that consumers can access. Hospitals, particularly academic medical centers, often have extensive Web sites that offer information to patients about specific conditions and how they are managed. U.S. organizations that advocate on behalf of the prevention and treatment of specific diseases and conditions, such as the American Cancer Society and the American Heart Association, offer extensive information about these conditions, and it is increasingly common for patients to approach health care providers with information about their conditions. Information shared by patients should be regarded with respect, and patients need to be viewed as collaborators in their own care. That does not mean that all health information is of high quality; therefore, all health professionals, including nurses, need to help patients understand which information is useful and why.

ALTERNATIVE HEALTH PRACTICES

Patients and families in the United States make extensive use of health practices that are outside the health care system, although increasingly, health care institutions are incorporating some of these strategies. These therapies often are referred to as complementary and alternative medicine.

According to a national survey conducted by the CDC's National Center for Health Statistics (2004), 36% of U.S. adults use some form of complementary therapy within a given year. When prayer is included, the number rises to 62%. The 10 most common modalities include prayer for own health (43%); prayer for health of another (24%); natural products including herbs, **botanicals,** and enzymes (19%); deep breathing exercises (12%); group prayer for own health (10%); meditation (8%); chiropractic (8%); yoga (5%); massage (5%); and diet therapies (4%).

Many prestigious medical centers have sought to integrate these modalities into conventional care. For example, Memorial Sloan-Kettering Cancer Center established its Integrative Medicine Service in 1999 to offer patients and their families a holistic approach to care that combines

alternative therapies with mainstream cancer care. The National Institutes of Health (NIH) also has a national center for complementary and alternative medicine that has been operating since 1999.

SUMMARY

While it is impossible to provide an exhaustive description of the U.S. health care system within the scope of a single article or chapter, this chapter is an attempt to offer a broad overview of issues that shape the way individual patients access health care services. There is much that is good about the U.S. health care system. Innovation in **biomedical research,** delivery of services, and health professions education has contributed to a high quality of life in the United States. Still, challenges associated with access to care and the financing of health care, as well as assurance of safe, high-quality care, remain to be solved.

REFERENCES

Agency for Healthcare Research and Quality. (2008). *AHRQ annual highlights, 2007.* Retrieved October 15, 2008, from http://www.ahrq.gov/about/highlt07.htm

Berwick, D. M., Calkins, D. R., McCannon, C. J., & Hackbarth, A. D. (2006). The 100,000 lives campaign: Setting a goal and a deadline for improving health care quality. *Journal of the American Medical Association, 295*(3), 324–327.

Bureau of Labor Statistics. (2008). *Occupational employment statistics. List of SOC occupations. U.S. Department of Labor Bureau of Labor Statistics.* Retrieved October 25, 2008, from http://www.bls.gov/oes/current/oes_stru.htm#29–0000

Centers for Disease Control and Prevention. (2008a). *About CDC.* Retrieved October 15, 2008, from http://www.cdc.gov/about/

Centers for Disease Control and Prevention. (2008b). *Chronic disease overview.* Retrieved January 29, 2009, from http://www.cdc.gov/NCCdphp/overview.htm

Centers for Disease Control and Prevention. (2008c). *Overweight and obesity.* Retrieved October 15, 2008, from http://cdc.gov/nccdphp/dnpa/obesity/

Centers for Medicare & Medicaid Services (CMS). (2008). *Center for Medicaid and State Operations. Letter of July 31, 2008.* Retrieved October 15, 2008, from http://www.cms.hhs.gov/SMDL/downloads/SMD073108.pdf

Chua, K.-P. (2006). *Overview of the U.S. health care system. American Medical Student Association.* Retrieved October 12, 2008, from http://www.amsa.org/uhc/HealthcareSystemOverview.pdf

Corporate Research Group. (2008). *Best practices of on-site employee health clinics: Strategies for success.* New Rochelle, NY: Corporate Research Group.

Health Care Without Harm. (2008). *About us.* Retrieved October 15, 2008, from http://www.noharm.org/us/aboutUs/missionGoals

Hospicenet. (2008). *Hospice.* Retrieved October 15, 2008, from http://www.hospicenet.org/index.html

Institute for Healthcare Improvement. (2008). *Protecting 5,000,000 lives.* Retrieved October 15, 2008, from http://www.ihi.org/IHI/Programs/Campaign/

Institute of Medicine (IOM). (1994). *Defining primary care: An interim report.* Washington, DC: National Academies Press.

Institute of Medicine. (1999). *To err is human: Building a safer health system.* Washington, DC: National Academies Press.

The Joint Commission. (2008). *Home care.* Retrieved October 15, 2008, from http://www.jointcommission.org/AccreditationPrograms/HomeCare

The Leapfrog Group. (2008). *The Leapfrog Group fact sheet.* Accessed on October 15, 2008, from http://www.leapfroggroup.org/about_us/leapfrog-factsheet

Medicare. (2008). *Long term care.* Retrieved October 15, 2008, from http://www.medicare.gov/longtermcare/static/home.asp

National Center for Health Statistics. (2004). *More than one-third of U.S. adults use complementary and alternative medicine.* Retrieved January 18, 2009, from http://www.cdc.gov/nchs/pressroom/04news/adultsmedicine/htm

Supportive Care Coalition. (2008). *About the coalition.* Retrieved October 15, 2008, from http://www.supportivecarecoalition.org/AboutCoalition/mission_statement.htm

Urgent Care Association of America. (2008). *About urgent care.* Retrieved October 15, 2008, from http://www.ucaoa.org/home_abouturgentcare.php

Veenema, T. G. (Ed.). (2007). *Disaster nursing and emergency preparedness for chemical, biological and radiological terrorism and other hazards* (2nd ed.). New York: Springer Publishing.

Zhan, C., & Miller, M. E. (2003). Excess length of stay, charges, and mortality attributable to medical injuries during hospitalization. *Journal of the American Medical Association, 290*(14), 1868–1874.

Health Care Professional Practice in the United States

6

DEBORAH McNEIL WHITEHOUSE, DAVID D. GALE, JAY LUBINSKY, KATHRYN M. DOIG, SCOTT McPHEE, BARBARA SANDERS, GERALDINE BUCK, NICOLE GARA, AND CAROLYN WILES HIGDON

In This Chapter

INTRODUCTION

DEBORAH McNEIL WHITEHOUSE
AND DAVID D. GALE

Keywords

CGFNS International: CGFNS International is an internationally recognized authority on credentials evaluation and verification pertaining to the education, registration, and licensure of nurses and health care professionals worldwide. The organization was named in the 1996 immigration law to screen all health professionals (except physicians) seeking an occupational visa to practice in the United States.

Cultural competence: An ability to interact effectively with people of different cultures.

Foreign Credentialing Commission on Physical Therapy (FCCPT): A nonprofit organization created to assist the U.S. Citizenship and Immigration Services (USCIS) and U.S. jurisdiction licensing authorities by evaluating the credentials of foreign-educated physical therapists who wish to immigrate and work in the United States.

National Board for Certification in Occupational Therapy (NBCOT): A not-for-profit credentialing agency that provides certification for the occupational therapy profession and federal screening for international occupational therapists seeking a visa to practice in the United States.

In the United States, the allied health professions include most health professions other than nursing, medicine, dentistry, and pharmacy and represent a large and increasingly important health care employment market. Physical therapy, medical laboratory technology, medical laboratory technician, occupational therapy, physician assistants, occupational therapy, speech-language pathology, and audiology are all identified as employment growth markets. Across these professions, the Bureau of Labor Statistics (BLS) has projected approximately 145,200 total new health care jobs by 2016 (see chapter 1, Table 1.3). The needs of a growing elderly population, the increased survival of high-risk patients, and a retiring health care workforce fuel this evolving market.

This chapter will first provide an overview of the education and practice of allied health professionals in the United States, highlighting the allied health professions named in the 1996 Illegal Immigration Reform and Immigrant Responsibility Act. The chapter will then focus on each of the allied health professions, discussing such topics as education for entry into practice, obtaining a license, licensure and certification requirements, scope of practice, ethical and legal considerations in practice, and professional resources for each profession.

IMMIGRATION OF ALLIED HEALTH PROFESSIONALS

Immigration is complex and the changing scope of practice, increased independence, and increasing education levels of health professionals in the United States have added to the challenges of entry and practice for the foreign-educated health professional. In order to work legally in the United States, all foreign-born health care providers must have a Health Care Worker Certificate. To obtain a certificate, the professional must have education that is comparable to that required for the profession in the United States. All foreign-educated health care workers also must meet state licensure and practice requirements, demonstrate English proficiency, and if already licensed, provide evidence of clear and unrestricted current and past licenses.

Three agencies are approved to review the credentials needed to obtain a certificate: **CGFNS International (CGFNS)** for all named professions; the **National Board for Certification in Occupational Therapy (NBCOT®)** for occupational therapists only; and the **Foreign Credentialing Commission on Physical Therapy (FCCPT)** for physical therapists only. In 2007, a little over 1,605 certificates were issued to allied health professionals. Physical therapists received the majority (1,196), followed by medical technologists (697), occupational therapists (255), and speech-language pathologists (154), with medical laboratory technicians, physician assistants, and audiologists each reported as receiving less than 15 certificates. The top countries of education reported for health care worker visa applicants were the Philippines, India, the United States, Canada, South Korea, Taiwan, and Australia (CGFNS International, 2008a; Foreign Credentialing Commission on Physical Therapy [FCCPT], 2008a; National Board for Certification in Occupational Therapy [NBCOT], 2008). By law, health care workers born outside of the United States but U.S.-educated must obtain a Health Care Worker Certificate (see chapter 3).

EDUCATION OF ALLIED HEALTH PROFESSIONALS

One of the evolving barriers to the immigration of foreign-educated health professions and to practice in the United States is the rapidly changing education market. The United States has made and is still making education changes, rapidly elevating degree requirements. Professional *entry* degree requirements have the greatest impact on immigration.

Degree Requirements

Audiology stopped accrediting master's level audiology programs in 2006 and now requires the doctorate, AuD, for entry into practice (Council on Academic Accreditation [CAA], 2008). Occupational therapy was originally offered at the baccalaureate level in the United States but the master's degree became the *entry* degree nationally in 2007 and the doctorate in occupational therapy (OTD) is becoming rapidly available (American Occupational Therapy Association [AOTA], 2008). While audiology and occupational therapy have actually changed the *entry* requirement, raising concerns about the educational comparability requirement for obtaining the Health Care Worker Certificate, other disciplines are moving rapidly toward future entry degree changes.

In 2000, the physical therapy professional organization, the American Physical Therapy Association (APTA), adopted the vision statement that all physical therapists would be educated at the doctorate level by 2020. Physical therapy stopped accrediting bachelor's programs in 2001, requiring the Master's in Physical Therapy (MPT) for entry into practice. In 2002, the Commission on Accreditation in Physical Therapy Education (CAPTE) changed its scope of accreditation to entry-level master's and doctorate programs (Commission on Accreditation in Physical Therapy Education [CAPTE], 2008a). Physical therapy graduate programs are converting to the doctorate in physical therapy (DPT) quickly, with over 85% of the schools offering the DPT and the profession seeking to have 99.5% of all U.S. physical therapy programs at the DPT level by 2010 (CAPTE, 2008b). If this occurs, the DPT may well be the entry requirement soon after the 2010 date.

Physician assistant programs, a product of the U.S. health care system, have converted most of their programs to a graduate entry with residencies available for specialization (American Academy of Physician Assistants [AAPA], 2008). Medical laboratory technologists are primarily educated at the baccalaureate level, but the profession is planning for a future professional doctorate (DCLS) to enhance education, which may eventually elevate their entry requirement at least to the master's level. While the occupational therapy doctorate (OTD), DPT, and DCLS are currently adding to educational opportunities for these professions, the availability of such degrees, the difference in practice areas, and the ability to practice more independently are forces likely to affect immigration and licensure issues throughout the United States in the future. The issue of comparable education, including clinical hours, has the potential to slow, or at least temporarily limit, the ability of foreign-educated health professionals to meet the comparable education criteria for obtaining an occupational visa.

HEALTH CARE DELIVERY IN THE UNITED STATES

The looming shortage of health care professionals places market pressure on clinical agencies and providers to find ways to deliver effective quality health care with different balances of providers. As roles expand, conflict often arises as professions overlap role boundaries and provide similar services. Health care agencies seek to find the right provider for the right health care need in the right setting. Much of U.S. health care has shifted from a hospital-based setting to a community or outpatient setting where different provider skill sets are emphasized. As a new employee in any of these settings, knowledge of agency policies and procedures and of professional practice guidelines is critical to successful safe practice.

Quality Health Care

The challenge of efficiently delivering individualized, effective care is one facing every health care provider. Hospitals, nursing homes, community clinics, and emergency rooms are often crowded. Waiting rooms may be overflowing and emergency rooms flooded with insured and uninsured individuals seeking needed health care. The use of emergency rooms for routine care is the most expensive delivery modality but guarantees that care will be provided.

The United States, even with its excellent technology and highly educated providers, has yet to master the challenge to provide quality health care to the full population. The country's public health challenges are many and continue to evolve as health care professionals and communities work with our elected leaders and government agencies to meet these tremendous needs and to discover and implement new and successful strategies.

Such health care challenges can be both energizing and rewarding. The exciting opportunity of delivering health care in the United States is afforded by the wealth of technology, expert colleagues and specialists, and the continually developing medical research that constantly leads to revolutionary new treatments and cures. An emphasis on evidence-based practice is pushing new, effective practices to the bedside and into the clinicians' hands quickly upon discovery. Pharmacology options and new procedures are being released at remarkable rates. Opportunities exist for interdisciplinary planning and development of collaborative new approaches for the delivery of quality health care. State-of-the-art technology combines with evidence-based practice delivery. Most work environments are energizing and exciting, with different patients and challenges every single day.

DIVERSITY IN HEALTH CARE

The United States is becoming rapidly more diverse. Because of this diversity, **cultural competence** is an integral part of health care practice in the United States and much has been written on cultural competence in health care since the 1990s. The U.S. Census Bureau projects that by 2050 no single racial or ethnic group will constitute a majority of the population (U.S. Census Bureau, 2004).

Cultural Competence

Madeline Leininger, the founder of transcultural nursing, defines human care in the context of culture, emphasizing that competent meaningful health care can occur only when cultural values are known and foundational to the care delivered (Leininger & McFarland, 2002). Cultural competence has been described as a process consisting of the five interrelated concepts of cultural desire, awareness, knowledge, skills, and encounters (Campinha-Bacote, 2007).

The American Psychiatric Association (2000) in its *Diagnostic and Statistical Manual of Mental Disorders,* fourth edition, with text revision (DSM-IV-TR), addresses the critical importance of consideration of cultural context in any assessment and treatment evaluation. It even includes an appendix for cultural formulation and a discussion on culturally bound syndromes, which denotes recurrent, locally specific behavioral variations that may not be linked to a diagnostic category.

Universities have focused on recruiting more diverse students into the health professions since the 1990s but the provider population still does not mirror the patient population in diversity. Most professional health care education programs specifically address cultural competence in their curriculums and their essential educational documents. Clinical agencies provide training in cultural sensitivity and competence. The government and many private entities offer online education in cultural competence. Most suggest that cultural competency training needs to occur early professionally and be repeated frequently (South-Paul & Like, 2008).

Language is an important part of cultural competence with any practice. Multilingual health care professionals are in greater demand and have a competitive advantage in most health care delivery systems because of the increasing patient diversity. The foreign-educated allied health professional adds diversity to the workforce and, like all providers, will need to strive to deliver culturally competent care to a diverse population.

ROLES OF ALLIED HEALTH PROFESSIONALS

As the population ages, new and more health services are needed. Many of these services fall clearly within the roles of audiologists, speech-language pathologists, occupational therapists, medical laboratory technologists/technicians, physical therapists, and physician assistants. Part of the new demand may be within the over-85-year-old patient population. Retirement communities, transitional living facilities, and long-term facilities are already part of American life. The need for qualified creative administrators, therapists, and other allied health care professionals with the new geriatric population is still evolving.

Care for Seniors

While traditional long-term care has been fraught with turnover, lower wages, and less pleasant environmental conditions, the new aging population is perhaps reforming that system. A shift from long-term institutional care to home-based and community care is already occurring. The new senior population is healthier and will be increasingly diverse and well educated (Stone, 2008). Thus, the new seniors will probably decide to live independently in the community longer and expect professional health services directed at enhancing their quality of life. Direct care and support services for healthy aging that incorporate exercise, diet, and activities of daily living will offer emerging avenues for enterprising health care professionals. Rewarding career opportunities will abound with this population.

SUMMARY

The allied health professions specifically designated in this book have tremendous opportunities in the United States and much to contribute to health care. Globalization will continue to strengthen and improve health care delivery. With increasing globalization, the United States will export as well as import health professionals, and professional roles and education curriculums will continue to merge. The evolving roles, challenges, opportunities, and professional development opportunities create an exciting present and future for the foreign-educated health professional in the United States.

AUDIOLOGY

JAY LUBINSKY

Keywords

Academy of Rehabilitative Audiology (ARA): An organization that promotes hearing care through the provision of comprehensive, rehabilitative, and habilitative services.

American Academy of Audiology (AAA): An organization that promotes quality hearing and balance care by advancing the profession of audiology through leadership, advocacy, education, public awareness, and support of research.

American Board of Audiology (ABA): An organization dedicated to enhancing audiologic services to the public by promulgating universally recognized standards in professional practice.

Bias: Term used to describe an action, judgment, or other outcome influenced by a prejudged perspective.

Certification: A process for verifying that an individual or institution has met predetermined standards.

Certificate of Clinical Competence in Audiology (CCC-A): The American Speech-Language-Hearing Association, ASHA, offers the Certificate of Clinical Competence in two areas: speech-language pathology and audiology. All applicants must possess an earned graduate degree (master's or doctoral degree) in order to meet application qualifications.

Council for Clinical Specialty Recognition (CCSR): An agency that implements, monitors, and revises as may become necessary the specialty recognition standards in audiology and in speech-language pathology.

Council of State Association Presidents (CSAP): An organization that provides leadership training for state speech-language-hearing association presidents and provides a forum for collaborating and networking.

Council on Academic Accreditation (CAA): The Council on Academic Accreditation in Audiology and Speech-Language Pathology (CAA) accredits eligible clinical doctoral programs in audiology and master's degree programs in speech-language pathology.

Endorsement: An amendment to a contract or license allowing a change in the original terms.

Mutual Recognition Agreement (MRA): An international agreement by which two or more countries agree to recognize one another's education, programs, licensure, and so forth, in an effort to increase mobility between and among the nations that sign the agreement.

Third-party payers: Any insurer, nonprofit hospital service plan, health care service plan, health maintenance organization, self-insurer, or any person or other entity that provides payment for medical and related services.

Audiology, at least in the United States, is a nonmedical clinical practice; that is, audiologists do not need to be medical doctors. The **American Academy of Audiology** *(AAA, 2008a) defines an audiologist as "a professional who diagnoses, treats, and manages individuals with hearing loss or balance problems." The American Speech-Language-Hearing Association (ASHA) says, "Audiologists are professionals engaged in autonomous [independent] practice to promote healthy hearing, communication competency, and quality of life for persons of all ages through the prevention, identification, assessment, and reha-bilitation of hearing, auditory function, balance, and other related systems" (ASHA, 2004a).*

AUDIOLOGY EDUCATION IN THE UNITED STATES

U.S. audiology education forms the basis for professional practice and also forms the basis for comparison with audiologists educated outside the United States. It becomes important, then, for foreign-educated au-diologists to understand the system. It also will be helpful to people in countries outside the United States who are thinking about coming to this country for audiology education.

Baccalaureate Education as Basis

Since 1962, the basis for professional practice has been a graduate degree. Education in U.S. colleges and universities offers first an undergraduate bachelor's degree (typically Bachelor of Arts or Bachelor of Science), which usually takes 4 years to achieve. Bachelor-level education most often includes studies in a wide range of subjects—literature, art, science, mathematics, social/behavioral sciences, and more. This is called general or liberal education.

Bachelor degrees usually include a *major*, which is a concentration of courses in a narrower field. Because audiology is part of the field of human communication sciences and disorders, undergraduate education is not limited to audiology, but will include basic processes for all communication sciences and disorders. Examples are courses in anatomy for speech and hearing, acoustic aspects of speech and hearing, phonetics, and normal language development. There are usually some courses in disorders of communication and clinical processes, such as an overview course of speech, language, and hearing disorders and courses in general clinical processes of diagnosis and treatment. Most often an introductory course in audiology is included. However, all these undergraduate, bachelor's-level courses do not prepare someone to work as an audiologist.

Graduate Degree for Entry into Practice

Following the bachelor's degree, to prepare to work as a professional audiologist, a person must achieve a graduate degree. Until recently, the degree was a master's degree, usually a Master of Arts or Master of Science. More recently, because of the expansion of knowledge and skill needed by audiologists, the great majority of audiology programs offer a professional (or clinical, as opposed to a research) doctoral degree. In fact, the requirements for **certification** in audiology (see the section on certification in this chapter) by ASHA will require a doctoral degree by 2012 (ASHA, 2008b). In practice, though, few programs still offer the master's degree and almost all programs now offer a professional doctoral degree, usually the Doctor of Audiology (AuD). Certification in audiology by the **American Board of Audiology** (ABA) requires a doctoral degree (ABA, 2005).

Theoretical Basis of Education

Education in audiology is based on a set of knowledge and skills considered to be the most important ones for entry into professional practice. The knowledge and skills required by ASHA are typical, and form the basis for their Certificate of Clinical Competence and for the license requirements for many states. These are stated in the standards for certification that went into effect in 2007 (ASHA, 2008b).

To meet these standards, someone who wants to be an audiologist must develop knowledge and skills in the following:

1. Prerequisite areas, such as the ability to write well and knowledge in areas of general education
2. Foundations of practice, such as ethics, anatomy, normal speech and language development, and characteristics of acoustic signals
3. Prevention, identification, assessment, and treatment of hearing and balance disorders (ASHA, 2008b)

These are only some examples from each of the categories of knowledge. You can see the full list in the certification standards on the ASHA Web site, www.asha.org.

Clinical Practicum

In addition to classes, audiology education includes requirements in practical application. Again, ASHA's standards are typical and require practical experience equal to 12 months of full-time work over the course of the program. In fact, most programs exceed this standard and require a fourth year in which students complete a full year of practicum after they have finished their courses and other practicum.

Finding an Audiology Program

If you are interested in studying for an audiology degree in the United States, there are a few sources you can go to for information. Probably the most complete one is the Web site of ASHA, www.asha.org, where you can find a list of all programs accredited by ASHA in speech-language pathology as well as in audiology. In addition, the Web site has answers to frequently asked questions about clinical doctoral programs (ASHA, 2008d). ASHA also has some advice on the best ways to be accepted into a graduate program (ASHA, 2008e). Finally, ASHA has a service called *EdFind* (ASHA, 2007b). On this page, you can search for a program by state, search for a program by areas of research interest, and ascertain whether a program offers courses or an entire degree by distance education. You also can find information about financial support. The listing of each program has a link to a page with more detail about the program, as well as the institution's Web site and the e-mail address of the program director.

The Web site of AAA also can help you find an academic program in audiology (AAA, 2008c). However, the listing of each program does not have the detail of the ASHA *EdFind* and you will need to contact the listed program director. You can also get some general information about what AAA thinks audiology programs should consist of and what to look for in a program.

No matter which source you use to find a program, make sure to carefully examine the Web site and any other available information about programs in which you are interested. Do not hesitate to contact the program director or other representative about questions you have.

CREDENTIALS IN AUDIOLOGY

Certification

Professions in the United States have a history and tradition of *certification*. Certification is a *voluntary* credential, reflecting the standards of a recognized professional association. It has no legal status, but may form the basis for government-issued credentials, especially licenses. It is offered to individuals, rather than to large entities such as academic programs or entire institutions (these receive *accreditation*). Certification should reflect high standards and a profession's responsibility to monitor the quality of service of its practitioners.

American Board of Audiology

In the United States, two certificates can be held by audiologists. One is offered by the American Board of Audiology (ABA). The ABA's purpose is "to identify and formally recognize those audiologists whose knowledge base and clinical skills are consistent with professionally established standards and who continue to enhance their knowledge, skills and abilities through advanced training and other educational activities" (ABA, 2008a). However, the ABA itself does not establish its own certification standards, but "verifies that an individual has successfully completed a course of graduate study in audiology from a regionally accredited university, and has earned a doctoral degree in audiology" (ABA, 2008b). The ABA also does not define standardized education, but instead relies on the accreditation of the parent college or university (not the audiology program) as the mark of quality. (Note: In the United States, the quality of colleges and universities is marked by approval, or *accreditation*, by one of several regional accrediting bodies approved by the U.S. Department of Education.)

Council on Clinical Certification

The other certificate is the **Certificate of Clinical Competence in Audiology (CCC-A)**, offered by the Council for Clinical Certification (CFCC), a semi-autonomous body of ASHA. Many more audiologists hold this certificate than the ABA certificate. In contrast to ABA's certificate, which relies on regional accreditation of the home institution, the CFCC has developed its own extensive *Standards for the Certificate of Clinical Competence in Audiology* (SCCC-A; ASHA, 2008b).

The current SCCC-A went into effect in 2007. The heart of the standards is the set of knowledge and skill statements in Standard IV. These are briefly described in this chapter's section on Education in Audiology in the United States. Besides the knowledge and skill outcomes, the SCCC-A contains standards relating to the degree (Standard I), the institution (Standard II), the program of study (Standard III), assessment (Standard V), and maintenance of certification (Standard VI).

You should be aware of the requirement in Standard V that, in order to be certified, you must pass a national examination in audiology. The examination used by ASHA is the Praxis Examination in Audiology, developed by the Educational Testing Service. The passing score is 600. The same examination is also used for the certificate of the ABA as well as for any states that require an examination for their license. The ABA also requires a passing score of 600, though the required passing score may be different for state licenses.

As a profession that is always growing, you should expect that standards will change from time to time. The CFCC has proposed changes to the audiology standards. As of this writing, they have been sent out for public comment. It is important that audiologists educated outside the United States, or individuals from outside the United States who want to study audiology in a U.S. university, keep up with these changes. Once approved, they will be on ASHA's Web site, www.asha.org.

Clinical Specialty Recognition

As audiologists develop their careers, they may become more skilled in a few areas of practice, or even one area. That is, they become specialized. Credentials exist to recognize specialization.

ASHA maintains a **Council for Clinical Specialty Recognition (CCSR).** According to ASHA, "Specialty recognition is a means by which audiologists or speech-language pathologists with advanced knowledge, skills and experience beyond the Certificate of Clinical Competence (CCC-A or CCC-SLP) can be recognized by consumers, colleagues, referral and payer sources, and the general public" (ASHA, 2007c). As of this writing (December, 2008), there are no recognized specialty areas in audiology by CCSR. The American Board of Audiology does have specialty recognition for audiologists who work with patients who have cochlear implants (ABA, 2008c).

Mutual Recognition Agreements

ASHA maintains a **mutual recognition agreement (MRA)** with several countries. This agreement allows a practitioner who becomes certified in a non-U.S. country to receive the ASHA Certificate of Clinical Competence upon applying and paying application fees. Currently, ASHA's MRA includes Canada, Great Britain, Australia, New Zealand, and Ireland. However, the MRA is only for speech-language pathologists; there are no MRAs for audiology.

Licensure

A license is a credential offered by a government agency. As such, it is a legal credential. You cannot legally practice in the jurisdiction of the licensing agency without it. In the United States, each state can require a license (or not) and, if you want to practice audiology in more than one state, you will need the license of each of those states. Many states, however, make the process quite simple (applying and paying fees) if you have a license from another state. Currently, 49 states and the District of Columbia require audiologists to have a license. Colorado has an *audiology registry,* which is not required to practice legally. However, if you are in Colorado and want to call yourself an audiologist, you must be registered (ASHA, 2008f).

The legal basis for selling hearing aids is particularly important for audiologists. Currently, 30 states allow audiologists to dispense hearing aids if they hold an audiology license (in New Mexico, audiologists must have an **endorsement** on their audiology license to dispense hearing aids; in Connecticut and Texas some other conditions apply). Twenty states and the District of Columbia require a separate hearing aid dispenser's license; that is, the audiology license will not allow you to dispense hearing aids (ASHA, 2008f).

The ASHA Certificate of Clinical Competence forms the basis for the requirements of many state licenses. However, states are free to have—and often do have—licensing requirements that differ from those of the ASHA CCC. This is especially true currently, as the CCC moves toward requiring a doctoral degree and many states have not made the change from requiring a master's degree.

Because of all the variations from state to state, it is critical that you find out the license requirements for any state(s) in which you are interested. The ASHA Web site has a link to each state's requirements (ASHA, 2008f).

Continuing Education

Part of being a professional is continuing to learn and develop throughout your lifetime. Continuing education is a requirement for almost all professional credentials. ASHA and ABA both require continuing education to maintain their certificates. Of the 50 states that regulate audiology through licensure or title registration, 41 require continuing education for licensure (ASHA, 2008f). Continuing education requirements for licensure differ from state to state and it is critical that, if you have a license in a particular state or states, you know—and abide by—the requirements of that state.

CGFNS/ICHP Requirements

If you are already an audiologist, but educated outside the United States, and you want to work in the United States, you must request a work visa from the U.S. Citizenship and Immigration Services. To be eligible for a visa, your education and other credentials must first be verified through the VisaScreen® Program administered by the International Commission on Healthcare Professions (ICHP), a division of CGFNS International (formerly the Commission on Graduates of Foreign Nursing Schools). The ICHP has a Speech-Language Pathology and Audiology Standards Committee, composed of members of the profession, that developed the education and clinical practicum standards that guide the VisaScreen process.

Because audiology is a growing and changing profession, and because ASHA's standards for certification in audiology are changing, ICHP is in the process of revising its audiology standards. The revisions are not yet complete or approved. For that reason, if you are considering working as an audiologist in the United States, you should contact CGFNS for details or visit their Web site at www.cgfns.org.

SCOPE OF PRACTICE

Every profession has a scope of practice that defines the areas in which the professional may legally and ethically practice his or her profession. Although scopes of practice are always developing, there is much agreement about what audiologists can do in the United States. Professional associations and state licensing bodies have statements about the scope of practice.

ASHA Statement

The ASHA (2004a) statement on scope of practice is typical and is based on a model of health developed by the World Health Organization of the United Nations into a system known as the International Classification of Functioning, Disability, and Health (ICF). The ICF is organized into two parts. One part is *Functioning and Disability* and the second part of the ICF is *Contextual Factors.*

Functioning and Disability

Functioning and Disability is further divided into two subparts: One subpart is *Body Functions and Structures,* which pays attention to anatomical structure and function and how these might be impaired. An audiologist would assess the function of various parts of the hearing mechanism. The other subpart of Functioning and Disability is *Activity/Participation.* It is not enough just to know in what ways or by how much someone's hearing mechanism is impaired. An audiologist must take into account what kinds of difficulties these impairments create for each person, because each person has different circumstances and will react to impairments differently.

Contextual Factors

Contextual factors are important because a person with a disability must function in a real environment. For that reason, the Contextual Factors include both *Environmental Factors* and *Personal Factors.* Environmental factors might include the particular sounds that a hearing-impaired person is exposed to daily. Personal factors include a person's willingness to live with a hearing loss, family support, and age, among other factors. Audiologists must take all of these into account at the same time to prevent, assess, and treat hearing and balance disorders.

Primary Functions of Audiologists

ASHA's (2004a) *Scope of Practice in Audiology* describes the services offered by qualified audiologists as primary service providers, case managers, and/or members of multidisciplinary and interdisciplinary teams. According to the scope of practice, audiologists have six primary functions:

- Prevention of hearing loss
- Identification of hearing and balance disorders
- Assessment
- Rehabilitation
- Advocacy and consultation
- Education, research, and administration

Prevention of Hearing Loss

Audiologists may accomplish prevention of hearing loss by publicizing the importance of quiet environments and the importance of reducing the loudness of sounds such as music. They also may work to prevent hearing loss by taking part in hearing conservation programs and making noise measurements in workplaces and other places where hearing may be at risk.

Identification of Hearing and Balance Disorders

A second primary function for audiologists is identification of people who may have hearing or balance disorders. Audiologists often do this through hearing screening programs, including programs for newborn babies.

Assessment

Assessment is one of the most common functions for audiologists. Audiologists use an extremely wide assortment of tests that rely on behavioral responses or automatic responses of the hearing anatomy to electrical and other types of input. From results of these tests, audiologists can measure and describe balance and hearing disorders.

Rehabilitation

The fourth function listed by ASHA is rehabilitation. An audiologist's work is not complete until he or she has taken all possible steps to help a person with a hearing or balance disorder regain communication or steadiness to the best of that person's ability. The most common way audiologists do this is by dispensing hearing aids. In fact, 81% of American audiologists dispense hearing aids or other devices to assist hearing (ASHA, 2007a). Rehabilitation also can include behavioral therapy to help communication (e.g., lip reading and auditory training), consultation about and programming of cochlear implants, nonmedical management of tinnitus (ringing in the ears), and taking part in setting up and helping people use large-area amplification systems, such as for classrooms.

Advocacy and Consultation

You might not think of advocacy and consultation as part of audiology practice, but they are—even though they are not direct services to a hearing- or balance-impaired person. Advocacy is a set of activities that supports or works for the causes of an individual or group, such as hearing-impaired people. An audiologist might be an advocate by contacting lawmakers about the importance of a law that would help hearing-impaired people. He or she might contact a lawmaker or government agency about reducing dangerous noise levels in a public area. Consultation is a set of activities, usually by an expert professional who is hired for a specific purpose. An audiologist might consult with a government agency for reducing public noise levels or even serve as an expert witness in a trial involving noise and hearing.

Education, Research and Administration

Finally, audiologists can be involved in education, research, and administration. Not all audiologists perform these functions, but they are within the scope of practice.

American Academy of Audiology Statement

The American Academy of Audiology (AAA) also has developed a scope of practice statement for audiologists (AAA, 2004). It too has six primary areas of function: (a) identification, (b) assessment and diagnosis, (c) treatment, (d) hearing conservation (the ASHA statement includes this under prevention), (e) intraoperative neurophysiological monitoring (monitoring hearing during surgery, included in assessment in the ASHA statement), and (f) research. You will note that the scopes defined by these two associations are quite similar.

State Licensure Boards Statement

Finally, you should note that licenses issued by individual states are defined by a scope of practice. Because of variation from state to state, there are too many to list here. Instead, you should review the licensure laws and scope of practice of any state(s) in which you are interested. Also see the section on licensure in this chapter.

WORK OPPORTUNITIES FOR AUDIOLOGISTS

As health care professionals, audiologists have a wide variety of places in which they can work. Traditionally, audiologists have worked for an institution, such as a hospital, where they receive a salary for their services. But in recent years, the opportunities for working in audiology have become more varied.

ASHA Surveys

ASHA (2007a) reported on a survey of 2,354 audiologists (responding out of 4,000 mailings) that requested information on work settings. About one-quarter of the respondents worked in hospitals (26%), one-quarter in private physicians' offices (26%), and one-quarter in other nonresidential health care facilities (25%). The remaining audiologists were employed in schools (10%), colleges or universities (8%), or some other facility (4%).

Although most of the 2,354 respondents reported receiving salaries, 346 (slightly under 15%) reported being the owner of a private practice. And, of the 952 audiologists who indicated that they worked in a private practice setting, 346, or about one-third, were owners of the practices.

ASHA (2008a) conducted a somewhat more recent survey of its members, including those who hold the Certificate of Clinical Competence in Audiology. From information gathered in 2006 they received responses from 10,230 audiologists. Of those, 9.4% worked in a school of some kind and 7.8% worked in a university. The great majority worked in a health care setting of some kind, including hospitals (23.6%), residential facilities, for example, a nursing home (1.2%), and nonresidential health care facilities (46.5%), with 2.1% working in a private physician's office. The remainder (11.4%) worked in a variety of other settings. In all these settings, 14.4% reported working full-time in private practice and 8.1% were working part-time in private practice.

The 2008 report showed that the great majority of audiologists (78.2%) primarily provide clinical service. However, audiologists did report several other work functions, such as college/university professor (4.4%), researcher (1.8%), and administrator (9.1%).

ETHICS IN AUDIOLOGY

No discussion of any profession is complete without a discussion of ethics. Ethics forms the guiding principles of a profession's behavior and reflects a set of values, especially moral values, held by members of that profession. The values often are summarized in codes of ethics. ASHA's (2003a) Code of Ethics is a good example. The AAA (2008b) also has a code of ethics. Any code of ethics in a health profession has basic and common language about several ethical issues, and the two codes previously mentioned are good examples.

Clients First

Health professions, including audiology, indicate that patients come first. The very first principle of the ASHA Code of Ethics states, "Individuals shall honor their responsibility to hold paramount the welfare of persons they serve professionally . . ." This means that any decisions an audiologist makes about client care must be, above all, to ensure the welfare of the client. Everything else follows from this principle.

Competence

One of the marks of a health profession is that practitioners must always try to be the best they can be. Audiologists must continue their education and development throughout their professional lives. This principle is echoed in certification and license requirements for continuing education.

Conflict of Interest

A conflict of interest arises when an audiologist is tempted to put his or her own financial or other self-interest above the patient's. In the Issues in Ethics Statement, *Conflicts of Professional Interest* (ASHA, 2003b), conflict of interest is defined as, "Situations where personal and/or financial considerations compromise judgment in any professional activity (e.g., clinical service, research, consultation, instruction, administration, etc.) or where the situation may appear to provide the potential for professional judgment to be compromised."

Because audiologists sell products, such as hearing aids, there is potential for conflict of interest. For example, an audiologist may be tempted to sell hearing aids to somebody who does not really need them. Or the audiologist may be tempted to sell somebody two hearing aids when one will do. However, the ethical audiologist will remember that the interest of the client comes first.

Self-Monitoring

Professionals must monitor their own behavior and decide when they should not or can not provide clinical services. This issue may arise in several situations. Because technology for audiology is developing so rapidly, a particular audiologist may not have kept up with latest developments. If the audiologist knows that a client could be helped with new technology, and the audiologist does not have enough expertise to use it, she or he should send the client to someone who does.

Another situation in which an audiologist must monitor his or her own abilities is in cases of illness, disability, or substance abuse that impair the audiologist's judgment or capabilities. In those cases, the audiologist must withdraw from clinical service and get professional help if it would be beneficial.

Bias

As professionals, audiologists must serve all populations equally. Audiologists should not discriminate against anybody based on such characteristics as race, age, socioeconomic status, sex or gender, national origin, ethnicity, or any other patient trait that cannot be justified.

Representation

Audiologists must represent themselves and people they supervise honestly. They should not call themselves "doctor" if they have a master's degree. They should not tell a client that their audiological assistant is an audiologist. They must represent their business or services honestly in advertising.

Charging for Services

Audiologists may receive payment from sources besides their clients (called **third-party payers**), such as insurance companies and government agencies. Ethical audiologists will always represent their services honestly to those agencies. For example, they will not tell the agency they gave a client two hearing aids (getting reimbursement for two), when they only dispensed one.

Confidentiality

Audiologists will be in a position to hear many personal things about their clients and their clients' families. This type of information is confidential, and is strictly between the audiologist and the client. The ethical audiologist will not reveal this information, except with the client's permission (or sometimes if ordered to do so by a court of law). This maintenance of confidential information is part of generally treating clients with the greatest respect.

Although the issues above are common ethical concerns, they are not the only ones. You should become familiar with ethics generally and with the code of ethics of any professional organizations to which you belong. A good place to start is with the ASHA and AAA Codes of Ethics mentioned above.

RESOURCES

If you are coming to the United States to work as an audiologist or study to become one, it will be very helpful to know about resources that can provide you with important information, help ease your transition, and support your professional activities. The ones described below are national associations but you also will find several others at more local levels once you are working.

American Speech-Language-Hearing Association (ASHA)

ASHA is the national association for all professionals—audiologists, speech-language pathologists, and speech-language-hearing scientists—concerned with the discipline of human communication sciences and disorders. At the end of 2007, ASHA had over 130,000 members and affiliates, with about 12,800 holding the Certificate in Clinical Competence (CCC) in Audiology only and another 1,200 certified in both audiology and speech-language pathology (ASHA, 2008g).

ASHA provides a wide range of services that are valuable to audiologists. To help further your education, the association publishes the *American Journal of Audiology,* which is of specific interest to audiologists. The association's several other journals regularly have articles aimed at audiologists. In addition, ASHA sponsors a large annual national convention and numerous other live conferences, Web-based seminars, and teleseminars.

As described above, ASHA, through the semi-autonomous Council on Clinical Certification, awards the Certificate of Clinical Competence, the only nationally recognized individual credential developed by a professional organization representing the whole field of communication disorders. Additionally, through its semi-autonomous **Council on Academic Accreditation (CAA),** the association develops standards for accreditation of academic programs in audiology, and awards accreditation to programs that meet those standards. CAA's accreditation is the only one recognized by the U.S. Department of Education.

Even though audiologists represent only about 10% of ASHA's membership, audiologists are represented in the association's governance structure equally with speech-language pathologists. ASHA's Board of Directors also has as many members who are audiologists as speech-language pathologists.

You should be aware of ASHA's Special Interest Divisions. Currently four of the divisions are specifically for ASHA members with an interest in hearing and balance: (a) Hearing and Hearing Disorders: Research and Diagnostics, (b) Aural Rehabilitation and Its Instrumentation,

(c) Hearing Conservation and Occupational Audiology, and (d) Hearing and Hearing Disorders in Childhood (ASHA, 2008h).

You may be particularly interested in ASHA's attention to international issues (ASHA, 2008i). You also may be interested in the support ASHA can give you to help you find a job, find an employer, advertise your business and make it prosper, and guide you through the process of billing governmental and private third-party payers for your services, as well as their guidelines and position papers for clinical practice in a variety of areas in audiology.

The list of ASHA's services and benefits is far too long to describe here. The association has an excellent Web site (www.asha.org), and helpful and knowledgeable staff to assist you.

American Academy of Audiology (AAA)

AAA is a professional association only for audiologists. At the end of June, 2008, AAA had just under 10,700 members. The Academy's mission is to "promote quality hearing and balance care by advancing the profession of audiology through leadership, advocacy, education, public awareness, and support of research" (AAA, 2005, p. 3). As such, its scope of interest is not the full range of knowledge and practice in communication sciences and disorders, but to be an association of audiologists, led only by audiologists.

The Academy publishes the excellent *Journal of the American Academy of Audiology* as its scholarly journal. It also publishes *Audiology Today*, a news magazine. The Academy sponsors an annual national convention that, along with its journal, can help you continue your audiology education. The Academy has developed several clinical practice guidelines to assist you. AAA can be a valuable resource for you. For a more complete description of its programs and services, see the Web site at www.audiology.org.

Academy of Rehabilitative Audiology (ARA)

Although a much smaller organization than either ASHA or AAA, ARA provides a connection for audiologists with special interest in rehabilitation. If you share that interest, you will find membership beneficial. ARA publishes an excellent journal, *The Journal of the Academy of Rehabilitative Audiology,* as well as the quarterly *Pinnacle* newsletter. In addition, the Academy sponsors an annual institute to help further your education. You can learn more at http://www.audrehab.org.

Council of State Association Presidents (CSAP)

If you come to the United States to work as an audiologist, you probably will be licensed in one or more states, and you will become involved in professional activities and issues in the state where you live and any others in which you hold a license. Just about every state has its own speech-language-hearing association. The members of CSAP are the presidents of each of those state associations. They can be very helpful to you, especially in your beginning time in the United States as you have questions about, or want to become involved in, professional activities at a statewide level. The association's Web site, http://www.csap.org/, can lead you to the right sources for the state information you need.

SUMMARY

You can see that audiology in the United States offers a dynamic career. Whether you come to the United States to study audiology and then work, or to work after your education in another country, you will find a growing community of talented professionals dedicated to the highest standards of clinical practice. You also will find a great variety of helpful resources and people willing to assist you. It is a truly satisfying profession.

MEDICAL TECHNOLOGISTS AND MEDICAL LABORATORY TECHNICIANS

KATHRYN M. DOIG

Keywords

Accrediting Bureau of Health Education Schools (ABHES): An independent, nonprofit agency recognized by the U.S. Secretary of Education for the accreditation of private, postsecondary institutions in the United States offering predominantly allied health education programs, and the programmatic accreditation of medical assistant, medical laboratory technician, and surgical technology programs.

American Medical Technologists (AMT): Established in 1939, the American Medical Technologists (AMT) is a national, not-for-profit agency that certifies health care professionals, such as medical technologists and medical technicians.

Board of Registry of the American Society for Clinical Pathology (BOR): The Board of Registry (BOR) was founded in 1928 by the American Society for Clinical Pathology (ASCP), 6 years after the society was founded in 1922. The BOR is a separate certifying body within the organizational structure of the ASCP. To date, over 430,000 individuals have been certified by the BOR, which is recognized as the preeminent certifying agency for clinical laboratory personnel.

National Accrediting Agency for Clinical Laboratory Sciences (NAACLS): An agency for the accreditation and approval of educational programs in the clinical laboratory sciences and related health care professions.

National Credentialing Agency for Laboratory Personnel (NCA): A voluntary, nonprofit, nongovernmental organization that conducts certification of medical laboratory personnel.

On-the-job training (OJT): Employee training at the place of work. On-the-job training takes place in a normal working situation, using the actual tools, equipment, documents, or materials that are part of the real-life job.

172

Phlebotomist: An individual trained to draw blood either for laboratory tests or blood banking.

Phlebotomy: The medical practice of opening a vein to draw blood, usually for diagnostic tests.

Reciprocity: Recognition by a state or territory of a license acquired in another state or territory.

The practice of medical laboratory testing in the United States is minimally regulated by the federal (U.S.) government. A few states add additional personnel regulations. But for the most part, qualifications for employment are set by employers that prefer to hire individuals who have passed national certification examinations validating their professional knowledge. Understanding this system requires familiarity with the differences between private-sector professional standards and governmental requirements and the terminology used to distinguish them. Navigating this complex regulatory system to be eligible for employment also depends on understanding the scope of practice for laboratory professionals in the United States, which may differ from that in other nations. Fortunately, there are many resources available to assist individuals seeking employment in U.S. medical laboratories. A list of professional resources is provided at the end of this chapter.

EDUCATION FOR ENTRY INTO PRACTICE

In the United States, individuals who perform testing in all areas of the *clinical pathology laboratory* are called *generalist laboratory professionals* because they work in all areas. Their scope of practice includes hematology, coagulation, clinical chemistry, immunohematology (blood typing), serology/immunology, urinalysis, and clinical microbiology. In recent years, the addition of molecular technologies to analyze DNA and RNA also has been included in the generalist's scope of practice. The tests performed by generalists are typically performed on blood, plasma, serum, urine or other body fluids.

There are multiple professional titles for generalist laboratory professionals. The most common is *medical technologist* (MT) for individuals with bachelor's degrees, which equates to clinical laboratory scientist (CLS). *Medical laboratory technician* (MLT) refers to individuals with associate degrees and equates to clinical laboratory technician (CLT).

Formal laboratory science education is the fastest way to achieve board certification and may be required for licensure in some states. Generalist laboratory professionals can be educated at either the *associate degree* (2-year) or *bachelor degree* (4-year) level. Both levels of programs should be *accredited,* which means a program meets specified standards. Graduation from an accredited program is a requirement for national certification when an individual is qualifying based on education without work experience. Accredited programs must meet stringent standards for how they conduct instruction, admit and evaluate students, select and train faculty, and conduct their overall operations.

Accreditation

There are two bodies that accredit educational programs. The one that accredits the largest number of laboratory science programs is the **National Accrediting Agency** for Clinical Laboratory Sciences (NAACLS). The second accrediting agency is the **Accrediting Bureau of Health Education Schools (ABHES)**, which accredits a broad array of health profession educational programs beyond just the laboratory.

National Accrediting Agency for Clinical Laboratory Sciences (NAACLS)

The National Accrediting Agency for Clinical Laboratory Sciences (NAACLS) is sponsored by various laboratory professional organizations representing the professions whose programs NAACLS accredits. That includes organizations representing medical technology, histology, cytotechnology, **phlebotomy,** and pathology assistancy. NAACLS requires that all students in accredited programs earn an academic degree before entering the accredited program or as part of the program. Thus, all graduates of NAACLS-accredited programs have either associate or bachelor degrees. Individuals completing educational programs accredited by NAACLS are eligible for the certification examinations provided by the **American Society for Clinical Pathology-Board of Registry (ASCP-BOR),** the **National Credentialing Agency for Laboratory Personnel (NCA),** or the **American Medical Technologists (AMT).** All NAACLS-accredited programs are listed on the agency's Web site (see the Professional Resources section at the end of this chapter) and the standards that programs must meet also can be accessed at the site.

Accrediting Bureau of Health Education Schools (ABHES)

The Accrediting Bureau of Health Education Schools (ABHES) accredits only medical laboratory technician programs including those in 2-year colleges that grant associate degrees. At this writing ABHES is not approved to accredit bachelor's degree programs. ABHES-accredited certificate programs (i.e., no degree is granted) may be sponsored by institutions that are not approved to grant academic degrees. These institutions may be associated with public high school (secondary school) systems or may be private technical schools.

Graduates of ABHES-accredited programs are eligible for certification by American Medical Technologists (AMT). All ABHES-accredited laboratory science programs and the standards the programs meet are listed on its Web site (www.abhes.org). Since there are relatively few ABHES-accredited educational programs in laboratory science, the remainder of this discussion will focus on those that meet NAACLS requirements.

Medical Laboratory Technician Programs

MLT programs are available at either 2-year colleges (also called community colleges or junior colleges) or less commonly, 4-year colleges. The degree conferred is an associate degree, abbreviated AD, or may be specifically an AS, for Associate of Science.

A typical AD curriculum in medical laboratory science will include general requirements (often called *liberal arts* requirements) in English composition and social sciences and/or humanities. Mathematics, including algebra and statistics, also will be required. Some institutions will include a basic physics requirement or will incorporate content on optics and electronics into some medical laboratory science courses. A course in biology and perhaps basic microbiology also can be expected in the preprofessional component of the curriculum. Once admitted to the professional phase of the curriculum, students should expect to study hematology, clinical chemistry, coagulation, urinalysis, immunology/serology, and clinical microbiology in lectures and laboratories. The program will culminate with rotations in medical laboratories in hospitals or other facilities affiliated with the college. These rotations typically last for up to one semester.

Medical Technology Programs

Accredited Medical Technology Programs are delivered in three general formats. For short, they are referred to as 2+2, 3+1, or 4+1. The first number refers to the number of years of college before entering the professional phase of the curriculum. The second number refers to the number of years spent in the professional phase.

2+2 Programs

A 2+2 program, also called an integrated program, is offered at a 4-year college where the major is typically called medical technology, clinical laboratory science, or medical laboratory science. The major is accredited by NAACLS. The first 2 years are spent studying basic sciences such as mathematics, chemistry, biology, and physics as well as the liberal arts, including English composition, social sciences, and humanities. This liberal arts component is a standard portion of any U.S. bachelor degree program and is intended to broaden an individual's view of the world beyond his/her selected major.

In the last 2 years, the students complete campus lectures and laboratories in hematology, clinical chemistry, coagulation, urinalysis, immunology/serology, clinical microbiology, and molecular diagnostics. NAACLS accreditation also requires courses in laboratory management and education since bachelor degree graduates may assume positions as supervisors, managers, and educators. The last 2 years will include rotations in hospital and other medical laboratories that have affiliations with the academic institution. There, students work alongside the laboratory staff learning to apply their student laboratory skills in the actual work setting.

The length of the rotation period is variable, usually not longer than 6 months, but sometimes as short at 16 weeks. Students pay tuition to the university and earn college credits for the rotations that apply to completion of the degree. Graduates of the 2+2 degree program are eligible for certification at the time they graduate from college, having earned their degree and completed the NAACLS-accredited program at the same time.

Variations. There is a variation of the 2+2 format. In some circumstances, the first 2 years and the second 2 years are not offered by the same institution. The first 2 years may be just 2 years of appropriate pre-requisites at any college or university that are then transferred to the institution offering the second 2 professional years and which holds the NAACLS accreditation. The first 2 years also may be an AD program, including medical laboratory technician programs. The bachelor degree is earned from the second institution.

3+1 Programs

Programs in the 3+1 format represent a close association between a college and an NAACLS-accredited professional program, usually based in a hospital. Students enroll at the college and spend the first 3 years studying basic sciences and liberal arts. For the fourth year, often called an internship, they go to a hospital laboratory. The experience at the hospital is accredited by NAACLS. There the students receive lectures on the clinical laboratory sciences of hematology, clinical chemistry, co-agulation, urinalysis, immunology/serology, clinical microbiology, and molecular diagnostics. Sometimes they also have student laboratory sessions, but more often, they learn the technical skills without prior student laboratories, by working "at the bench" alongside the laboratory staff. They also receive their NAACLS-required education and management training in the hospital.

The students continue to pay tuition to the university for the fourth year (i.e., the "+1" year) and earn college credit for the hospital experience. Upon successful completion of the hospital year, the bachelor's degree is granted from the college and the student is eligible to take the certifying examination by virtue of earning the degree and completing a NAACLS-accredited program.

4+1 Programs

Hospital-based NAACLS-accredited programs may admit students who already possess a bachelor's degree, that is, postbaccalaureate applicants. For individuals with international bachelor's degrees, this is the most common educational route into medical laboratory employment in the United States. In such a circumstance, the educational format is described as 4+1, with the 4 referring to a completed bachelor's degree and the 1 referring to the internship year. That internship year is the same as the internship for 3+1 students as previously described; thus a hospital-based internship may have both 3+1 and 4+1 students in the same class.

Since the bachelor's degree may have been earned anywhere, each NAACLS-accredited internship will determine what prerequisites a postbaccalaureate applicant must present to be eligible for admission. Typically they will require a bachelor's degree in chemistry or some aspect of biology. The title of the degree is less important than the content of particular courses and science credits, which must conform to certification specifications. Individuals with international bachelor's degrees will be expected to provide an evaluation from an international transcript review agency for comparability to U.S. degrees.

Students completing an internship in a 4+1 format will not earn a second degree but they also will not pay tuition to any college for the internship. There may be a modest tuition charged by the hospital, typically less than U.S. $2,000. Upon completion of the internship, the graduate receives a certificate of completion and is eligible for the national certification examinations based on his/her prior bachelor's degree plus completion of a NAACLS-accredited program.

General Comments on Bachelor's Degree Programs

When viewing the online list of NAACLS-accredited educational programs, the distinction between 2+2, 3+1, and 4+1 programs is not clearly noted. In general, programs listed in hospitals will provide a hospital-based, "+1" internship. Institutions listed as colleges or universities will provide 2+2 programs. The college portion of a 3+1 program cannot be determined at the NAACLS Web site since the college does not hold NAACLS accreditation. Those programs will be discovered by inquiries to the hospital-based programs about their affiliated colleges.

Although conferring with an immigration expert at a college or university is advised, in general, U.S. noncitizens seeking to complete all of the necessary education for job entry should consider 2+2 or 3+1 programs. Since one is an enrolled college student throughout the educational process, a student visa will cover the entire experience. The year of *optional practical training* (OPT) on the F-1 visa can then apply to a year of employment in the United States following graduation. For individuals already possessing a bachelor's degree, applying the OPT to an internship is possible. However, gaining admission can be difficult. Internship programs may hesitate to admit U.S. noncitizens or nonpermanent residents since they cannot readily hire the individuals after graduation. Institutions vary in their willingness to sponsor immigrants for employment.

Articulation Agreements

An AD in medical laboratory technology does not automatically apply to one-half of a bachelor's degree program in medical technology. Accepting transfer of credits is at the discretion of the bachelor's degree institution. Some credits may not transfer or may not apply to specific courses. Yet some 2-year institutions have what are called articulation agreements with 4-year institutions to facilitate transfer without loss of credits. When considering an AD program, asking about possible transfer and articulation is advised.

Online Education

Online educational programs are available. Programs vary in how this is conducted, but in general, the equivalent of lectures is provided on the Internet. Then students must find laboratories near their homes that will be willing to train them in the technical phase of the curriculum. Another option is to move temporarily to be near a laboratory affiliated with the college for the short time required for the clinical experience. A listing of online degree programs is available on the Web site of the American Society for Clinical Laboratory Science (www.ascls.org).

QUALIFICATIONS FOR ENTRY INTO LABORATORY PRACTICE

There are minimal standards for laboratory professionals set by the federal government. Only a few states add specific additional *license* requirements for laboratory professionals. As a result, employment qualifications beyond minimums are the prerogative of the employer in nonlicensing states. Although most prefer to hire *board-certified* professionals with formal laboratory science education, they can hire individuals without formal education in laboratory science for whom they then provide **on-the-job training (OJT).** Each of these routes to qualify for employment will be described following an introduction to terminology that is pertinent to the regulation of laboratory professionals and laboratories.

Federal Government Regulations Effective in All States

The U.S. Congress passed the Clinical Laboratory Improvement Amendments of 1988 (CLIA 88) to insure that laboratory testing performed in any site in the United States would meet quality standards. The Congress wanted to insure that money was well spent for laboratory tests paid by the Medicare health insurance program for senior citizens.

CLIA 88 includes provisions governing personnel qualifications for what the law calls testing personnel as well as for supervisory personnel. The qualifications for testing personnel are correlated to the complexity of the test performed—with more complex tests requiring more highly qualified personnel. Employers who receive Medicare reimbursement (and most do) are responsible for insuring that individuals have the necessary qualifications (education and training) for the complexity of testing they perform.

Individual State Licensing

CLIA 88 is the only federal-level personnel regulation for medical laboratory professionals. As a federal personnel regulation it is somewhat unusual. Most governmentally imposed personnel standards are set at the state level. This is a state's right as granted under the U.S. Constitution. Although states routinely license physicians, nurses, pharmacists, and optometrists, for example, state licensing of medical laboratory professionals is infrequent, and for the most part, relatively recent. In those states with a personnel licensing requirement, it is illegal to perform medical laboratory testing without a valid license.

At this writing there are 13 states, plus Puerto Rico, that require personnel licensure for medical laboratory professionals. A list of the states with links to their licensing divisions is available on the Web sites of the American Society for Clinical Laboratory Sciences (www.ascls.org) and the American Society for Clinical Pathology (www.ascp.org). More information on these organizations may be found under Professional Resources included at the end of this section on medical technicians and medical laboratory technologists.

The states typically do not recognize a license from another state; that is, there is no **reciprocity** between the states. Most of the state licensing laws will recognize national certification as a qualification for the license; however, some states may require prospective licensees to take a state-specific test. Individuals seeking employment in a licensing state must investigate the state's requirements carefully. States may provide temporary licenses to allow employment while training or before completing the full license requirements.

Licensure Renewal

Licenses are typically limited in duration and must be renewed after several years. Renewal often requires documentation of *continuing education* (CE) such as attendance at conferences or workshops during the license period. Acceptable CE providers may include professional organizations, educational institutions, manufacturers, employers, and others. The states will specify those they will accept as well as how many *continuing education units* (CEUs) or hours of instruction must be accumulated.

On-the-Job Training for Entry Into Practice

In states that do not license, employers are free to hire any individual that meets CLIA's minimum requirements. Employers must provide specific job training pertinent to the tests the individual will perform. The willingness of employers to do on-the-job training will vary. Although being trained on the job allows employment by that institution without a formal credential, job mobility and advancement are limited. However, work experience can apply toward certification.

VOLUNTARY PROFESSIONAL REGULATION OF LABORATORY OCCUPATIONS

Board Certification

Although mandatory state licensing is not routine for medical laboratory professionals, voluntary *board certification* is a routine and a commonly expected method for individuals to demonstrate their knowledge and qualifications for employment. As mentioned previously, most medical laboratory employers prefer to hire certified individuals.

Board certification is offered by certifying agencies sponsored by professional membership organizations. In order to achieve board certification in the generalist laboratory professions, there are three basic requirements:

1. Meet the agency's specified educational requirements including minimum credits in sciences and mathematics (see details below).
2. Complete a practical experience in a laboratory.
3. Pass the agency's certifying examination.

Educational Requirements

Individuals applying for board certification must meet the educational requirements for a medical technologist or a medical technician and have graduated from an accredited institution. For a more in-depth description of the required education, see the section in this chapter entitled, "Education of Medical Laboratory Personnel in the United States."

Practical Experience

The practical experience can be achieved in either of two ways. The fastest way is to complete an *accredited educational program* that incorporates laboratory experience into the curriculum. However, each certifying agency also allows individuals to qualify for the examination by work experience. Because the work requirement may be as much as 4–5 years, qualifying by this *experiential route* is not as fast as using formal education. Nevertheless, individuals with international credentials who are able to find employment in the United States may qualify for the U.S. certifying examinations by an experiential route. Even though an individual has found employment without U.S. certification, achieving certification is desirable because it will enlarge an individual's employment options and enhance geographic mobility and job advancement.

Certifying Examinations

The certifying examinations are offered throughout the United States at specific locations that differ by agency. Typically there are several sites for each agency within each state. When offered by computer, the examinations can be taken virtually any day of the year. Some agencies will provide results at the time the applicant completes the examination. Details such as these, as well as policies governing the testing and eligibility routes, are provided in what is typically called the *candidate handbook* available on the Web site of the certifying agency. Anyone contemplating a certifying examination should read the candidate handbook thoroughly.

Eligibility Criteria

The eligibility criteria for certification vary from one agency to the next. These differences mean that an individual may qualify for the medical technologist/clinical laboratory scientist examination from one agency, but not the others. Therefore, individuals seeking certification should investigate each agency's requirements to see if they qualify.

As a result of the variability in qualifications for certification among the agencies, some employers have a preference for certification from particular agencies. Even though a job advertisement specifies the employer's preference for a particular agency's credential, applications may still be considered without it. This is especially true when there is a shortage of qualified personnel and no one with the preferred credential applies for a given job.

Special Considerations for International Certification Applicants' Academic Degrees

Individuals with international academic degrees must have their transcripts evaluated by a *credential evaluation service* to determine comparability to a U.S. degree. The candidate handbook for a given certifying agency will list acceptable transcript evaluation firms, although almost any reputable firm is accepted. Reputable transcript evaluation agencies can be found through the National Association of Credential Evaluation Services (NACES) at www.naces.org.

Qualifying by Work Experience

Individuals educated outside the United States may be eligible for examinations offered by NCA without any additional education or experience. To be eligible they must possess an academic degree comparable to a U.S. degree and have work experience in an international laboratory that is accredited through a U.S. *laboratory accrediting agency,* such as the College of American Pathologists (CAP). The NCA Candidate Handbook lists acceptable U.S. laboratory accrediting agencies. The Web sites of the agencies will usually list accredited laboratories so individuals can determine if their experience was in one of those laboratories.

Certifying Agencies

The three certifying agencies most widely recognized in the United States have been the **Board of Registry of the American Society for Clinical Pathology (BOR),** the National Credentialing Agency for Laboratory Personnel (NCA), and American Medical Technologists (AMT). Each agency had different standards and administered different examinations. Effective October 23, 2009, the BOR and NCA unified their certification programs into a single agency, known as the ASCP Board of Certification (BOC). NCA was dissolved as a corporation. Current and active certifications at the time of the merger were transferred to the ASCP BOC; no examination was required for the transfer. The "ASCP" suffix is attached to all BOC certifications. Medical technologists (MT) and clinical laboratory scientists (CLS) are called Medical Laboratory Scientists (MLS) and the designation is MLS(ASCP).

Board certification is typically granted for a limited period, like 3 years. In order to maintain active certification beyond that period, certificants must document completion of continuing education units (CEUs). The number of CEUs required annually is specified by the particular agency, as are acceptable providers and topics.

BOR Examination

The Board of Registry (BOR) offers in-country examinations in a number of countries such as Korea and the Philippines. These examinations are the same as the U.S. BOR exams with the exception of any country-specific regulatory questions. Individuals possessing an international BOR certificate may find U.S. employers that consider this equivalent to U.S. certification. Such recognition of international BOR certificates is at the discretion of each employer, however, and some may not accept it as equivalent to the U.S. certification. Individuals may still gain initial employment so they can complete U.S. practical experience and then qualify for the U.S. version of the BOR certifying examination, if required by their employer. Current information on the BOC examination can be found at http://www.ascp.org.

NCA Examination

Individuals with international degrees comparable to U.S. degrees plus international work experience, even in nonaccredited laboratories, may be eligible to sit for the NCA examination through a program called Temporary Status by Qualification (TSQ). If they are determined to be eligible and they pass the examination, these individuals earn TSQ status for a limited period of time. During the TSQ period they may find U.S. employment by virtue of being able to prove they have passed a U.S. credentialing examination. Then the TSQ holders can complete the experience requirement for their credentials and convert their TSQ to full certification. However, employers will vary in their willingness to recognize TSQ. Check the ASCP website at http://www.ascp.org to confirm continuation of this policy.

AMT Examination

American Medical Technologists (AMT) is the only agency that will accept international experience as fully equivalent to U.S. experience for candidates qualifying by experiential routes. Thus, international candidates may not need to augment recent international experience at all to be eligible for AMT examinations.

SCOPE OF PRACTICE FOR U.S. MEDICAL LABORATORY PROFESSIONALS

The distinction between the scope of practice of MTs and MLTs has been based on the difference in educational level. The background provided to MTs by virtue of a baccalaureate degree is meant to support the application of independent judgment to solve unfamiliar problems and develop new techniques. They may act as supervisors and laboratory managers or conduct training and education for other laboratory staff members. MTs will typically perform the more unusual and complicated tests. MLTs perform the bulk of routine tests under the supervision of MTs and solve common problems using preestablished protocols.

Categorical Certifications

At the baccalaureate level, some individuals may be educated or trained in just one area of clinical pathology testing such as clinical chemistry or clinical microbiology. They can then earn a professional credential in that single area. These credentials are known as *categorical certifications* since they qualify an individual to work in just that one category of the generalist's scope of practice. The U.S. scope of practice for medical technologists/technicians does not include *histology* (tissue processing), *cytology* (examination of cells for cancer detection), *cytogenetics* (examination of karyotypes), or *histocompatibility* (tissue typing) testing. Individuals specialize in these separate areas of laboratory testing and a separate credential is available in each discipline.

Relationships With Other Health Care Providers

In addition to the specialists previously mentioned, medical technologists and technicians work closely with *pathologists* who are medical doctors specializing in laboratory testing and often acting as the director of the laboratory. In larger laboratories there are also nonphysicians who hold doctor of philosophy (PhD) degrees. Most often these individuals are responsible for the management and supervision of individual departments of clinical chemistry, clinical microbiology, molecular diagnostics, or immunology.

One other group of professionals on whom medical technologists and technicians rely heavily is **phlebotomists.** Though phlebotomy (i.e., venesection) and capillary puncture are part of the scope of practice for generalist professionals, most institutions hire high school (secondary school) educated individuals and train them to specialize in blood collections.

ETHICAL PRACTICE

The trust patients must place in professionals is the foundation of the professional relationship. The professional practitioner has the obligation to perform his or her duties in a manner that is worthy of that trust and that places the well-being of the patient in the forefront. To do so, professionals are expected to adhere to the highest principles of ethical conduct. Veatch and Flack (1997) list five principles of ethics to which health professionals must adhere. For laboratory professionals, those that are most directly applicable are:

- Benefiting the client and others, which means doing the best job possible including performing tasks according to procedures and staying current in one's knowledge with continuing education.
- Autonomy, which means respecting patients' right to make their own decisions, such as not having a test drawn or having access to their medical records.
- Veracity, which means telling the truth if a patient asks about the purpose of a test.
- Fidelity, which means being trustworthy, especially in maintaining patient confidentiality.

Patient Confidentiality

In the United States, the issue of patient confidentiality is so important that it has been incorporated into a federal law as part of the Health Information Portability and Accountability Act of 1996 (HIPAA). In short, HIPAA forbids the disclosure of patient health information to others, including family members, unless the patient grants permission for the disclosure. Professionals involved in the patient's direct care are permitted access to the information that they need in order to perform their duties, but may not have access to all information; that is, they can access what they "need to know." Employee orientation at any health care institution will include training on the details of the HIPAA privacy rule and the manner in which the institution complies with it.

Responsibility to Colleagues

Beyond their ethical responsibilities to patients, health professionals have responsibilities to their colleagues to:

- help perpetuate the profession by teaching the next generation of professionals;
- participate in establishing standards for entry to the profession and enforcing those standards through professional credentialing mechanisms;
- conduct research to advance the body of knowledge in the profession while protecting the current scope of practice; and
- advocate for the profession in public arenas, such as influencing government regulations, and in private areas as with employers, to influence the compensation and respect for the profession.

As an example, the Code of Ethics of the American Society for Clinical Laboratory Science (http://www.ascls.org/about/ethics.asp) embodies these ethical obligations to patients and colleagues.

Each person will not be able to participate in every one of these professional roles. That is one reason why professionals join *professional organizations (associations or societies)*. Professional societies are involved in each of these areas, so members participate indirectly through their membership. Then if a member wants to take an active role in any of these, the opportunity is available for more active and direct participation.

SUMMARY

Navigating the complexities of clinical laboratory employment in the United States can be simplified by consulting the resources provided by state licensing authorities, national certifying agencies, and professional associations. The directors of NAACLS-accredited educational programs are excellent resources for employment advice as well as education and certification information. The good news is that a shortage of qualified clinical laboratory professionals in the United States offers international professionals improved opportunities for employment.

PROFESSIONAL RESOURCES

National Accrediting Bodies for Educational Programs

Accrediting Bureau of Health Education Schools (ABHES)

7777 Leesburg Pike, Suite 314
N. Falls Church, VA 22043
Phone 703-917-9503
Fax 703-917-4109
www.abhes.org

National Accrediting Agency for Clinical Laboratory Sciences (NAACLS)

5600 N. River Rd., Suite 720
Rosemont, IL 60018-5119
Phone 773-714-8880
Fax 773-714-8886
www.naacls.org

Certification Agencies for Generalist Laboratory Professionals

American Medical Technologists

10700 West Higgins Rd, Suite 150
Rosemont, IL 60018
Phone 847-823-5169
Fax 847-823-0458
www.amt1.com

Board of Registry of the American Society for Clinical Pathology

33 West Monroe Street, Suite 1600
Chicago, IL 60603
Phone 800-267-2727, option 2, 2
Fax 312-541-4845
http://www.ascp.org/FunctionalNavigation/certification.aspx

National Credentialing Agency for Laboratory Personnel

PO Box 15945-289
Lenexa, KS 66285
Phone 913-895-4613
Fax 913-895-4652
www.nca-info.org

Professional Associations for Generalist Laboratory Professionals

American Medical Technologists and its active state chapters

10700 West Higgins Rd, Suite 150
Rosemont, IL 60018
Phone 847-823-5169
Fax 847-823-0458
www.amt1.com

American Society for Clinical Laboratory Science and its active state chapters

6701 Democracy Boulevard, Suite 300
Bethesda, MD 20817
Phone 301-657-2768
Fax 301-657-2909
www.ascls.org

American Society for Clinical Pathology

33 West Monroe Street, Suite 1600
Chicago, IL 60603
Phone 800-267-2727, option 2
Fax 312-541-4472
www.ascp.org

Organizations Establishing and Enforcing Laboratory Standards

Centers for Medicare and Medicaid Services (CMS) (enforces the Clinical Laboratory Improvement Amendments of 1988)

CMS Baltimore Headquarters Telephone Numbers

Toll-Free: 877-267-2323 (Employee directory available)
Local: 410-785-3000
http://www.cms.hhs.gov/clia/

College of American Pathologists (Laboratory Accreditation Program)

325 Waukegan Road
Northfield, IL 60093-2750
Phone 800-323-4040
Fax 847-832-8000
http://www.cap.org/apps/cap.portal?_nfpb=true&_pageLabel=accreditation

Clinical and Laboratory Standards Institute (establishes U.S. and international standards for laboratory testing procedures)

940 West Valley Road, Suite 1400
Wayne, PA 19087
Phone 610-688-0100
Fax 610-688-0700
www.clsi.org

State Licensing Authorities

Links for state licensing authorities are available on the Web site of the American Society for Clinical Laboratory Science at http://www.ascls.org/jobs/grads/personnellicensure.pdf and also at the Web site of the American Society for Clinical Pathology, which is http://www.ascp.org/FunctionalNavigation/certification/International/StateLicensureAgencies.aspx.

Agencies Conducting Academic Transcript Evaluations

Links are available to individual agencies conducting academic transcript evaluations from the National Association of Credential Evaluation Services (NACES) at http://www.naces.org/members.htm.

Online Clinical Laboratory Educational Programs

Directory available at the Web site of the American Society for Clinical Laboratory Science at http://www.ascls.org/leadership/sa/esa.asp#CLEP-Online.

OCCUPATIONAL THERAPY

SCOTT McPHEE

Keywords

Accreditation Council for Occupational Therapy Education (ACOTE): The accrediting body of the American Occupational Therapy Association. ACOTE accredits approximately 275 occupational therapy and occupational therapy assistant educational programs.

American Occupational Therapy Association (AOTA): The national professional association established in 1917 to represent the interests and concerns of occupational therapy practitioners and students of occupational therapy and to improve the quality of occupational therapy services.

National Board for Certification in Occupational Therapy, Inc. (NBCOT®): A not-for-profit credentialing agency that provides certification for the occupational therapy profession.

Occupation: The means through which a client achieves therapeutic goals for maximum independence and life satisfaction.

Occupational therapist (OT): Occupational therapists use treatments to develop, recover, or maintain the daily living and work skills of their patients. They work with individuals, families, groups, and populations to facilitate health and well-being through engagement or reengagement in occupation.

Occupational therapy assistant (OTA): Occupational therapy assistants work under the direction of occupational therapists to provide rehabilitative services to persons with mental, physical, emotional, or developmental impairments.

Trademark: A distinctive sign or indicator used by an individual to identify that the services provided by the individual are unique. The trademark distinguishes the services provided from those of other entities. Occupational Therapist Registered (OTR) and Certified Occupational Therapy Assistant (COTA) are examples of trademarks.

World Federation of Occupational Therapists (WFOT): Key international representative organization for occupational therapists and occupational therapy around the world and the official international organization for the promotion of occupational therapy. Founded in 1952, WFOT currently has 66 member associations.

Occupational therapy is a profession that provides skilled treatment to help individuals attain independence in performing activities of daily living. Occupational therapists work with individuals and groups who have experienced impairment in bodily functioning to enhance their ability to participate in everyday life and to modify their environment so that participation can be achieved.

HISTORY OF OCCUPATIONAL THERAPY IN THE UNITED STATES

A relatively new profession, occupational therapy's U.S. roots can be traced back to just the first part of the 20th century. However, the idea behind the healing effects of purposeful activity (**occupation**) has been taught for several centuries by such notables as Asclepiades, Celsus, and Pinel (Licht, 1983). The first recorded evidence of occupation as a healing form dates to the ancient Egyptians. The healing arts of that time used various forms of work, music, exercise, and recreation as part of the recuperative process.

Occupational therapy's philosophical base is firmly established in the moral treatment movement of the early 19th century (Licht, 1983). During the late 18th century, the use of physical exercises and manual occupations were prescribed for the treatment of mental disorders. Following World War II, the profession saw a major shift in services provided. Three areas of occupational therapy evolved: physical dysfunction, psychosocial dysfunction, and pediatrics. Along with this delineation of specialization there was a corresponding development of theories, frames of reference, and models of practice to demonstrate the unique qualities associated with occupational therapy practice (Schwartz, 2003).

EDUCATION FOR ENTRY INTO PRACTICE

The **occupational therapist (OT)** and the **occupational therapy assistant (OTA)** make up the two professional levels within the field of occupational therapy. Each level requires completion of a professional curriculum that meets the education standards set by the **Accreditation Council for Occupational Therapy Education (ACOTE).** The ACOTE establishes the educational standards for all education programs. Education comprises both the didactic as well as the clinical education requirements. Upon successful completion of an accredited course of instruction, the graduate is eligible to take a national certification examination, which is a requirement by most states before being allowed to practice occupational therapy.

Occupational Therapists

An occupational therapist (OT) has two educational entry options by which to prepare to practice occupational therapy. Beginning in 2007, a postbaccalaureate degree in occupational therapy was the lowest level of degree required of individuals entering the profession. This is generally a 2-year course of instruction with an emphasis on clinical training. Beginning in 2008, a clinical doctorate degree was approved as an alternate way to enter the profession. Completion of a clinical Doctor of Occupational Therapy entails 3 years of full-time study. The doctoral degree focuses on clinical practice skills, research skills, administration, leadership, program and policy development, advocacy, education, and theory development. Both degree paths are offered at universities and must meet the educational standards set by ACOTE.

Occupational therapists are skilled practitioners whose education includes the study of human growth and development with specific emphasis on the social, emotional, and physiological effects of illness and injury. Coursework in occupational therapy programs include the physical, biological, and behavioral sciences as well as the application of occupational therapy theory and skills. Programs also require the completion of 6 months of supervised fieldwork (Bureau of Labor Statistics, 2009a).

Occupational Therapy Assistant

An occupational therapy assistant (OTA) works under the direction of an occupational therapist to provide services to persons with mental, physical, emotional, or developmental impairments. After high (secondary) school, an OTA completes a 2-year education program, accredited by ACOTE, and typically offered through community colleges.

The first year of study typically involves an introduction to health care, basic medical terminology, anatomy, and physiology. In the second year, courses are more rigorous and usually include occupational therapist courses in areas such as mental health, adult physical disabilities, gerontology, and pediatrics. Students also must complete 16 weeks of supervised fieldwork in a clinic or community setting (Bureau of Labor Statistics, 2009b).

OBTAINING A LICENSE

Graduates of an accredited occupational therapy program are eligible to take a national certification examination as part of their requirement to practice occupational therapy. The **National Board for Certification in Occupational Therapy, Inc. (NBCOT®)** is the national certification organization that offers the certification examination. The NBCOT was established as a means to protect the public as well as to ensure that individuals entering the profession of occupational therapy meet minimum standards that demonstrate their readiness to practice in the profession. NBCOT monitors the development, administration, and review of standards that represent reliable indicators of competence for entry into practice. The organization has certified over 175,000 OT and OTA practitioners and their examination is used by all 50 states, Guam, Puerto Rico, and the District of Columbia as a basis for licensing these practitioners (National Board for Certification in Occupational Therapy, 2009a).

Philosophy of States' Rights

Each state sets its own rules and regulations for occupational therapy practice regardless if it is by licensure, registration, certification, or **trademark.** Each occupational therapy practitioner has the responsibility to be aware of and comply with all state laws and regulations. Although each state establishes its own regulations for the practice of occupational therapy within its jurisdiction, most will use the **American Occupational Therapy Association (AOTA)** guidelines as a way to define standards for practice and the NBCOT examination to determine competency for entry-level practice.

Licensure Renewal

Each state will determine its licensure renewal requirements. Many will require demonstration of continued competence to practice as evidenced by completion of continuing education programs. Each state sets the number of required hours of continuing education. Individual state rules and regulations governing occupational therapy practice can be viewed at the AOTA Web site: http://www1.AOTA.org/state_law/lawprofile.asp. Addresses and Web sites for each state occupational therapy licensing or registration organization can be found at http://www1.AOTA.org/state_law/reglist.asp.

STATUTORY LICENSE AND CERTIFICATION REQUIREMENTS

Certification Examination

As previously noted, all 50 states, Guam, Puerto Rico, and the District of Columbia require NBCOT certification for licensure of occupational therapy practitioners. Candidates seeking certification as an occupational therapist (OTR) or an occupational therapy assistant (COTA) must satisfy the following criteria to be granted certification:

- OTR candidates must graduate from an NBCOT-recognized occupational therapy education program at the postbaccalaureate degree level. COTA candidates must graduate from an accredited U.S. occupational therapy education program at the associate or technical degree level.
- Candidates must complete appropriate clinical fieldwork requirements.
- Candidates must apply for and attain a passing score on the OTR or COTA national certification examination.
- Candidates must agree to adhere to the standards of the NBCOT Candidate/Certificant Code of Conduct.

To maintain the OTR or COTA certification status, certificants must satisfy a 36-unit requirement of professional development activities every three years (NBCOT, 2009b).

Foreign-Educated Occupational Therapists

Foreign-educated occupational therapists with baccalaureate degrees seeking eligibility to take the Certification Examination for Occupational Therapist Registered OTR® must first be approved through the NBCOT Occupational Therapist Eligibility Determination (OTED) Program. OTED applicants are classified as either Category A or Category B.

- *Category A:* Has been awarded a postbaccalaureate degree from an occupational therapy education program recognized by NBCOT (**World Federation of Occupational Therapists [WFOT]** approved).
- *Category B:* Has graduated from an accredited occupational therapy education program recognized by NBCOT (ACOTE or WFOT approved) *and* must present evidence of academic equivalence to U.S. occupational therapy educational standards.

Examination Administration

The NBCOT certification examination is administered at Prometric Test Centers worldwide. To insure the integrity of its testing process, Prometric maintains stringent security standards in its test centers and across its network.

In order to obtain authorization to take the certification examination, eligible applicants must submit a Certification Examination Application to NBCOT. Once approved, applicants will be instructed to contact Prometric to schedule their examination (NBCOT does not schedule exams). The examinations are computer-delivered and candidates are provided 4 hours to take the examination (NBCOT, 2009).

Since June 15, 2009, NBCOT only accepts credit card payments (MasterCard and Visa) for examination applications and related services such as score transfer and confirmation of examination eligibility notices. Candidates applying for the examination (OTR® or COTA®) must pay by submitting a credit card at the time of application submission. No off-line payments will be accepted. NBCOT made this change to increase security and decrease processing time—enabling candidates to move through the eligibility process in a shorter period of time. Additional information and an applicant handbook may be accessed at the NBCOT Web site, http://www.nbcot.org.

SCOPE OF PRACTICE

Occupational therapy is "the art and science of helping people do the day-to-day activities that are important and meaningful to their health and well-being" (Crepeau, Cohn, & Schell, 2009, p. 217). Occupational therapy practitioners help patients improve their ability to perform tasks of daily living (such as dressing, grooming, meal preparation, child care, etc.) and their work environments (such as job performance). Occupational therapists work with individuals who suffer from mental, physical, developmental, or emotionally disabling conditions. The focus is on the ability to perform activities of daily living (ADL).

Activities of daily living can include such activities as dressing, cooking, eating, bathing, using a computer, and other functional tasks. These tasks are meaningful activities that are important to the client as determined by the client-centered intervention model used in occupational therapy practice. This model stresses the importance of including the client in the decision-making process who then becomes an active contributor to the intervention process and goals.

Patient Self-Care

The occupational therapy practitioner evaluates the self-care, work, and leisure skills of individuals and then, in collaboration with the client, plans for and implements treatment programs that emphasize social and interpersonal activities to develop, restore, and/or maintain that individual's ability to perform their daily living activities. The therapist's primary goal is to improve basic motor functions and cognitive reasoning abilities. If this is unattainable, individuals can be taught to compensate for permanent loss of function. An example of this might be to modify one's home to make it wheelchair accessible. The ultimate goal is to return the person to a productive and satisfying lifestyle.

Physical Rehabilitation

Occupational therapy intervention in physical rehabilitation might include activities to increase strength and dexterity or training in daily living skills through adaptive or compensatory measures. For individuals with a cognitive or perceptual disability, activities may be chosen to improve recall, visual acuity, or the ability to discern patterns. Examples of such activities may take various forms:

- A patient who has had a stroke makes a sandwich with adapted tools that increase independence and promote improvement in perceptual motor skills.

- A child with developmental delays plays with toys/games selected by the occupational therapist to improve fine motor coordination and strength so that the child can function well in school.
- A person with short-term memory loss makes lists to aid recall.
- A person with coordination problems might undertake craft activities to improve eye-hand coordination.
- Elders with decreased energy or endurance benefit from environmental modifications.
- Children with learning disabilities are involved in play sessions to help enhance their sensory integration ability.

Occupational therapy practitioners working with individuals who have traumatic brain injuries might use specially designed computer programs to help improve decision making, abstract reasoning, problem solving, and perceptual skills, as well as memory, sequencing, and coordination, all of which are important for independent living. Other treatments can include the fitting and training in the proper use of wheelchairs, prosthetic appliances, assistive devices for eating, dressing, ambulation, and communication. Also important is consulting for the designing or building of the special equipment needed to improve independence at home or at work, for example, modification of bathrooms for safety, or rearranging workspace environments to decrease energy consumption.

Practice Settings

Fisher and Keehn (2007) report that there are approximately 104,000 licensed occupational therapists and 32,000 licensed certified occupational therapy assistants practicing in the United States. These occupational therapy practitioners can be found working in a wide range of areas, including physical rehabilitation (inpatient/outpatient hospitals and private practices), pediatrics (i.e., early intervention, sensory integration, school systems, etc.), special assistive technology clinics, consulting with work and industry, home health, mental health hospitals/clinics, and administration, to name a few. AOTA (2006a) reports that the three top states that employ occupational therapy practitioners are California, New York, and Pennsylvania. The majority (52.6%) of practicing therapists are employed in schools, early intervention programs, and hospitals. Practitioners who work with children (birth to 21 years) make up 35% of the workforce while 29.6% of practitioners work with adults over the age of 65 years.

Growth and Shortage Areas

Currently, there is a shortage of occupational therapy practitioners in the United States and a predicted future shortage. The median age of OTs in the United States has increased from 36 in 1990 to 42 in 2006. Shortages have been identified in acute care hospitals, inpatient rehabilitation, skilled nursing facilities, and home health care (Fisher & Keehn, 2007). Shortages are more severe in rural areas than in urban or suburban areas. The strongest growth areas for occupational therapy are in the South Atlantic, North Central, and South Central geographic regions of the United States, which have averaged a 4% annual increase since 2000. Steady growth and a demand for occupational therapy services have been seen in school systems and early intervention programs. Further, the need for rehabilitation services is growing in assisted living facilities. Salaries for entry-level occupational therapists in the United States for full-time, 12-month contracts generally fall in the $55,000–$62,000 range. Salaries will differ depending upon the geographic region and area of practice (AOTA, 2006a).

ETHICAL AND LEGAL CONSIDERATIONS IN PRACTICE

AOTA has publicly stated its ethical principles that promote high standards of conduct for occupational therapy practitioners. These principles demonstrate a commitment by practitioners to "promoting inclusion, diversity, independence, and safety for all recipients in various stages of life, health, and illness" (AOTA, 2005, p. 639). Occupational therapy practitioners have a responsibility to provide ethical treatment to recipients of care and to society as a whole. The following excerpt is from the official statement of commitment to seven ethical principles as established by AOTA:

Occupational Therapy Personnel Shall:

Principle 1. Demonstrate a concern for the safety and well-being of the recipients of their services (*Beneficence*).

Principle 2. Take measures to ensure a recipient's safety and avoid imposing or inflicting harm (*Nonmaleficence*).

Principle 3. Respect recipients to assure their rights (*Autonomy, Confidentiality*).

Principle 4. Achieve and continually maintain high standards of competence (*Duty*).

Principle 5. Comply with laws and association policies guiding the profession of occupational therapy (*Procedural Justice*).

Principle 6. Provide accurate information when representing the profession (*Veracity*).

Principle 7. Treat colleagues and other professionals with respect, fairness, discretion, and integrity (*Fidelity*). (American Occupational Therapy Association, 2005).

Commitment to ethical practice can be demonstrated through professional behaviors. As a guideline, AOTA has presented the following professional behaviors that reflect a high level of ethics.

Honesty: Professionals must be honest with themselves, must be honest with all with whom they come in contact, and must know their strengths and limitations.

Communication: Communication is important in all aspects of occupational therapy. Individuals must be conscientious and truthful in all facets of written, verbal, and electronic communication.

Ensuring the common good: Occupational therapy personnel are expected to increase awareness of the profession's social responsibilities to help ensure the common good.

Competence: Occupational therapy personnel are expected to work within their areas of competence and to pursue opportunities to update, increase, and expand their competence.

Confidential and protected information: Information that is confidential must remain confidential. This information cannot be shared verbally, electronically, or in writing without appropriate consent. Information must be shared on a need-to-know basis only with those having primary responsibilities for decision making.

Conflict of interest: Avoidance of real or perceived conflict of interest is imperative to maintaining the integrity of interactions.

Impaired practitioner: Occupational therapy personnel who cannot competently perform their duties after reasonable accommodation are considered to be impaired. The occupational therapy practitioner's basic duty to students, patients, colleagues, and research subjects is to ensure that no harm is done. It is difficult to report a professional colleague who is impaired. The motive for this action must be to provide for the protection and safety of all, including the person who is impaired.

Sexual relationships: Sexual relationships that occur during any professional interaction are forms of misconduct.

Payment for services and other financial arrangements: Occupational therapy personnel shall not guarantee or promise specific outcomes for occupational therapy services. Payment for occupational therapy services shall not be contingent on successful outcomes.

Resolving ethical issues: Occupational therapy personnel should utilize any and all resources available to them to identify and resolve conflicts and/or ethical dilemmas (AOTA, 2006b).

PROFESSIONAL RESOURCES

American Occupational Therapy Association

In 1917, notables such as Doctors Adolf Meyer and William Rush Dunton (both psychiatrists), Thomas Kidner and George Barton (both architects), and Eleanor Clarke Slagle (a reformer and early occupational therapist) influenced the formation of an organization that would become the American Occupational Therapy Association (AOTA). This group of occupational therapy pioneers came to the realization that engaging in meaningful activity is healing.

Today, AOTA represents the interests of occupational therapy practitioners in the United States. Several commissions are established within AOTA to manage the affairs of occupational therapy. These include the Commissions on Education, Practice, Ethics, and Professional Development. These commissions, in turn, provide oversight for the profession within each of their areas to ensure that occupational therapy education and practice comply with a set of standards believed to be in the best interest of the profession as well as the public for whom it serves. Information about AOTA can be found at http:www.AOTA.org.

AOTA will be 100 years old in 2017. Its centennial vision states that by the year 2017 occupation therapy will be recognized as "a powerful, widely recognized, science-driven, and evidence-based profession with a globally connected and diverse workforce meeting society's occupational needs" (AOTA, 2007, p. 613). This statement demonstrates the intent of the profession to continue to base evaluations and intervention strategies on available research. It also seeks to collaborate with international partners to work to meet the occupational needs of clients.

World Federation of Occupational Therapists (WFOT)

The **World Federation of Occupational Therapists (WFOT)** was established formally at meetings held in England in 1952 by representatives from seven countries with occupational therapy associations. In 1959 WFOT joined the World Health Organization (WHO) and in 1963 it was recognized as a nongovernmental organization (NGO) by the United Nations (UN). Today there are 57 country member associations. The WFOT mission is that it "promotes occupational therapy as an art and science internationally. The Federation supports the development, use and practice of occupational therapy worldwide, demonstrating its relevance and contribution to society" (WFOT, 2007).

WFOT manages five distinct programs: education and research, promotion and development, standards and quality, international cooperation, and executive programs. To meet its education and research mandate, it developed minimal standards for the education of occupational therapists in 2002 and a companion guide explaining the process for approving education programs in 2004. The American Occupational Therapy Association recognizes WFOT and graduates of approved WFOT education programs have been eligible to apply for visas to practice in the United States. Information on WFOT may be accessed at http://www.wfot.org.

SUMMARY

Occupational therapists help patients improve their ability to perform tasks in living and working environments. They work with individuals who suffer from a mentally, physically, developmentally, or emotionally disabling condition. Occupational therapists use treatments to develop, recover, or maintain the daily living and work skills of their patients. The practitioner helps clients not only to improve their basic motor functions and reasoning abilities, but also to compensate for permanent loss of function. The goal is to help clients have independent, productive, and satisfying lives.

Employment of occupational therapists is expected to grow much faster than the average for all occupations, with the increasing elderly population driving growth in the demand for occupational therapy services.

PHYSICAL THERAPY

BARBARA SANDERS

Keywords

American Physical Therapy Association (APTA): The national professional organization for physical therapists representing more than 72,000 members. Its goal is to advocate for the advancement of physical therapy practice, research, and education.

Americans with Disabilities Act: The 1990 civil rights law that prohibits, under certain circumstances, discrimination based on disability.

Commission on Accreditation in Physical Therapy (CAPTE): The accreditation agency recognized by the U.S. Department of Education and the Council for Higher Education Accreditation to accredit entry-level physical therapist and physical therapist assistant education programs.

Federation of State Boards of Physical Therapy (FSBPT): Organization that develops and administers the National Physical Therapy Examinations for both physical therapists (PT) and physical therapist assistants (PTA).

National Physical Therapy Examinations: Examinations that assess the basic, entry-level competence for first-time licensure or registration as a physical therapist (PT) or physical therapist assistant (PTA) within 53 U.S. states and jurisdictions.

Physical therapists (PTs): Physical therapists provide services that help restore function, improve mobility, relieve pain, and prevent or limit permanent physical disabilities of patients suffering from injuries or disease. They restore, maintain, and promote overall fitness and health.

Physical therapist assistants (PTAs): Physical therapist assistants and aides help physical therapists to provide treatment that improves patient mobility, relieves pain, and prevents or lessens physical disabilities of patients.

Physical therapy: A health care profession that provides services to clients in order to develop, maintain, and restore maximum movement and functional ability throughout life.

Physical therapy is a profession that is dynamic and interactive. *Physical therapy is provided by* **physical therapists (PTs)** *who are essential members of the health care delivery system. PTs provide diagnosis and management of movement dysfunction and work to enhance physical and functional abilities and performance. They also play a role in the promotion of fitness and wellness to enhance quality of life as it relates to movement and health. In most states, physical therapy can be provided only by qualified PTs or by* **physical therapist assistants (PTAs)** *working under the supervision of a PT (American Physical Therapy Association, 2008; Federation of State Boards of Physical Therapy, 2008).*

EDUCATION FOR ENTRY INTO PRACTICE

Physical therapists (PTs) must hold a degree from an accredited entry-level (professional) program and a license in order to practice. The degrees currently offered are master's degrees and the Doctor of Physical Therapy (DPT) degree. There are 210 accredited PT education programs in the United States and over 190 of these programs currently provide entry-level education with the DPT. It is anticipated that by 2010, almost all programs will have made the transition from the master's degree to the DPT.

PT education programs require prerequisite courses that generally include the basic sciences of anatomy and physiology, chemistry, and physics as well as social science and liberal arts courses. Students interested in a career in physical therapy are encouraged to have strong interpersonal skills because they will be required to communicate with patients, patients' families and other caregivers, and other health care professionals. They also provide education about patients' physical therapy treatment and goals. PTs are expected to continue their professional development by participating in continuing education courses and other professional development activities such as residencies and fellowships.

Accreditation

Accreditation of physical therapy education for both PTs and physical therapist assistants (PTAs) is under the auspices of the **Commission on Accreditation in Physical Therapy Education (CAPTE).** An accredited program must meet certain standards and criteria established by CAPTE. Additional information is available at the CAPTE Web site, www.apta.org/capte. The role of CAPTE is to establish and apply standards for quality education through the constant evaluation and consideration of the state of practice and the health care needs of the public (CAPTE, 2008a).

OBTAINING A LICENSE

In most states, health care practitioners must be licensed to provide clinical services, and this is true for PTs: a license is required to practice in all U.S. jurisdictions. A license is evidence that the state (or other jurisdiction) has recognized an individual's qualification to practice within the parameters of the state law (i.e., state statute, practice act). A license is not guaranteed; rather, one must apply for the license and show evidence that he or she is qualified under the requirements of each jurisdiction.

States' Rights

Each state reserves the right to determine the legal basis for the practice of physical therapy and for the protection of the residents within that state. There is a provision within the Constitution of the United States for states' rights. Each state enacts the legislation through the state's legislative process to provide protection of residents within the state from incompetent or unscrupulous health care practitioners. The state legislators are the lawmakers and have control over the licensure legislation in each state.

State Practice Acts

The scope of practice of the PT is statutorily defined in each state's laws in the form of a practice act. State legislatures have the authority to adopt or change practice acts and thus provide the legal definition and requirements for the practice of physical therapy in that state. State statutes are enacted by each of the state legislatures and those groups are entitled to tailor the law to meet the needs of their citizens. As a result, laws vary from state to state. State statutes can affect the practice of physical therapy in a number of ways, including regulation of the insurance industry, state funding for health care, and state health department requirements. However, the single most important factor for state statute is the physical therapy practice act. It is the legal foundation for the scope and protection of physical therapy practice.

Practice acts generally include a definition of physical therapy practice, identification of who may legally provide physical therapy, identification of the tasks that may be delegated and to whom they may be delegated, and supervisory requirements. The state practice act is the highest authority for the practice of physical therapy for that state and thus supersedes provisions of other states or organizations. Note that in protecting the public, practice acts also protect the profession of physical therapy from infringement by those who are not licensed PTs and from encroachment on its scope of practice by other health care professions. For example, only PTs may use the initials "PT" after their name.

State Licensure Boards

Typically, each state identifies a governing board with the authority in the practice act to issue and renew licenses to individuals who are qualified and to discipline those who do not comply with the law. Rules and regulations are generally put in place to interpret and assist in the administration of the practice act. Enforcement is in the category of administrative law in which decisions are governed by a hearing panel composed of health care professionals and the public. Administrative law procedures differ from typical civil or criminal law procedures in that strict rules of evidence are not required. Courts will generally not overturn a licensure board's decision unless the hearing panel has violated due process or the regulation is unconstitutional.

Many states require a regular review of state regulatory bodies, termed "sunset review." Sunset review entails a detailed review that may lead to elimination of regulatory boards if the boards cannot provide compelling evidence that they are meeting their mission of public protection. It is not unusual for regulatory changes in the statutes to occur through the sunset review process.

Licensure Criteria

A PT must apply for licensure in each state in which he or she will practice. Each state practice act differs. Some states do not allow practice by qualified PT license applicants (new-graduate PTs) until they have taken and passed the state licensure examination and received a license to practice. Some states offer temporary licenses to new graduates who are in the process of becoming licensed.

Each of the 50 states, the District of Columbia, Puerto Rico, and the U.S. Virgin Islands has specific requirements for licensure of PTs. Each jurisdiction has established its own criteria for licensure and eligibility for the licensure examination, the **National Physical Therapy Examination (NPTE).** Many include a jurisprudence examination (a test of state law) as well. The following Web site provides links to each of these licensing boards: www.fsbpt.org/LicensingAuthorities/index.asp (Federation of State Boards of Physical Therapy, 2008). With all of the jurisdictions licensing PTs, a license cannot be automatically transferred from one to another; rather, an individual must apply for a license in each state. All states do require graduation from an accredited PT education program and a passing score on the NPTE, but the exact procedures, forms, costs, and other requirements vary.

Eligibility for Licensure

The NPTE is only one part of the process of obtaining a license to practice. Eligibility for licensure is determined after review of many documents in addition to the NPTE score. Licensing requirements also may include an extensive review of educational preparation and transcripts, experience in the field, recommendations of licensed PTs, passing jurisprudence examinations, screening for a criminal record (criminal background checks), and review of prior convictions. The application process and fees involved for initial licensure often costs the candidate hundreds of dollars.

Each licensing authority establishes its own criteria for eligibility to sit for the NPTE. The candidate should review the materials distributed by the licensing authority to determine eligibility in that state. The NPTE may be taken for initial licensure or relicensure. It also may be taken by candidates who are not licensed in that jurisdiction and do not have a qualifying NPTE score for that jurisdiction.

Federation of State Boards of Physical Therapy

Once the candidate is determined to be eligible by the state authority, the candidate's materials are forwarded to the **Federation of State Boards of Physical Therapy (FSBPT),** the organization that administers the

NPTE. The FSBPT sends the candidate an "Authorization To Test" letter that includes instructions for scheduling the NPTE at a testing center in the United States, U.S. territories, and Canada.

The computer-based examination is administered by FSBPT through Prometric®, its test vendor. The FSBPT receives the scores for the NPTE and reports the score to the licensing authority. The individual licensing authority then makes a decision about the score and other paperwork to determine licensure. All jurisdictions have adopted the FSBPT criterion-referenced passing score on the NPTE, so the minimum passing score is the same in all jurisdictions (Federation of State Boards of Physical Therapy, 2008).

Foreign-Educated Physical Therapists

Requirements for licensure of PTs vary from state to state for the foreign-educated PT as well. All 50 states require an educational credentials review. Thirty-seven states require graduation from a program comparable to a CAPTE-accredited program. Forty-two states require verification of English language proficiency, and 13 require a clinical internship. The FSBPT maintains a jurisdictional licensure reference guide at www.fsbpt.org/RegulatoryTools/ReferenceGuide/index.asp (Federation of State Boards of Physical Therapy, 2008). Additional information for foreign-educated PTs may be found on the Web site of the **American Physical Therapy Association (APTA)** at http://www.apta.org/AM/Template.cfm?Section=Core_Documents1&TEMPLATE=/CM/ContentDisplay.cfm&CONTENTID=50262.

The National Physical Therapy Examination (NPTE)

The purpose of the NPTE is to protect the public by providing a mechanism to ensure that licensees are minimally competent. The NPTE program also provides examination services to the regulatory authorities in the states and other legal jurisdictions and provides a common means for evaluating licensee applicants across those jurisdictions. The NPTE measures the knowledge and skill required for safe and effective practice as an entry-level PT. The content outline for the NPTE (Table 6.1) is revised every 5 years at a minimum. This outline determines the content of the NPTE and assures that the content is relevant to current practice (Federation of State Boards of Physical Therapy, 2008).

Table 6.1

NPTE TEST CONTENT OUTLINE FOR PHYSICAL THERAPISTS (FEDERATION OF STATE BOARDS OF PHYSICAL THERAPY)

CONTENT AREA	SPECIFIC AREAS	% OF ITEMS
Clinical application of foundational sciences	Cardiac, vascular and pulmonary Musculoskeletal Neuromuscular and nervous Integumentary Other	14.5
Examination/foundations for evaluation, differential diagnosis, and prognosis	Examination Foundations for evaluation, differential diagnosis, and prognosis	36.5
Interventions/equipment and devices; therapeutic modalities	Interventions Equipment and devices; therapeutic modalities	29.5
Safety, protection, and professional roles; teaching and learning; and research and evidence-based practice	Safety, protection and professional roles Teaching and learning Research and evidence-based practice	19.5
Total		**100**

Note: Adapted from 2008 *NPTE Candidate Handbook,* Federation of State Boards of Physical Therapy. The full content outline may be accessed at http://www.fsbpt.org/download/Candi dateHandbook20090406.pdf

Practice Analysis

The process used to determine the content of the NPTE is called an "analysis of practice" and identifies the work requirements for entry-level practitioners. The product is a formal set of test specifications that delineates the knowledge and skills related to safe and effective entry-level practice. This analysis is conducted periodically to be sure that it reflects the nature of current practice.

Examination Content

The NPTE consists of 250 items developed to measure the knowledge and skill required of the entry-level PT. The content outline delineates the major content areas of the NPTE. The items for the NPTE are written by PTs representing a broad spectrum of practice across the United States. The item writers are trained to produce high-quality, sound, multiple-choice test questions that cover the major areas of PT practice and address the identified content areas. The items are reviewed by an independent panel of experts and pretested prior to being included in the scored portion of the NPTE (Federation of State Boards of Physical Therapy, 2008).

There are a number of resources available to support candidates seeking successful completion of the NPTE. These are available in the form of test-preparation books, on-line practice examinations, and review courses. Also, the American Physical Therapy Association (APTA) maintains a list of resources on its Web site (www.apta.org).

Licensure Renewal

License renewal is also governed by each jurisdiction and there may be significant differences in requirements, so the licensee should be well versed in the requirements of his or her state. For example, many states require continuing education units (CEUs) in specific areas and specific amounts. Others may require the passing of a jurisprudence examination. Most states no longer issue a temporary license to practice due to the processing of licenses.

Continued Competence

Historically, continuing education has been the standard for proof of **continued competence.** However, this philosophy is in review in many jurisdictions and in other health care professions as well, including medicine. Several jurisdictions have adopted mechanisms for more conclusive evidence of continued competence such as retesting or clinical assessment.

SCOPE OF PRACTICE

Physical therapy is defined as the care and services provided by or under the direction of a PT. PTs are the only professionals who provide physical therapy. PTs practice in diverse health care settings, including hospitals, outpatient offices or clinics, private offices, rehabilitation facilities, intermediate and long-term care facilities, education centers, patients' homes, and many other settings. They are integral members of the health care delivery team (American Physical Therapy Association, 2001).

Physical Therapists

The scope of practice for the PT is initially defined by the professional guiding documents but then specifically defined by the practice act in each state. In general, the role of the PT includes the examination and development of a plan of care for each patient. When a PT sees a patient for the first time, he or she examines that individual and develops the plan of care. The goal is to promote the patient's ability to move, reduce pain, restore function, and prevent disability. PTs also work with individuals to prevent the loss of mobility by developing fitness and wellness programs for healthier, more active lifestyles. Therapeutic exercise and functional training are hallmarks of the PT intervention program. PTs may use other techniques and modalities in addition to exercise to accomplish individual patient goals. Depending on the needs of the patient, the PT may perform such hands-on modalities as mobilizing a joint or massaging a muscle to promote proper movement and function.

Physical Therapist Assistants

PTs are assisted in the patient care process by physical therapist assistants (PTAs). The PTA provides services under the direction and supervision of a PT. Care provided by the PTA may include teaching patients exercises for mobility, strength, and coordination; training for activities such as walking with assistive devices; and the use of physical agents. In most states, PTAs are required to be licensed or certified.

Guide to Physical Therapist Practice

In defining physical therapy, the scope of practice is defined by the APTA (HOD P06-99-19-23) in this way:

> Physical therapy is a health profession whose primary purpose is the promotion of optimal health and function. This purpose is accomplished through the application of scientific principles to the processes of examination, evaluation, diagnosis, prognosis, and intervention to prevent or remediate

impairments, functional limitations, and disabilities as related to movement and health. Physical therapy encompasses areas of specialized competence and includes the development of new principles and applications to meet existing and emerging health needs. Other professional activities that serve the purpose of physical therapy are research, education, consultation and administration. (American Physical Therapy Association, 2008)

The *Guide to Physical Therapist Practice* (*Guide*) has been a critical tool in defining and describing what PTs do as clinicians in the health care arena. These activities have been summarized in the patient/client management model (Figure 6.1).

This model identifies the elements of data collection, plan of care development, and implementation of the plan for the best outcomes for the patient/client. Components of the patient/client management model are examination, evaluation, diagnosis, prognosis, and intervention.

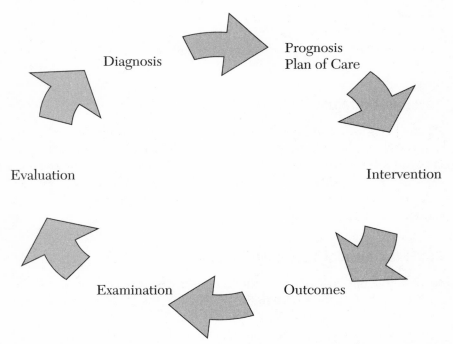

Figure 6.1 Elements of the patient/client management model (adapted from American Physical Therapy Association, 2001).

Examination and Evaluation

Examination is the process of gathering information about the past and current status of the patient/client. It includes the history, systems review, and selected tests and measures that allow the PT to ascertain the physical and functional status of the patient/client. The next element is evaluation. Evaluation is the process by which the PT makes clinical judgments based on the examination (American Physical Therapy Association, 2001).

Diagnosis

The diagnosis is established based on the examination and evaluation of the patient/client. It is a categorization of the findings through a defined process, a label encompassing a cluster of signs and symptoms commonly associated with a disorder or syndrome or category of impairment, functional limitation, or disability. The APTA Guide (p. 37) defines diagnosis as follows:

> Diagnostic labels may be used to describe multiple dimensions of the patient/client, ranging from the most basic cellular level to the highest level of functioning—as a person in society. Although physicians typically use labels that identify disease, disorder, or condition at the level of the cell, tissue, organ, or system, physical therapists use labels that identify the *impact of a condition on function at the level of the system (especially the movement system) and at the level of the whole person.* (American Physical Therapy Association, 2001)

Thus, diagnosis by PTs is distinct from diagnosis by physicians in that the diagnostic labels pertain to different levels of disablement. While diagnosis by physicians concerns identifying or determining the nature and cause of a disease or injury, Sahrmann defined physical therapy diagnosis as "the term that names the primary dysfunction toward which the physical therapist directs treatment. The dysfunction is identified by the physical therapist based on the information obtained from the history, signs, symptoms, examination, and tests the physical therapist performs or requests" (Sahrmann, 1988, p. 1905).

The Guide (p. 37) identifies the objective of the PT diagnostic process as "the identification of discrepancies that exist between the level of function that is desired by the patient/client and the capacity of the patient/client to achieve that level." Further, "[i]f the diagnostic process reveals findings that are outside the scope of the physical therapist's knowledge, experience, or expertise, the physical therapist refers the patient/client to an appropriate practitioner" (American Physical Therapy Association, 2001).

Prognosis

Once the diagnosis has been made, the PT's attention shifts to the establishment of a prognosis—a prediction of the level of improvement and the time required to reach that point. The PT also designs a plan of care that incorporates the expectations of the patient/client in the establishment of short- and long-term goals.

Intervention

The final element is intervention, which occurs when the PT conducts procedures with the patient/client to achieve the desired outcomes. There are three activities in this process:

- coordination, communication, and documentation;
- patient instruction; and
- procedural intervention.

Ultimately physical therapy goals will be reached or the services will be terminated. This termination occurs with discharge (when goals are met) or discontinuation of services (when goals are not met, which can occur for a variety of reasons). The PT ultimately decides the status of the patient/client at that time and makes any recommendations for follow-up care.

Additional Roles

Other professional roles for the PT include consultation, education, critical inquiry, and administration. Consultation may be patient/client-centered or aimed at the level of the community and health policy. Examples of consultation include court testimony, architectural recommendations, academic and clinical program evaluation, and suggestions for health policy. The role of the PT in education can range from a formal appointment as a faculty member in an educational program to patient education in a clinical setting, student supervision in a clinical setting, and professional development and instruction in continuing education.

Critical inquiry is an essential element for the future of the profession. Research is the key to critical inquiry and thus PTs may be involved in clinical or laboratory research activities. PTs may also function in administrative positions, which can include planning, communicating, delegating, managing, directing, supervising, budgeting, and evaluating (Pagliarulo, 2007).

ETHICAL AND LEGAL CONSIDERATIONS IN PRACTICE

There are many types of legal and regulatory influences that control health care practice. Their interpretation is generally through judicial bodies and review boards. Ethical standards deal with the conduct and moral choice that arise from the profession. Table 6.2 provides a summary of the types of laws affecting physical therapy practice. The primary purpose of laws, regulations, and policies affecting the practice of physical therapy is the protection of the public by ensuring that providers are competent and services are provided in accordance with the wise use of taxpayer dollars.

Laws, regulations, and policies that impact physical therapy practice vary from state to state and program to program. Various aspects of practice may be governed by both state and federal law; federal law

Table 6.2

SUMMARY OF TYPES OF LAWS AFFECTING PHYSICAL THERAPY PRACTICE

LICENSE	INSURANCE	TORTS	HEALTH CARE	CRIMINAL	EMPLOYMENT	CONTRACTS
Administrative law	Insurance and contract law	Civil law	Medicare-Medicaid	Criminal law	Labor law, ADA, worker's compensation	Contract law
States' rights	State and federal	State and federal	State and federal	State and federal	State and federal	State and federal

prevails over state law. Some laws, regulations, and policies address how PT services are reimbursed. Regulations are developed by government agencies, not through the legislative process, and are considered rules controlling the practice of physical therapy.

Federal Laws

Federal regulations come from a variety of sources, including the Centers for Medicare and Medicaid Services (CMS), which are responsible for administering the Medicare and Medicaid programs. Federal statutes that address physical therapy practice include the following:

- The **Americans with Disabilities Act (ADA)** requires that goods and services available to the public be made accessible to persons with disabilities.
- The Individuals with Disabilities Education Act (IDEA) requires that special education and related services be provided at public expense to students with disabilities when needed for the student to benefit from an educational program.
- The Social Security Amendments of 1965 contain the provisions for the Medicare program, a federally subsidized health insurance program for people 65 years of age and older, and Medicaid, jointly funded by the state and federal governments to provide health care services to the poor.
- The Health Insurance Portability and Accountability Act (HIPAA) requires that all health care providers adhere to federal guidelines as to the type of patient information that they disclose, to whom they disclose it, and how they store it in order to protect patient confidentiality.

State Laws

State regulations also provide rules for physical therapy; each state has a board of physical therapy that determines the rules under which a PT can be licensed and can practice in that jurisdiction. State statutes generally include the practice act that serves as the legal foundation for the scope and protection of physical therapy practice. State statutes are enacted by each state and may be tailored to meet the needs of that state's citizens. For this reason, state laws vary from state to state.

Common, Criminal, and Civil Laws

Other legal issues will be managed under common law, criminal law, or civil law. Common law is the law that has been created by court decisions, written by judges and passed down. *Negligence* is an area of common law. Criminal law involves prosecution in a court of law for acts done in violation of duties that an individual owes to the community—in other words, infractions committed against society. The state prosecutes these violations on behalf of the public. An example of a criminal prosecution would be *insurance fraud.* Civil law is concerned with wrongs committed among private parties. This is generally where most *malpractice* issues fall. The act of negligence is defined as the failure to act as a reasonable and prudent person would act in the same circumstance. Malpractice is professional negligence—an injury caused by the failure to do something a member in good standing of the profession would have done. It is a failure to meet a professional standard of care.

Professional Guidelines

The American Physical Therapy Association (APTA) has developed several documents that provide for the legal and ethical practice of physical therapy. One is the *Standards of Practice for Physical Therapy,* which includes two documents: the *Code of Ethics* and the *Guide for Professional Conduct.* These are established policies of the APTA (see Exhibit 6.1) (American Physical Therapy Association, 2008a, Ethics).

PROFESSIONAL RESOURCES

American Physical Therapy Association (APTA)

The APTA is a national professional organization that represents more than 64,000 PTs, PTAs, and students. APTA members are automatically members of a chapter. The chapter is based either on the home address of the individual or the individual's primary work address. There are 52 chapters: the 50 states, Puerto Rico, and the District of Columbia. A listing of the chapters can be found on the APTA Web site (www.apta.org). The APTA also offers voluntary membership to special-interest groups called sections. There are 18 sections that address specialty practice areas, such as orthopedics and pediatrics, and interest areas such as

Exhibit 6.1

CODE OF ETHICS OF THE AMERICAN PHYSICAL THERAPY ASSOCIATION (APTA, 2008)

PREAMBLE
This *Code of Ethics* of the American Physical Therapy Association sets forth principles for the ethical practice of physical therapy. All physical therapists are responsible for maintaining and promoting ethical practice. To this end, the physical therapist shall act in the best interest of the patient/client. This *Code of Ethics* shall be binding on all physical therapists.

PRINCIPLE 1. A physical therapist shall respect the rights and dignity of all individuals and shall provide compassionate care.

PRINCIPLE 2. A physical therapist shall act in a trustworthy manner toward patients/clients, and in all other aspects of physical therapy practice.

PRINCIPLE 3. A physical therapist shall comply with laws and regulations governing physical therapy and shall strive to effect changes that benefit patients/clients.

PRINCIPLE 4. A physical therapist shall exercise sound professional judgment.

PRINCIPLE 5. A physical therapist shall achieve and maintain professional competence.

PRINCIPLE 6. A physical therapist shall maintain and promote high standards for physical therapy practice, education, and research.

PRINCIPLE 7. A physical therapist shall seek only such remuneration as is deserved and reasonable for physical therapy services.

PRINCIPLE 8. A physical therapist shall provide and make available accurate and relevant information to patients/clients about their care and to the public about physical therapy services.

PRINCIPLE 9. A physical therapist shall protect the public and the profession from unethical, incompetent, and illegal acts.

PRINCIPLE 10. A physical therapist shall endeavor to address the health needs of society.

PRINCIPLE 11. A physical therapist shall respect the rights, knowledge, and skills of colleagues and other health care professionals.

CODE OF ETHICS HOD S06-00-12-23 (Program 17) [Amended HOD 06-91-05-05; HOD 06-87-11-17; HOD 06-81-06-18; HOD 06-78-06-08; HOD 06-78-06-07; HOD 06-77-18-30; HOD 06-77-17-27; Initial HOD 06-73-13-24] **[Standard]**

education and federal regulation. They also can be found on the APTA Web site.

Federation of State Boards of Physical Therapy (FSBPT)

The FSBPT develops and administers the NPTE for PTs and PTAs in 53 jurisdictions. The FSBPT is a federation of the state regulatory agencies that protects the public by providing service and leadership to promote safe and competent physical therapy practice. The vision of the FSBPT is "that the organization will achieve a high level of public protection through a strong foundation of laws and regulatory standards in physical therapy; effective tools and systems to assess entry-level and continuing competence, and public and professional awareness of resources for public protection" (Federation of State Boards of Physical Therapy, 2008).

Foreign Credentialing Commission on Physical Therapy

The Foreign Credentialing Commission on Physical Therapy (FCCPT) is a nonprofit organization created to assist the U.S. Citizenship and Immigration Services (USCIS) and U.S. state licensing agencies by evaluating the credentials of foreign-educated PTs who wish to immigrate to, and work in, the United States (Foreign Credentialing Commission on Physical Therapy, 2008b). Extensive information concerning licensure for the foreign-educated PT can be found at the FCCPT Web site (www. fccpt.org).

Planned Learning and Assistance Network

The *Planned Learning and Assistance Network* (PLAN) is a new service provided by the FCCPT that will assist foreign applicants whose credentials have been evaluated and are not found to be comparable to the physical therapy education in the United States or who have not met specific requirements for that jurisdiction. The service assists applicants in identifying resources that will allow them to complete the educational coursework that will bring them into compliance with the requirements for comparability. PLAN offers a consultation to review and interpret the coursework evaluation and assist in developing a study plan to meet the requirements; and it provides a list of institutions within the United States that will offer the required content (Foreign Credentialing Commission on Physical Therapy, 2008).

CGFNS International

CGFNS International is a nonprofit organization that provides services that validate international professional credentials and supports international regulatory and educational standards for health care professionals. It is recognized as an authority on credentials evaluation related to the education, registration, and licensure of health professionals worldwide. This organization offers both the VisaScreen® Program, which evaluates the credentials of foreign-educated PTs seeking an occupational visa to practice in the United States, and the Credentials Evaluation Service (CES), which provides an analysis of international credentials for licensure and academic purposes (CGFNS International, 2008b).

Citizen Advocacy Center

The Citizen Advocacy Center (CAC) is a unique support program for the thousands of public members serving on health care regulatory, credentialing, oversight, and governing boards as representatives of consumer interest (Federation of State Boards of Physical Therapy, 2008).

SUMMARY

Physical therapists provide services that help restore function, improve mobility, relieve pain, and prevent or limit permanent physical disabilities of patients suffering from injuries or disease. They restore, maintain, and promote overall fitness and health. Physical therapists practice in hospitals, clinics, and private offices that have specially equipped facilities. They also treat patients in hospital rooms, homes, or schools. Employment of physical therapists is expected to grow much faster than average. Job opportunities will be good, especially in acute hospital, rehabilitation, and orthopedic settings (Bureau of Labor Statistics, 2009c).

PHYSICIAN ASSISTANTS

GERALDINE BUCK AND NICOLE GARA

Keywords

Accreditation Review Commission on Education for Physician Assistants (ARC-PA): The accrediting agency that defines the standards for physician assistant education and evaluates physician assistant educational programs within the United States to ensure their compliance with those standards.

American Academy of Physician Assistants (AAPA): National professional society, founded in 1968, that represents physician assistants in all 50 states, the District of Columbia, Guam, and the Federal Services.

Clinical privileges: Official permission to treat patients in a health care setting, usually a hospital.

House staff: Individuals employed directly by a health care institution, usually a hospital.

National Commission on Certification of Physician Assistants (NCCPA): The credentialing organization for physician assistants in the United States that administers the Physician Assistant National Certifying Exam (PANCE).

Physician Assistant National Certifying Exam (PANCE): Credentialing examination for physician assistants that entitles those who pass it to use the designation PA-C.

Physician Assistant National Recertifying Exam (PANRE): Examination required to maintain certification as a physician assistant.

Prescriptive authority: Right granted by law to prescribe medications, usually under the supervision of a physician.

Reimbursement: Payment by government or private insurers for services provided by certain allied health professionals.

The physician assistant (PA) profession is relatively new to the United States. The first class of four physician assistants graduated from Duke University in 1967. In 2008 there were approximately 80,000 PAs eligible to practice in the United States, and 12,000 students enrolled in PA programs (AAPA, 2008a). A physician assistant provides a broad range of health care services that are traditionally performed by physicians.

EDUCATION FOR ENTRY INTO PRACTICE

Physician assistant (PA) programs produce health professionals who practice under the supervision of a physician and who are committed to working as part of the physician/physician assistant team. PAs may exercise autonomy in decision making but they are not independent health care providers. In clinical practice, PAs work within the supervising physician's scope of practice, and complement the practice style of the supervising physician(s). PAs work in all medical and surgical specialties providing medical care to patients by collecting medical data via the patient's medical history, physical examination, and diagnostic testing; diagnosing patients; and providing patients with therapies such as medications, counseling, and patient education.

PAs are lifelong learners who build upon their generalist education by training and experience in the clinical work environment and through continuing medical education. Additionally, a relatively small number of postgraduate training programs are available to PAs in specialty areas such as neonatology, emergency medicine, and surgery. Notably, all 50 states in the United States require PAs to be board certified and approved by a state licensing agency for clinical practice privileges.

Academic Degree Requirements

As the PA profession has evolved over the past 40 years, so has the educational process for PAs. At the inception of the PA profession in the mid-1960s, a certificate of completion was awarded. By 1970 the first academic degree for PA training was awarded (Cawley, 2007; Joslin et al., 2006), and throughout the 40-year history of the profession the academic degree associated with PA education has advanced.

Although the first PA master's degree was offered in 1973, by 1990 there were only five (5) master's degree granting PA programs (Joslin et al., 2006). In 2001, the second edition of the *Accreditation Standards for Physician Assistant Education,* published by the **Accreditation Review Commission on Education for Physician Assistants (ARC-PA),** recommended awarding a graduate degree to reflect the level of academic rigor and intensity of PA training (p. 5). PA programs quickly adopted this recommendation—by 2002 more than half of all PA programs awarded the master's degree (Cawley, 2007; Joslin et al., 2006). As of October 2008, 80% of U.S.-accredited PA training programs (113 of 142) award the master's degree, and the remaining 29 programs award BS/BA degrees (15%), AS/AA degrees (2%), or certificates only (3%) (ARC-PA, 2008).

Prerequisites

Applicants to PA programs must complete at least 2 years of college courses in basic science and behavioral science as prerequisites, similar to the premed studies required of medical students. Preference in selection of candidates is usually given to those who have prior experience in health care. Most currently enrolled PA students have earned at least a bachelor's degree and accrued nearly three years of health care experience prior to admission to a PA program (**American Academy of Physician Assistants [AAPA],** 2008b; Physician Assistant Education Association [PAEA], 2008).

Physician Assistant Curriculum

Physician assistant (PA) education programs in the United States offer an intense but abbreviated medical school-type curriculum with a primary care focus. Classroom and laboratory components of training are complemented by supervised clinical practice. The mean length of PA education programs is 26.8 months (PAEA, 2008).

The first year of PA education typically provides a classroom-based, broad grounding in medical principles with a focus on their clinical applicability. This curriculum consists of coursework in the basic sciences, including anatomy, physiology, biochemistry, pharmacology, physical diagnosis, pathophysiology, microbiology, clinical laboratory sciences, behavioral sciences, health policy and practice issues, and medical ethics. In the second year, students receive hands-on clinical training through a series of clerkships or rotations in a variety of inpatient, outpatient, and long-term care settings. Clinical rotations include family medicine, internal medicine, obstetrics and gynecology, pediatrics, general surgery, emergency medicine, and psychiatry. Physician assistant students complete on average more than 2,000 hours of supervised clinical practice prior to graduation (AAPA, 2008c).

Program Accreditation

Physician assistant programs are accredited by the independent Accreditation Review Commission on Education for the Physician Assistant (ARC-PA). The ARC-PA accredits only those programs located in the United States (http://www.arc-pa.org/Acc_Programs/acc_programs.html). It awards accreditation to programs through a peer review process that includes documentation and periodic site visit evaluation to substantiate compliance with the Accreditation Standards for Physician Assistant Education.

The accreditation process is designed to encourage sound educational practices and innovation by programs and to stimulate continuous self-study and improvement (ARC-PA, 2009). PA program accreditation standards are rigorous, and only graduates of accredited programs are eligible to sit for the **Physician Assistant National Certifying Exam (PANCE)** administered by the independent **National Commission on Certification of Physician Assistants (NCCPA).**

OBTAINING A LICENSE

In the United States, each individual state, plus the District of Columbia, has its own set of laws and regulations governing the practice of medicine by physicians and physician assistants. These laws and regulations specify the qualifications for licensure as a PA, the application and renewal process, and requirements for supervision. They also describe the scope of practice for PAs and how that is determined.

Initial Licensure

All states except Illinois, Minnesota, and North Dakota specify that physician assistants must be graduates of accredited PA programs. A baccalaureate degree also is required by Arkansas, Connecticut, Idaho, Maryland, Massachusetts, and Pennsylvania. A master's degree is required in Mississippi, Missouri, and Ohio.

In every state, it is mandatory that applicants for PA licensure have passed the Physician Assistant National Certifying Exam (PANCE). PANCE serves as a *de facto* licensing exam because states do not administer their own, separate examinations.

Physician assistants must have one or more licensed supervising physicians before starting clinical practice. Supervising physicians, who are medical doctors (MDs) or doctors of osteopathy (DOs), may be required to submit applications to supervise PAs or to acknowledge their supervisory role in the practice of PAs.

Licensure Renewal

Once a license is granted, it must be renewed on a regular basis. States generally specify renewal and payment of a fee every 2 or 3 years. There may be other requirements as well, such as proof of current national certification by the NCCPA or completion of a certain number of continuing medical education hours.

CERTIFICATION REQUIREMENTS

The NCCPA is the only national certifying organization for PAs in the United States. Established as a not-for-profit organization in 1975, NCCPA is dedicated to assuring the public that certified PAs meet established standards of knowledge and clinical skills throughout their careers. All 50 states, the District of Columbia, and the majority of U.S. territories rely on NCCPA certification criteria for initial and continued licensure of PAs.

To obtain initial NCCPA certification, all PAs must successfully complete the PANCE, a national board examination. PANCE is designed to assess general medical and surgical knowledge and is administered by computer at testing centers throughout the United States continually during the year. The NCCPA exam is open only to graduates of ARC-PA accredited physician assistant programs. There are no exceptions. After passing the PANCE examination, PAs are issued an NCCPA certificate, entitling them to use the PA-C designation until the expiration date printed on the certification (approximately 2 years). Individuals who have never been certified and who graduated from an ARC-PA accredited physician assistant program on or after January 1, 2003, will be eligible to take PANCE for up to 6 years after completing the requirements for graduation from that program. During that 6-year period, the examination may be taken a maximum of six times. When either the six attempts or 6 years is exhausted, whichever occurs sooner, the individual loses eligibility to take PANCE. The only way to establish new eligibility to take PANCE is to enter into and complete an unabridged ARC-PA accredited physician assistant educational program.

To maintain a valid NCCPA certificate, PAs must complete an ongoing 6-year process of certification maintenance that involves two steps: continuing medical education and a recertification exam.

Continuing Medical Education

Every 2 years, a minimum of 100 hours of continuing medical education credit must be earned to maintain certification, including at least 50 hours of Category I (Preapproved) credit. Category I activities are preapproved because they have been reviewed in advance by particular medical organizations. All Category I activities must be documented with certificates of completion or attendance or some other official verification from the program's provider.

Category II activities are elective and may be used in addition to required Category I activities to maintain certification. Because Category II activities have not been reviewed for educational content, they should be chosen according to the following guidelines:

- Any practice-related program that is not eligible for Category I credit, such as educational programs provided by pharmaceutical companies or medical device manufacturers
- Any practice-related, voluntary, self-learning activity, such as reading medical texts or medical journals, or precepting students
- Any practice-related postgraduate course, excluding courses taken in an actual PA program

Recertification Exam

To maintain NCCPA certification, a PA must pass either the **Physician Assistant National Recertifying Exam (PANRE)** or Pathway II before the expiration date at the end of the 6th year of the certification maintenance cycle. PANRE is a 5-hour, computer-based exam administered at testing centers throughout the United States. To be eligible to take the PANRE, you must hold valid NCCPA certification and be in the 5th or 6th year of the certification maintenance cycle.

Pathway II, which will no longer be an option after 2010, is an alternative that involves completing an elective component requirement prior to receiving a Web-based take-home exam. The elective component involves earning 100 points within the following categories.

- Extra clinical Category I Continuing Medical Education (CME)
- Medical teaching

- Postgraduate coursework
- Self-assessment and specialty review
- Clinical skills training
- Publications
- Professionally relevant postgraduate degree
- Other professional activities

Elective component activities may be completed at any time during the current 6-year NCCPA certification maintenance cycle. PAs also must complete the 100-hour CME requirements for each CME logging cycle within the NCCPA certification maintenance cycle. For complete details, visit the NCCPA Web site, www.nccpa.net.

SCOPE OF PRACTICE

Physician assistant scope of practice is determined by the fund of knowledge and clinical skills gained from education in a PA program, from working with physicians in the patient care environment, and from formal continuing medical education courses. It is also determined by the delegatory decisions made by supervising physicians. State laws allow physicians to delegate patient care tasks within the physician's specialty to the PAs he or she supervises. The physician remains responsible for coordinating and managing the care of patients and ensuring the quality of care provided to them. The role of the PA depends in large measure on his or her skills, the needs of the patient, and the understanding or guidelines developed by the physician and PA.

In licensed health care facilities, such as hospitals, nursing homes, and surgical centers, providers may have to apply for **clinical privileges.** The privileges for PAs, such as assisting at surgery, are generally granted in accordance with community needs and norms, and in accordance with state law.

Relationship of PAs to Other Providers

Physician assistants are most closely aligned with physicians and work as part of physician-directed teams. Legally, they serve as an extension of the physician, so that orders written by a PA are considered to be the orders of the physician and may be carried out by nurses, therapists, and other personnel.

In hospitals, PAs frequently work as **house staff,** providing continuity of care to inpatients. Their experience and expertise can be useful to residents (physicians in training) who move through medical and surgical departments on a regular basis. PAs are frequently the providers who respond initially to a physician's request for a specialty consultation. Their assessment and recommended treatment would then be shared with their supervising physician. PAs, as part of patient care teams, also provide consultative services for other physicians.

Specialties and Role Options

PAs practice in more than 60 different specialty fields. Slightly more than one-third of PAs work in family medicine, general internal medicine, obstetrics/gynecology, and pediatrics. Other prevalent specialties for PAs include general surgery and surgical subspecialties; emergency medicine; internal medicine subspecialties such as cardiology, oncology, and gastroenterology; and dermatology (AAPA, 2008d).

With their generalist medical backgrounds, PAs are able to adapt to any specialty practice. By functioning as part of physician-directed teams, PAs have the flexibility to learn new tasks and assume new responsibilities. PAs may change specialties by changing supervising physicians. There are no specialty-specific certifications required to practice in a particular area of medicine.

ETHICAL AND LEGAL CONSIDERATIONS IN PRACTICE

The *Guidelines for Ethical Conduct for the Physician Assistant Profession,* available at http://www.aapa.org/manual/22-EthicalConduct.pdf (AAPA, 2008e), describe the four main bioethical principles that govern PA practice: autonomy, beneficence, nonmalfeasance, and justice. For example, patients have the right to make autonomous (self) decisions and choices, and physician assistants should respect these decisions and choices. To display beneficence, PAs should always act in the patient's best interest. Nonmaleficence means that PAs should do no harm and should impose no unnecessary or unacceptable burden upon the patient. To be just, PAs should provide similar care to patients in similar circumstances, using norms for fair distribution of resources, risks, and costs.

Physician assistants are expected to behave both legally and ethically. They should know and understand the laws governing their practice, as well as the ethical responsibilities of being a health care professional. The law may describe minimum standards of behavior, while ethical principles delineate the highest moral standards of behavior.

Statement of Values of the PA Profession

The **American Academy of Physician Assistants (AAPA)** has issued value statements to which all PAs are expected to adhere (AAPA, 2008e).

- Physician assistants hold as their primary responsibility the health, safety, welfare, and dignity of all human beings.
- Physician assistants uphold the tenets of patient autonomy, beneficence, nonmaleficence, and justice.
- Physician assistants treat equally all persons who seek their care.
- Physician assistants hold in confidence the information shared in the course of practicing medicine.
- Physician assistants assess their personal capabilities and limitations, striving always to improve their medical practice.
- Physician assistants actively seek to expand their knowledge and skills, keeping abreast of advances in medicine.
- Physician assistants work with other members of the health care team to provide compassionate and effective care of patients.
- Physician assistants use their knowledge and experience to contribute to an improved community.
- Physician assistants respect their professional relationship with physicians.
- Physician assistants share and expand knowledge within the profession.

Legal Considerations

Physician assistant practice is the delegated practice of medicine and as such, is subject to laws and regulations on both the federal and state level. PAs must be aware of the requirements contained in the law and regulations covering licensure, practice, **prescriptive authority,** informed consent, liability, peer review, **reimbursement,** confidentiality, public health reporting, and so forth. In addition, they must abide by policies set by the hospitals, nursing homes, or other facilities in which they may work.

PROFESSIONAL RESOURCES

National Professional Association

The American Academy of Physician Assistants (AAPA; www.aapa.org) is the national professional society for physician assistants. Its mission is to ensure the professional growth, personal excellence, and recognition of physician assistants and to support their efforts to improve the quality, accessibility, and cost-effectiveness of patient-centered health care. AAPA has chapters in all 50 states and the District of Columbia. It is located at 950 North Washington Street, Alexandria, VA 22314. Telephone 703/826-2272.

State Regulatory Bodies

Each state plus the District of Columbia has regulations governing the practice of PAs. See Table 6.3.

Table 6.3

STATE REGULATORY BODIES

AGENCY NAME ALPHABETICALLY BY STATE	AGENCY ADDRESS
Alaska Medical Licensing Board	550 West 7th Ave., Anchorage, AK 99501
Alabama Board of Medical Examiners	PO Box 946, Montgomery, AL 36101
Arizona Regulatory Board of Physician Assistants	9545 E. Doubletree Ranch Rd., Scottsdale, AZ 85258
Arkansas State Medical Board	2100 Riverfront Dr., Little Rock, AR 72202
California Physician Assistant Committee	2005 Evergreen St., Sacramento, CA 95815
Colorado Board of Medical Examiners	1560 Broadway, Denver, CO 80202
Connecticut Division of Medical Quality Assurance - PA Licensing	PO Box 340308, Hartford, CT 06134
Delaware Board of Medical Practice	861 Silver Lake Blvd., Dover, DE 19904
District of Columbia Board of Medicine	717 14th St NW, Washington, DC 20005

(Continued)

STATE REGULATORY BODIES (*CONTINUED*)

AGENCY NAME ALPHABETICALLY BY STATE	AGENCY ADDRESS
Florida Board of Medical Examiners	4052 Bald Cypress Way, Bin #C03, Tallahassee, FL 32399
Georgia State Board of Medical Examiners	2 Peachtree St. NW, Atlanta, GA 30303
Hawaii Board of Medical Examiners	PO Box 3469, Honolulu, HI 96801
Idaho Board of Medicine	PO Box 83720, Boise, ID 83720
Illinois Div. of Professional Regulation	320 W. Washington St., Springfield, IL 62786
Indiana Health Professions Bureau, Attn: PA Committee	402 W. Washington St., Indianapolis, IN 46204
Iowa Board of Physician Assistants	321 East 12th St., Des Moines, IA 50319
Kansas Board of Healing Arts	235 SW Topeka Blvd, Topeka, KS 66603
Kentucky Board of Medical Licensure	310 Whittington Parkway, Louisville, KY 40222
Louisiana Board of Medical Examiners	PO Box 30250, New Orleans, LA 70190
Maine Board of Licensure in Medicine	137 State House Station, 161 Capitol St., Augusta, ME 04333
Maryland Board of Physicians	4201 Patterson Ave., Baltimore, MD 21215
Massachusetts Board of PA Registration	239 Causeway St., Boston, MA 02114
Michigan PA Task Force	PO Box 30670, Lansing, MI 48909
Minnesota Board of Medical Practice	2829 University Ave. SE, Minneapolis, MN 55414
Mississippi Board of Medical Licensure	1867 Crane Ridge Dr., Jackson, MS 39216
Missouri Board of Registration for the Healing Arts	PO Box 4, Jefferson City, MO 65102
Montana Board of Medical Examiners	PO Box 200513, Helena, MT 59620
Nebraska Board of Examiners in Medicine & Surgery	PO Box 94986, Lincoln, NE 68509
Nevada Board of Medical Examiners	PO Box 7238, Reno, NV 89510

(Continued)

STATE REGULATORY BODIES *(CONTINUED)*

AGENCY NAME ALPHABETICALLY BY STATE	AGENCY ADDRESS
New Hampshire Board of Medicine	2 Industrial Park Dr., Concord, NH 03301
New Jersey PA Advisory Committee	PO Box 45035, Newark, NJ 07101
New Mexico Medical Board	2055 S. Pacheco St., Santa Fe, NM 87505
New York State Board for Medicine	89 Washington Ave, Albany, NY 12234
North Carolina Medical Board	PO Box 20007, Raleigh, NC 27619
North Dakota Board of Medical Examiners	418 E. Broadway Ave, Bismarck, ND 58501
Ohio State Medical Board	77 South High St., Columbus, OH 43215
Oklahoma Board of Medical Licensure & Supervision	PO Box 18256, Oklahoma City, OK 73154
Oregon Board of Medical Examiners	1500 SW First Ave., Portland, OR 97201
Pennsylvania Board of Medicine	PO Box 2649, Harrisburg, PA 17105
Rhode Island Board of PAs	3 Capitol Hill, Rm. 104, Providence, RI 02908
South Carolina Board of Medical Examiners	PO Box 11289, Columbia, SC 29211
South Dakota Board of Medical & Osteopathic Examiners	125 S. Main Ave., Sioux Falls, SD 57104
Tennessee PA Committee, Department of Health-Related Boards	227 French Landing, Nashville, TN 37243
Texas Physician Assistant Board	PO Box 2018, Austin, TX 78768
Utah PA Licensing Board	PO Box 146741, Salt Lake City, UT 84114
Vermont Board of Medical Practice	PO Box 70, Burlington, VT 05402
Virginia Board of Medicine	9960 Mayland Dr., Richmond, VA 23233
Washington Medical Quality Assurance Commission	PO Box 47865, Olympia, WA 98504
West Virginia Board of Medicine	101 Dee Dr., Charleston, WV 25311
Wisconsin Medical Examining Board	PO Box 8935, Madison, WI 53708
Wyoming Board of Medicine	211 W. 19th St., Cheyenne, WY 82002

State Professional Organizations

The AAPA has a federated structure of 57 chartered chapters representing PAs in all 50 states, the District of Columbia, Guam, and the federal services. A list of state physician assistant associations may be obtained by visiting https://members.aapa.org/extra/constituents/chapter-menu.cfm.

SUMMARY

A PA is a licensed health professional who practices under the supervision of a physician. As part of the physician/physician assistant team, a PA exercises considerable autonomy in diagnosing and treating illnesses. PAs, depending on the practice act in their state, can perform physical exams, diagnose illnesses, develop and carry out treatment plans, order and interpret lab tests, suture wounds, assist in surgery, provide preventive health care counseling, and write prescriptions. Physician assistants receive a broad education in primary care medicine. Their education is ongoing after graduation through continuing medical education programs that are required and through continual interaction with physicians and other health care providers. Employment of PAs is expected to grow much faster than the average as health care establishments increasingly use physician assistants to contain costs (Bureau of Labor Statistics, 2009d).

SPEECH-LANGUAGE PATHOLOGY

CAROLYN WILES HIGDON

Keywords

American Speech-Language-Hearing Association (ASHA): The professional, scientific, and credentialing association for audiologists, speech-language pathologists, and speech, language, and hearing scientists.

Certificate of Clinical Competence (CCL): ASHA offers the Certificate of Clinical Competence in two areas: speech-language pathology and audiology. All applicants must possess an earned graduate degree (master's or doctoral degree) in order to meet application qualifications.

Council for Clinical Certification (CFCC): ASHA council that defines the standards for clinical certification and applies those standards in the certification of individuals; may also develop and administer a credentialing program for speech-language pathology assistants.

Council for Clinical Specialty Recognition (CCSR): ASHA council that implements, monitors, and revises as necessary, ASHA's Specialty Recognition Standards; formulates procedures for applications from petitioning groups for creation of specialty commissions; ensures that each specialty commission administers its requirements with efficiency and fairness and imposes equitable requirements for proper documentation from applicants; and establishes procedures to hear appeals from individuals who were denied recognition by a specialty commission.

Council on Academic Accreditation (CAA): The Council on Academic Accreditation in Audiology and Speech-Language Pathology (CAA) accredits eligible clinical doctoral programs in audiology and master's degree programs in speech-language pathology.

Praxis examination: The national examination in speech-language pathology and audiology required for certification.

Preceptor: A specialist in a profession, especially health care, who gives practical training to a student or novice in the profession.

Speech-language pathologists provide clinical services that include prevention and prereferral, screening, assessment, evaluation, consultation, diagnosis, treatment, intervention, management, counseling, collaboration, documentation, and referral. Speech-language pathologists work with people who cannot produce speech sounds or cannot produce them clearly; those with speech rhythm and fluency problems, such as stuttering; people with voice disorders, such as inappropriate pitch or harsh voice; those with problems understanding and producing language; those who wish to improve their communication skills by modifying an accent; and those with cognitive communication impairments, such as attention, memory, and problem-solving disorders. They also work with people who have swallowing difficulties (Bureau of Labor Statistics, 2009e).

EDUCATION FOR ENTRY INTO PRACTICE

Training programs in Communication Sciences and Disorders (formal name of the training programs for speech-language pathology and audiology) provide a curriculum leading to a master's or other entry-level graduate clinical degree with a major emphasis in speech-language pathology. The program must offer appropriate courses and clinical experiences on a regular basis so that students may satisfy the degree requirements within the published time frame. The intent is to ensure that program graduates are able to acquire the knowledge and skills needed for entry into professional practice and to meet relevant licensure and certification standards.

Programs of study in speech-language pathology must be sufficient in depth and breadth for graduates to achieve the knowledge and skills outcomes identified for entry into professional practice. Typically, the achievement of these outcomes requires the completion of 2 years of graduate education or the equivalent.

Educational Programs

Educational programs in speech-language pathology adhere to the Standards for Accreditation of Graduate Education Programs in Audiology and Speech-Language Pathology as defined by the **American Speech-Language-Hearing Association (ASHA).** Programs must provide an academic and clinical curriculum that is sufficient for students to acquire and demonstrate, at a minimum, knowledge of basic human communication and swallowing processes—including their biological, neurological, acoustic, psychological, developmental, and linguistic and cultural bases.

The program also must provide opportunities for students to acquire and demonstrate knowledge of the nature of speech, language, hearing, and communication disorders and differences, as well as swallowing disorders, including etiologies, characteristics, and anatomical, physiological, acoustic, psychological, developmental, linguistic, and cultural aspects. These opportunities must be provided in nine areas:

1. Articulation
2. Fluency
3. Voice and resonance, including respiration and phonation
4. Receptive and expressive language (phonology, morphology, syntax, semantics, and pragmatics) in speaking, listening, reading, writing, and manual modalities
5. Hearing, including the impact on speech and language
6. Swallowing (oral, pharyngeal, esophageal, and related functions and orofacial myofunction)
7. Cognitive aspects of communication (e.g., attention, memory, sequencing, problem solving, executive functioning)
8. Social aspects of communication (e.g., behavioral and social skills affecting communication)
9. Communication modalities (e.g., oral, manual, and augmentative and alternative communication techniques and assistive technology)

Appendix D presents a detailed list of speech-language treatment areas and provides a list of potential etiologies that speech-language pathologists address.

Clinical Education

The curriculum in speech-language pathology must provide the opportunity for students to complete a minimum of 400 clinical education hours, 325 of which must be attained at the graduate level. The program must provide sufficient breadth and depth of opportunities for students to obtain a variety of clinical education experiences in different work settings, with different populations, and with appropriate equipment and resources. This allows students to acquire and demonstrate skills across the scope of practice in speech-language pathology, sufficient to enter professional practice.

It is the responsibility of the program to plan a clinical program of study for each student. The program must demonstrate that it has sufficient agreements with supervisors or **preceptors** and clinical sites to provide each student with the clinical experience necessary to prepare them for independent professional practice. It is the program's responsibility to design, organize, administer, and evaluate the overall clinical education of each student.

The program must provide opportunities for students to acquire and demonstrate *knowledge* in the following areas:

- Principles and methods of prevention, assessment, and intervention for people with communication and swallowing disorders across the life span, including consideration of anatomical, physiological, psychological, developmental, linguistic, and cultural aspects of the disorders
- Standards of ethical conduct
- Interaction and interdependence of speech, language, and hearing in the discipline of human communication sciences and disorders
- Processes used in research and the integration of research principles into evidence-based clinical practice
- Contemporary professional issues
- Certification, specialty recognition, licensure, and other relevant professional credentials

The program also must provide opportunities for students to acquire and demonstrate *skills* in the following areas:

- Oral and written or other forms of communication
- Prevention, evaluation, and intervention of communication disorders and swallowing disorders
- Interaction and personal qualities, including counseling, collaboration, ethical practice, and professional behavior
- Effective interaction with patients, families, professionals, and other individuals, as appropriate

- Delivery of services to culturally and linguistically diverse populations
- Application of the principles of evidence-based practice
- Self-evaluation of effectiveness of practice

OBTAINING A LICENSE

Philosophy of States' Rights

Forty-eight states and the District of Columbia regulate the profession of speech-language pathology (ASHA, 2008). Most states with licensure laws have professional standards based on ASHA's Code of Ethics. Because state licensure laws may reflect the ASHA **Certificate of Clinical Competence,** most of the rules and/or regulations used by states either adopt the wording of ASHA's Code of Ethics exactly or use it as the basis for the state's professional conduct. When state licensure laws adopt nationally recognized standards of professional conduct, one can move from state to state with less confusion. Readers are referred to Table 6.4 for a list of the states that license speech-language pathologists.

Initial Licensure

Licensure for speech-language pathology may have three components. The first is the national association certification known as the Certificate of Clinical Competence (CCC), the second is state (health) licensure as an SLP, and the third is state Department of Education certification for those working as salaried employees in schools in a number of states.

ASHA Certification

The American Speech-Language Hearing Association (ASHA) certification is a voluntary credential that verifies an SLP's achievement of rigorous, uniform, and validated standards that are nationally recognized.

Requirements. Individuals applying for certification in speech-language pathology must have completed a course in each of the following

Table 6.4

STATE LICENSURE FOR SLPs AND AUDIOLOGISTS

Alabama	Kentucky	Ohio
Alaska	Louisiana	Oklahoma
Arizona	Maine	Oregon
Arkansas	Massachusetts	Pennsylvania
California	Michigan[a]	Rhode Island
Colorado[a]	Minnesota	South Carolina
Connecticut	Mississippi	South Dakota
Delaware	Missouri	Tennessee
District of Columbia	Montana	Texas
Florida	Nebraska	Utah
Georgia	Nevada	Vermont
Hawaii	New Hampshire	Virginia
Idaho	New Jersey	Washington
Illinois	New Mexico	West Virginia
Indiana	New York	Wisconsin
Iowa	North Carolina	
Kansas	North Dakota	

[a]Regulates only audiology.

areas: biological sciences, physical sciences, mathematics, and behavioral/social sciences. Applicants also must have been assessed to ensure that they have achieved the knowledge and skills outlined in the Standards of Certification in Speech-Language Pathology (ASHA, 2005) in a graduate program accredited by the **Council on Academic Accreditation** in Audiology and Speech-Language Pathology (CAA).

Knowledge in the areas outlined in the standards is typically achieved through participation in the clinical practicum (400 clock hours total, including 25 hours of clinical observation and 375 clock hours in direct client/patient contact, of which 325 are at the graduate level); however, academic programs may assess compliance with the standards in any manner they wish.

Clinical Fellowship. Upon completion of the academic course work and clinical practicum requirements, individuals applying for certification in speech-language pathology must complete a Speech-Language Pathology Clinical Fellowship (SLPCF) experience under the mentorship of an individual holding ASHA certification. This experience must consist of the equivalent of 36 weeks of full-time clinical practice, with *full-time* defined as 35 hours per week.

Praxis Examination. Applicants for certification in speech-language pathology also must successfully complete the **Praxis Examination** in Speech-Language Pathology that is administered by the Educational Testing Service (ETS). Results of the examination must be submitted to ASHA directly from ETS no more than 5 years prior to submission of the application for certification and no less than 2 years following completion of the knowledge and skills required for certification. Once certification has been granted, individuals must comply with the certification maintenance requirements outlined in the 2005 standards and must also remit a yearly certification fee.

State (Health) License

Forty-eight (48) of 50 states and the District of Columbia have a mandatory credential, a state license that grants the SLP permission to practice in a particular state in any setting. The license demonstrates minimal competence for entry into practice. There are added requirements to work in the public education system in the United States. Only 12 states require this same license to practice in the public schools. The other states issue a teaching license or certificate that typically requires a master's degree from an approved college or university. Some states will grant a provisional teaching license or certificate to applicants with a bachelor's degree, but a master's degree must be earned within 3 to 5 years. A few states grant a full teacher's certificate or license to bachelor's degree applicants.

State Department of Education Certification

Certification by a state Department of Education (DOE), which is mandatory in certain states, regulates SLPs who work in public schools and are salaried employees of that school system. Readers should note that there is a difference between a salaried employee of a school system and a contract employee who contracts for certain hours and services to the schools and is required to have a state (health) license only.

At this time (early 2009) there are 12 states in which individuals must hold a state license in speech-language pathology to work in any setting, including the schools. These states are Connecticut, Delaware, Hawaii, Kansas, Indiana, Louisiana, Massachusetts, Montana, New Mexico, Ohio, Texas, and Vermont. In the remaining states, individuals must obtain a separate credential issued by each state's department of education to provide services in the public schools.

In some cases, speech-language pathologists are contract employees and do not fall under the purview of the state department of education. State (health) licensure is, then, typically required for practice. The following tables may be helpful to the reader to explain speech-language pathology requirements for initial employment in the schools in the United States. Tables 6.5, 6.6, 6.7, and 6.8 provide additional information on states' requirements for licensure and certification. Appendix D compares ASHA certification, state (health) licensure, and department of education certification.

Support Personnel

At this point, it is necessary to discuss support personnel, whose regulation has recently gained more attention. According to ASHA (2004b), there are 33 states that officially regulate the use of support personnel. Nine of those states require licensure; the other 24 states regulate support personnel through registration. Four states do not directly regulate support personnel; however, SLPs who use support personnel are

Table 6.5

STATE (HEALTH) LICENSURE REQUIRED TO PRACTICE SPEECH-LANGUAGE PATHOLOGY IN THE SCHOOLS

Connecticut	Massachusetts
Delaware	Montana
Hawaii	New Mexico
Indiana	Ohio
Kansas	Texas
Louisiana	Vermont

Table 6.6

MASTER'S DEGREE REQUIRED TO PRACTICE SPEECH-LANGUAGE PATHOLOGY IN THE SCHOOLS

Alaska	Iowa	New Hampshire	Utah
Arkansas	Kentucky	New Jersey	Vermont
California	Maryland	North Carolina	Virginia
District of	Michigan	North Dakota	Washington
Columbia	Minnesota	Oklahoma	West Virginia
Georgia	Mississippi	Rhode Island	Wisconsin
Idaho	Missouri	South Dakota	Wyoming
Illinois	Nebraska	Tennessee	

Table 6.7

PROVISIONAL LICENSE (EDUCATIONAL) WITH A BACHELOR'S DEGREE TO PRACTICE SPEECH-LANGUAGE PATHOLOGY IN U.S. SCHOOLS*

Colorado

Florida

Maine

New York

South Carolina

*A master's degree must be attained within 3 to 5 years.

Table 6.8

FULL (EDUCATIONAL) LICENSE WITH A BACHELOR'S DEGREE TO PRACTICE SPEECH-LANGUAGE PATHOLOGY IN THE SCHOOLS

Alabama

Arizona

Nevada

Pennsylvania

required to observe specific supervisory guidelines (ASHA, 2004c). Regardless of the type of education, experience, and amount of supervision required for support personnel, ethical issues and dilemmas that arise in practice are ultimately the responsibility of the supervising SLP.

Licensure Renewal

To maintain ASHA certification, an individual is required to complete 30 hours of continuing education every 3 years following initial receipt of the Certificate of Clinical Competence. The requirements for the Department of Education certificate and specific state (health) licensure renewal vary by state. Individuals interested in specific state requirements should review that state's speech and hearing association, Department of Education, or state licensure Web sites. Table 6.9 provides a listing of continuing education and state licensure renewal requirements.

STATUTORY LICENSE AND CERTIFICATION REQUIREMENTS

Licensing Examination

The national licensing examination for SLPs is a comprehensive examination of learning outcomes at the culmination of professional preparation. Evidence of a passing score on the ASHA-approved national examination in speech-language pathology must be submitted to ASHA by the testing agency administering the examination. ASHA's **Council for Clinical Certification (CFCC)** requires that all applicants must pass the national examination in the area for which the certificate is sought. It is recommended that individuals register and take the Praxis examination *no earlier* than the completion of their graduate coursework and graduate clinical practicum or during their first year of clinical practice following graduation. Applicants should take into consideration any state licensing requirements regarding completion of the exam.

Since January 1, 2005, the CFCC has required that the results of the Praxis Examinations in Speech-Language Pathology and Audiology submitted for initial certification in either speech-language pathology or audiology must have been obtained no more than 5 years prior to the submission of the certification application. Scores older than 5 years will not be accepted for certification.

Table 6.9

CONTINUING EDUCATION REQUIREMENTS BY STATE

10 CLOCK HOURS PER 1-YEAR RENEWAL PERIOD	20 CLOCK HOURS PER 2-YEAR RENEWAL PERIOD	
Arkansas	Delaware	New Jersey
Idaho	Georgia	Ohio
Louisiana	Illinois	Oklahoma
New Mexico	Kansas	Pennsylvania
North Dakota	Maryland	Rhode Island
Tennessee	Massachusetts	Utah
Texas	Michigan	West Virginia
	Mississippi	Wisconsin
	Nebraska	

30 CLOCK HOURS PER 2-YEAR RENEWAL PERIOD	OTHER CATEGORIES	
Florida	Alabama - 12 hours per year	Montana - 40 hours per 2-year renewal period
Iowa	Arizona - 8 hours per year	Nevada - 15 hours per year
Minnesota	California - 24 hours per 2-year renewal period	New York - 30 hours per triennial renewal period
Missouri	Idaho - Guidelines and criteria to be developed	Oregon - 40 hours per 2-year renewal period
New Hampshire	Indiana - 36 hours per biennial renewal period	South Carolina - 16 hours per biennial renewal period
Virginia	Kentucky - 15 hours per year	South Dakota - 12 hours per year
	Maine - 25 hours per 2-year renewal period	Vermont - 30 credits per every 3 years
		Wyoming - 20 hours per year

STATES WITHOUT CONTINUING EDUCATION REQUIREMENTS:

Alaska, Colorado, Connecticut, Hawaii, North Carolina

Practice Analysis

Approximately every 5–7 years, ASHA commissions an independent skills validation study, also called a practice analysis, for both audiology and speech-language pathology. Each practice analysis incorporates a multimethod approach that involves a number of independent expert panels and a large-scale survey of practitioners, educators, clinical supervisors, and clinic directors. This process can take up to 12 months to complete. The results of the practice analysis provide descriptive information about the tasks performed on the job and the knowledge, skills, and abilities thought necessary to perform those tasks by new graduates entering independent professional practice.

Evaluation of current certification standards is then undertaken using the practice analysis results as well as

- A review of practice-specific literature (e.g., scopes of practice, practice policy guidelines and position statements, preferred practice patterns, and publications from related professional organizations); and
- Widespread peer review from the ASHA membership, state licensure boards, academic programs, and related professional organizations.

Any recommendation for changes in the standards by ASHA's Council for Clinical Certification (CFCC) is made following the comprehensive analysis of findings.

Test Blueprint

The blueprint for the Praxis exams is derived from the certification standards, which reflect the results of the comprehensive practice analysis study. ASHA nominates subject matter experts to serve on Praxis Committees that work with the Educational Testing System (ETS), a test vendor, to develop the examinations. Subject matter experts are ASHA-certified individuals from both academic and clinical backgrounds. The speech-language pathology exam is developed by speech-language pathologists along with audiologists who write questions about hearing and hearing science.

Standard Setting

Standard setting studies are performed periodically to evaluate each question for its relevance to beginning clinicians and to determine how many questions a beginning clinician should be able to answer correctly. A recommended passing score for the examination is then approved by the CFCC.

Examination Retakes

All applicants who fail the examination may retake it. If the examination is not successfully passed within the 2-year period, the applicant's certification file will be closed. If the examination is passed at a later date, the individual will have to reapply for certification under the standards in effect at the time of reapplication and will be required to pay the appropriate application fees.

SCOPE OF PRACTICE

The *Scope of Practice in Speech-Language Pathology* (ASHA, 2007d) includes a statement of purpose, a framework for research and clinical practice, qualifications of the speech-language pathologist, professional roles and activities, and practice settings. The speech-language pathologist is the professional who engages in clinical services, prevention, advocacy, education, administration, and research in the areas of communication and swallowing across the life span from infancy through geriatrics.

Given the diversity of the client population, ASHA policy requires that these activities are conducted in a manner that takes into consideration the impact of cultural and linguistic exposure/acquisition and uses the best available evidence for practice to ensure optimal outcomes for persons with communication and/or swallowing disorders or differences.

Relationship to Other Health Care Providers

Speech-language pathologists are the primary care providers for communication and swallowing disorders. They are autonomous professionals, that is, their services are not prescribed or supervised by another professional. However, individuals frequently benefit from services that include speech-language pathologist collaborations with other professionals.

SLPs are trained to be team members, although the definition of different teams does vary. SLPs team with health care providers in medical, home-based, community-based, and educationally based settings. SLPs understand how the areas of communication, language, and swallowing interface with other medical and clinical fields. An understanding of services provided by other health care workers, terminology, projected outcomes, and the process of building a strong successful treatment plan with the support and involvement of the other health care providers is included in training programs. It is also included in continuing education following graduation.

Specialty Recognition

ASHA provides specialty recognition for individuals with advanced knowledge, skills, and experience beyond the Certificate of Clinical Competence (CCC-SLP) so that these individuals may be recognized by consumers, colleagues, referral and payer sources, and the general public. ASHA initiated specialty recognition in 1995 and established a **Council for Clinical Specialty Recognition (CCSR)** that reviews and votes on petitions to establish specialty boards in specific areas of clinical practice. Once approved, a specialty board is responsible for operating the specialty recognition program in that area, including review of individual applications and conferring of specialist status on qualified applicants.

Specialty Recognition Program

The key components of ASHA's Specialty Recognition Program are that it is (a) completely voluntary, (b) nonexclusionary (holding specialty recognition in an area is not required in order to practice in the area), and (c) member-driven.

Establishment of specialty boards in areas of specialized clinical practice depends on the initiative of groups of ASHA members to submit petitions to the CSSR. The following areas of clinical practice have established specialty boards and are available for application for specialty recognition: child language, fluency disorders, and swallowing disorders. Each specialty board is responsible for identifying the specific educational, experiential, and clinical experience requirements beyond the CCC-SLP that must be met to qualify for specialty recognition in a given area of practice.

Special Interest Divisions

ASHA also has 16 Special Interest Divisions. Membership in any of the special interest divisions is open to ASHA members, ASHA international affiliates, consumers (individuals receiving services or family members or nonprofessional caregivers), and students (members of the National Student Speech-Language-Hearing Association and full-time doctoral students). A listing of the Special Interest Divisions may be found on the ASHA Web site at www.asha.org.

ETHICAL AND LEGAL CONSIDERATIONS IN PRACTICE

Code of Ethics

For over 70 years, the profession has had a Code of Ethics developed by ASHA and interpreted, administered, and enforced by a board of ethics. The ASHA Code of Ethics contains four Principles of Ethics that provide the underlying moral basis for decision making.

- *Principle of Ethics I* focuses primarily upon the welfare of persons served, both professionally and in research, as well as the humane treatment of animals.
- *Principle of Ethics II* relates to achieving and maintaining the highest level of professional competence, including holding the appropriate Certificate of Clinical Competence.
- *Principle of Ethics III* primarily involves promoting public understanding about the professions, including the dissemination of research findings and scholarly activities.
- *Principle of Ethics IV* focuses primarily upon the relationships that professionals often encounter, and acceptance of the self-imposed standards (ASHA, 2003b).

State Associations

State speech-language-hearing associations have the option of being affiliated with ASHA. If the state affiliates with ASHA, then it is required to adopt a code of ethics. All 50 states, the District of Columbia, and the Overseas Association of Communication Sciences have an official affiliation with ASHA (ASHA, 2003a). State associations vary in governing structure, and the process for enforcing the code of ethics for a particular state will depend on the structure. Because state associations do not award certification or licensure, the most severe penalty imposed is revocation of membership; however, other types of reprimand may follow the procedures outlined by ASHA.

SUMMARY

Employment of speech-language pathologists is expected to grow 11% from 2006 to 2016, which is about average for all occupations. As members of the baby boom generation (those born between 1946 and 1964) continue to age, the possibility of neurological disorders and associated speech, language, and swallowing impairments increases. Medical advances also are improving the survival rate of premature infants and trauma and stroke victims, who then need assessment and sometimes treatment. The combination of growth in the occupation and an expected increase in retirements over the coming years should create excellent job opportunities for speech-language pathologists. Opportunities should be particularly favorable for those with the ability to speak a second language, such as Spanish (Bureau of Labor Statistics, 2009e).

PROFESSIONAL RESOURCES

This section contains a list of select professional resources for speech-language pathologists including national regulatory bodies, national associations, state speech, language, and hearing associations, interdisciplinary associations, and advocacy associations. It is impossible to include everything in this type of document, but the writer has attempted to identify the primary ones, and to provide either a ground address or a Web site to contact for further information.

National Regulatory Bodies

ASHA, the individual state boards of examiners (for state health licenses), and the department of education (for individuals who wish to practice in education settings) are the primary regulatory bodies for speech-language pathologists. The National Association of Credential Evaluation Services (NACES) is an association of private foreign credential evaluation services dedicated to promoting excellence in independent foreign credential evaluation.

American Speech-Language-Hearing Association (www.asha.org)

2200 Research Blvd.
Rockville, MD 20805
301-897-5700

The American Speech-Language-Hearing Association is the professional, scientific, and credentialing association for 135,000 members and affiliates who are speech-language pathologists, audiologists, and speech, language, and hearing scientists in the United States and internationally.

National Council of State Boards of Examiners (www.ncsbe.org)

The mission of the National Council of State Boards of Examiners for Speech-Language Pathology and Audiology (NCSB) is to facilitate the role of state licensure boards by promoting more uniform national standards for licensure, by providing information or services to related professional organizations, by aiding licensing boards in fulfilling statutory, professional, and ethical obligations, and by advocating for the passage of licensure statutes.

National Association of Credential Evaluation Services (www.naces.org)

In applying for ASHA certification, an individual will need to complete the official ASHA application and submit the application, along with an official copy of the translation received from an agency that conducts credentials evaluation of international credentials. A list of NACES approved private credentials evaluation services may be found on the NACES Web site.

National Professional Bodies

The following is a partial list of national professional bodies and organizations for speech-language pathologists. In addition to a description of the organization, the organization name and Web site are given, and a ground mailing address, if available.

American Speech-Language-Hearing Association (www.asha.org)

2200 Research Blvd.
Rockville, MD 20805
301-897-5700

The American Speech-Language-Hearing Association is the professional, scientific, and credentialing association for 135,000 members and affiliates who are speech-language pathologists, audiologists, and speech, language, and hearing scientists in the United States and internationally.

Council of Academic Programs in Communication Sciences and Disorders (www.capcsd.org)

The Council's mission is to support programs worldwide that educate undergraduate and graduate students in the communication sciences and disorders.

National Stuttering Association (www.nsastuttering.org)

The largest self-help support organization in the United States for people who stutter. Its mission is to bring hope and empowerment to children and adults who stutter, their families, and professionals through support, education, advocacy, and research.

National Association of Parents with Children in Special Education (www.napcse.org)

A national membership organization dedicated to rendering support and assistance to parents whose children receive special education services, both in and outside of school. It was founded for parents of children with special needs to promote a sense of community and provide a national forum for their ideas.

National Information Center on Deafness, Gallaudet University (www.gallaudet.edu/~nicd/)

800 Florida Ave., NE
Washington, D.C. 20002
202-651-5051 (V); 202-651-5052 (TTY)

The National Information Center on Deafness at Gallaudet University responds to a wide range of questions received from the general public, deaf and hard of hearing people, their families, and professionals who work with them.

American Association for the Deaf-Blind (www.aadb.org)

814 Thayer Avenue, Room 302
Silver Spring, MD 20910
301-588-6545 (V/TTY)

AADB is a national consumer organization of, by, and for deaf-blind Americans and their supporters. Membership consists of deaf-blind individuals from diverse backgrounds, as well as family members, professionals, interpreters, and other interested supporters.

USA Deaf Sports Federation (www.usdeafsports.org)

PO Box 910338
Lexington, KY 40591-0338
605-367-5760 (V); 605-367-5761 (TTY)

The USA Deaf Sports Federation (USADSF) is the American sports organization for athletes who are deaf. The organization was established as the American Athletic Association for the Deaf (AAAD) in Ohio in 1945. The name change to USADSF was adopted in 1998. Its purpose is to foster and regulate uniform rules of competition and provide social outlets for deaf members and their friends; serve as a parent organization of national sports organizations; conduct annual athletic competitions; and assist in the participation of U.S. teams in international competition.

National Association for the Deaf (www.nad.org)

814 Thayer Ave., Room 302
Silver Spring, MD 20910
301-587-1788; 301-587-1789 (TTY)

As a nonprofit federation, the mission of the NAD is to preserve, protect, and promote the civil, human, and linguistic rights of deaf and hard of hearing individuals in the United States of America. The advocacy scope of the NAD is broad, covering the breadth of a lifetime and impacting future generations in the areas of early intervention, education, employment, health care, technology, telecommunications, youth leadership, and more.

State Regulatory Bodies (Licensing and Education)

The following is a list of each state's board of examiner's office and each state's department of education office.

Alabama

Alabama Board of Examiners for Speech-Language Pathology and Audiology

PO Box 304760
Montgomery, AL 36130-4760

State of Alabama Department of Education

PO Box 3021101
50 North Ripley Street
Montgomery, AL 36104

Alaska

Alaska Professional Licensing

Audiology and Speech Pathology
PO Box 110806
Juneau, AK 99811-0806

Alaska Department of Education and Early Development

West 10th Street, Suite 200
Juneau, AK 99801-1894

Arizona

Arizona Department of Health Services, Division of Licensing

Office of Special Licensing
Hearing Aid Dispensers, Audiologists and
    Speech-Language Pathologists

150 North 18th, Suite 460
Phoenix, AZ 85007

Arizona Department of Education

Exceptional Student Services
Department of Education
1535 West Jefferson
Phoenix, AZ 85007-3280

Arkansas

Arkansas Board of Examiners in Speech-Language Pathology and Audiology

101 E. Capitol, Suite 211
Little Rock, AR 72201

Arkansas Department of Education

Special Education Unit
4 Capitol Mall
Little Rock, AR 72201

California

California Speech-Language Pathology and Audiology Board

2005 Evergreen Street, Suite 2100
Sacramento, CA 95815

California Department of Education

Special Education Division
PO Box 944272
Sacramento, CA 94244-2720

Colorado (Colorado only regulates audiology)

Colorado Audiologists and Hearing Aid Providers Registration

1560 Broadway, Suite 1350
Denver, CO 80202

Colorado Department of Education

Exceptional Student Services Unit
201 East Colfax Avenue
Denver, CO 80203-1799

Connecticut

Connecticut Speech-Language Pathology and Audiology Licensure Department of Public Health

410 Capitol Avenue—MS #12APP
PO Box 340308
Hartford, CT 06134-0308

Connecticut State Department of Education

Bureau of Special Education
165 Capitol Avenue
PO Box 2219
Hartford, CT 06145-2219

Delaware

Delaware Audiology, Speech/Language Pathology and Hearing Aid Dispensing Board

Canon Building, Suite 203
861 Silver Lake Boulevard
Dover, DE 19904

Delaware Department of Public Instruction

PO Box 1402
Dover, DE 19903

District of Columbia

District of Columbia Health Professional Licensing Administration Department of Health

717 14th Street, NW, Suite 600
Washington, DC 20005

District of Columbia Office of Special Education

825 North Capitol Street, NE, 6th Floor
Washington, DC 20002

Florida

Florida Board of Speech-Language Pathology and Audiology

Department of Professional Regulation
4052 Bald Cypress Way, Bin C06
Tallahassee, FL 32399

Florida Department of Education

Speech and Language Impaired/Deaf and Hard of Hearing
Bureau of Education for Exceptional Students
Florida Education Center, Room 601
325 West Gaines Street
Tallahassee, FL 32399-0400

Georgia

Georgia Board of Examiners for Speech-Language Pathology and Audiology

237 Coliseum Drive
Macon, GA 31217

Georgia Department of Education

Division for Exceptional Students
State Office Building
1870 Twin Towers East
Atlanta, GA 30334-5040

Hawaii

Hawaii Board of Speech-Language Pathology and Audiology

Department of Commerce and Consumer Affairs-PVL
PO Box 3469
Honolulu, HI 96801

Hawaii Department of Education

3430 Leahi Avenue
Honolulu, HI 96815

Idaho

Idaho Speech and Hearing Services Licensure Board

Idaho Bureau of Occupational Licenses
1109 Main Street, Suite 220
Boise, ID 83702-5642

Idaho Department of Education Bureau of Special Education

PO Box 83720
Boise, ID 83720-0027

Illinois

Illinois Department of Professional Regulations

320 West Washington Street
Springfield, IL 62786

Illinois State Board of Education

Center for Educational Innovation and Reform
100 North First Street
Springfield, IL 62777-0001

Indiana

Indiana Speech-Language Pathology and Audiology Board

Indiana Health Profession Service Bureau
402 West Washington Street, Room W072
Indianapolis, IN 46204-2758

Indiana State Department of Education

Center for Community Relations and Special Education
Populations
Division of Special Education

State House, Room 229
Indianapolis, IN 46204-2798

Iowa

Iowa State Board of Speech Pathology and Audiology Bureau of Professional Licensure

Lucas State Office Building, 5th Floor
321 E. 12th Street
Des Moines, IA 50319-0075

Iowa Department of Education

Grimes State Office Building
Des Moines, IA 50319-0146

Kansas

Kansas Department of Health and Environment

Health Occupations Credentialing
1000 SW Jackson, Suite 200
Topeka, KS 66612-1365

Kansas State Department of Education

Student Support Services
120 SE 10th Avenue
Topeka, KS 66612-1102

Kentucky

Kentucky Board of Speech-Language Pathology and Audiology

PO Box 1360
Frankfort, KY 40602-1360

Kentucky Department of Education

Office of Education for Exceptional Children
Capitol Plaza Tower, Room 820
Frankfort, KY 40601

Louisiana

Louisiana Board of Examiners for Speech-Language Pathology and Audiology

18550 Highland Road, Suite B
Baton Rouge, LA 70809

Louisiana State Department of Education

Office of Special Education
PO Box 94064
Baton Rouge, LA 70804-9064

Maine

Maine Office of Licensing and Registration Board of Examiners on Speech-Language Pathology and Audiology

35 State House Station
Augusta, ME 04333-0035

Maine Department of Education

State House State #23
Augusta, ME 04333

Maryland

Maryland Board of Examiners for Audiology, Hearing Aid Dispensers, and Speech-Language Pathologists

4201 Patterson Avenue, Room 308
Baltimore, MD 21215

Maryland Department of Education

200 West Baltimore Street
Baltimore, MD 21201-2592

Massachusetts

Massachusetts Board of Speech-Language Pathology and Audiology

239 Causeway Street, Suite 500
Boston, MA 02114

Massachusetts Department of Education

1385 Hancock Street
Quincy, MA 02169-5183

Michigan (Michigan regulates only audiology)

Michigan Board of Audiology

Bureau of Health Professions
611 W. Ottawa Street
Lansing, MI 48933

Michigan Department of Education

608 W. Allegan Street
Lansing, MI 48933

Minnesota

Minnesota Department of Health

Speech-Language Pathologists and Audiologists Licensing
PO Box 64882
St. Paul, MN 55164-0882

Minnesota Department of Education

818 Capitol Square
St. Paul, MN 55101

Mississippi

Mississippi Department of Health and Professional Licensure

Speech Language Pathology and Audiology Council
PO Box 1700
Jackson, MS 39215

Mississippi Department of Education

Office of Special Education
PO Box 771
Jackson, MS 39205-0771

Missouri

Missouri Board of Registration for the Healing Arts Advisory Commission of Professional Speech-Language Pathologists and Audiologists

3605 Missouri Boulevard
Jefferson City, MO 65102

Missouri Department of Elementary and Secondary Education

Division of Special Education
PO Box 480
Jefferson City, MO 65102

Montana

Montana Board of Speech-Language Pathologists and Audiologists

301 S. Park Avenue, 4th Floor
Helena, MT 59620

Montana Office of Public Instruction

Division of Special Education
PO Box 202501
State Capitol
Helena, MT 59620-2501

Nebraska

Nebraska Department of Health and Human Services Board of Audiology and Speech-Language Pathology

PO Box 94986
301 Centennial Mall South
Lincoln, NE 68509-4986

Nebraska Department of Education

Special Education Office
6949 South 110th Street
Omaha, NE 68128

Nevada

Nevada State Board of Examiners for Audiology and Speech Pathology

PO Box 70550
Reno, NV 89570-0550

Nevada State Department of Education

4604 Carriage Lane
Las Vegas, NV 89119

New Hampshire

New Hampshire Allied Health Professionals, Speech-Language Pathologists

2 Industrial Park Drive
Concord, NH 03301-8520

New Hampshire Department of Education

101 Pleasant Street
Concord, NH 03301-3860

New Jersey

New Jersey Audiology and Speech-Language Advisory Committee

124 Halsey Street, 6th Floor
PO Box 45002
Newark, NJ 07102

New Jersey Department of Education

Division of Special Education
PO Box CN 500
225 West State Street
Trenton, NJ 08625-0001

New Mexico

New Mexico Regulation and Licensing Department

Speech Language Pathology, Audiology and Hearing Aid
Dispensers Board
2550 Cerrillos Road
Santa Fe, NM 87505

New Mexico State Public Education Department

300 Don Gasper Avenue
Santa Fe, NM 87501-2786

New York

New York State Education Department, Office of the Professions
State Board for Speech-Language Pathology and Audiology

89 Washington Avenue
Education Building, 2nd Floor, West Wing
Albany, NY 12234-1000

New York State Education Department

Vocational and Educational Services for Individuals with
Disabilities
One Commerce Plaza
Albany, NY 12234

North Carolina

North Carolina Board of Examiners for Speech-Language
Pathology and Audiology

PO Box 16885
Greensboro, NC 27416-0885

North Carolina State Department of Public Instruction

301 N. Wilmington Street
Raleigh, NC 27601

North Dakota

North Dakota State Board of Examiners on Audiology and Speech-Language Pathology

Education Building, Room 212
231 Centennial Drive, Stop 7189
Grand Forks, ND 58202-7189

North Dakota Department of Public Instruction

600 East Boulevard, Dept. 201
Bismarck, ND 58505-0440

Ohio

Ohio Board of Speech-Language Pathology and Audiology

77 South Height Street, 16th Floor
Columbus, OH 43215

Ohio Department of Education

Office for Exceptional Children
25 South Front Street
Columbus, OH 43215-4183

Oklahoma

Oklahoma State Board of Examiners for Speech-Language Pathology and Audiology

PO Box 53592
3700 North Classen Boulevard, Suite 2248
Oklahoma City, OK 73152

Oklahoma Department of Education

2500 Lincoln Boulevard
Oklahoma City, OK 73105-4599

Oregon

Oregon Board of Examiners for Speech-Language Pathology and Audiology

800 NE Oregon Street, Suite 407
Portland, OR 97232-2162

Oregon Department of Education

255 Capitol Street, NE
Salem, OR 97310-0203

Overseas Association of Communication Sciences (OSACS)

CMR 437, Box 956
APO AE 09267

Pennsylvania

Pennsylvania Bureau of Professional and Occupational Affairs Board of Examiners in Speech-Language and Hearing

PO Box 2649
Harrisburg, PA 17105-2649

Pennsylvania Department of Education

Bureau of Special Education
333 Market Street
Harrisburg, PA 17126

Rhode Island

Rhode Island Department of Health, Office of Health Professional Regulation Board of Examiners in Speech-Language Pathology and Audiology

3 Capitol Hill, Room 104
Providence, RI 02908-5097

Rhode Island Department of Education

Office of Special Needs
255 Westminster Street
Providence, RI 02903

South Carolina

South Carolina Board of Examiners in Speech Pathology and Audiology

PO Box 11329
Columbia, SC 29211-1329

South Carolina Department of Education

503 Rutledge Building
1429 Senate Street
Columbia, SC 29201-6123

South Dakota

South Dakota Board of Hearing Aid Dispensers and Audiologists

135 East Illinois, Suite 214
Spearfish, SD 57783-2446

South Dakota Section for Special Education

South Dakota Department of Education
700 Governor's Drive
Pierre, SD 57501

Tennessee

Tennessee State Board of Communication Disorders and Sciences

Speech Pathology and Audiology
227 French Landing, Suite 300
Nashville, TN 37243

Tennessee Department of Education

Division of Special Education
Andrew Johnson Tower, 6th Floor
Nashville, TN 37243-0375

Texas

Texas State Board of Examiners for Speech-Language Pathology and Audiology

1100 W. 49th Street
Austin, TX 78756-3183

Texas Special Education Division

Texas Education Agency
1701 North Congress
Austin, TX 78701

Utah

Utah Division of Occupational and Professional Licensing Speech-Language Pathology and Audiology Licensing Board

PO Box 146741
Salt Lake City, UT 84114-6741

Utah Specialist Communication Disorders and Learning Disabilities

Special Education Services Unit
Utah State Office of Education
250 East 500 South
Salt Lake City, UT 84114-4200

Vermont

Vermont Department of Education Licensing Office

Speech-Language Pathologist and Audiologist
120 State Street
Montpelier, VT 05620-2501

Vermont Department of Education

120 State Street
Montpelier, VT 05620-2501

Virginia

Virginia Department of Health Professions, State Board of Audiology and Speech Pathology

Perimeter Center
9960 Maryland Drive, Suite 300
Richmond, VA 23233-1463

Virginia Department of Education

PO Box 2120
Richmond, VA 23210-2120

Washington

Washington Department of Health, Health Professions Quality Assurance

Board of Hearing and Speech
PO Box 47869
Olympia, WA 98504-7869

Washington Special Education, Washington Department of Public Instruction

Old Capitol Building
PO Box 47200
Olympia, WA 98504-7200

West Virginia

West Virginia Board of Examiners for Speech-Language Pathology and Audiology

Route 1, Box 191
Buckhannon, WV 26201

West Virginia Department of Education

Building #6, Room 304
1900 Kanawha Boulevard East
Charleston, WV 25305

Wisconsin

Wisconsin Department of Regulation and Licensing

Wisconsin Hearing and Speech Examining Board
PO Box 8935
Madison, WI 53708-8935

Wisconsin Department of Public Instruction

Special Education
125 South Webster Street, 4th Floor
PO Box 7841
Madison, WI 53707-7841

Wyoming

Wyoming Board of Speech Pathology and Audiology

1800 Carey Avenue, 4th Floor
Cheyenne, WY 82002

Wyoming Department of Education

Hathaway Building, Second Floor
2300 Capitol Avenue
Cheyenne, WY 82002-0050

State Speech-Language-Hearing Professional Associations

The following is a list of state speech-language pathology associations
and each current website.

- Alabama Speech and Hearing Association: www.alabamashaa.org
- Alaska Speech-Language-Hearing Association: www.aksha.org

- Arizona Speech-Language-Hearing Association: www.arsha.org
- California Speech-Language-Hearing Association: www.CSHA. org
- Colorado Speech-Language-Hearing Association: www.cshassoc. org
- Connecticut Speech-Language-Hearing Association Inc.: www. ctspeechhearing.org
- Delaware Speech-Language-Hearing Association: www.dsha.org
- Florida Association of Speech-Language Pathologists and Audiologists: www.flasha.org
- Georgia Speech-Language-Hearing Association: www.gsha.org
- Hawaii Speech-Language-Hearing Association: www.hsha.org
- Idaho Speech-Language-Hearing Association: www.idahosha.org
- Illinois Speech-Language-Hearing Association: www.ishail.org
- Indiana Speech-Language-Hearing Association: www.islha.org
- Iowa Speech-Language-Hearing Association: www.isha.org
- Kansas Speech-Language-Hearing Association: www.ksha.org
- Kentucky Speech-Language-Hearing Association: www.kysha. org
- Louisiana Speech-Language-Hearing Association: www.lsha.org
- Maine Speech-Language-Hearing Association: www.mslha.org
- Maryland Speech-Language-Hearing Association: www.mdslha. org
- Massachusetts Speech-Language-Hearing Association: www. mshahearsay.org
- Michigan Speech-Language-Hearing Association: www.michigan speechhearing.org
- Minnesota Speech-Language-Hearing Association: www.msha. net
- Mississippi Speech-Language-Hearing Association: www.mshausa. org
- Missouri Speech-Language-Hearing Association: www.show memsha.org
- Montana Speech-Language-Hearing Association: www.mshaon line.org
- Nebraska Speech-Language-Hearing Association: www.nslha.org
- Nevada Speech-Language-Hearing Association: www.nvsha.org
- New Hampshire Speech-Language-Hearing Association Inc.: www.nhslha.org

- New Jersey Speech-Language-Hearing Association: www.njsha. org
- New Mexico Speech-Language-Hearing Association: www.nmsha. net
- New York Speech-Language-Hearing Association: www.nysslha. org
- North Carolina Speech-Language-Hearing Association: www. ncshla.org
- North Dakota Speech-Language-Hearing Association: www. ncshla.org
- Ohio Speech-Language-Hearing Association: www.ohioslha.org
- Oklahoma Speech-Language-Hearing Association: www.oslha. org
- Oregon Speech-Language-Hearing Association: www.oregon speechandhearing.org
- Pennsylvania Speech-Language-Hearing Association: www.psha. org
- Rhode Island Speech-Language-Hearing Association: www.risha. info
- South Carolina Speech-Language-Hearing Association: www. scsha.com
- South Dakota Speech-Language-Hearing Association: www. sdslha.org
- Tennessee Association of Audiologists and Speech-Language Pathologists: www.taaslp.org
- Texas Speech-Language-Hearing Association: www.txsha.org
- Utah Speech-Language-Hearing Association: www.ushaonline. net
- Vermont Speech-Language-Hearing Association: www.vslha.org
- Virginia Speech-Language-Hearing Association: www.shav.org
- Washington Speech and Hearing Association: www.wslha.org
- West Virginia Speech-Language-Hearing Association: www. wvsha.org
- Wisconsin Speech-Language-Hearing Association: www.wisha. org
- Wyoming Speech-Language-Hearing Association: www.wsha. info
- District of Columbia Speech-Language-Hearing Association: www.dcsha.org

Interdisciplinary

Listed below are several interdisciplinary organizations that include speech-language pathologists as members. Such a list is too lengthy to complete in this document.

Communication Independence for the Neurologically Impaired (http://www.cini.org)

Founded by speech pathologists, people with amyotrophic lateral sclerosis (ALS) and family members, Communication Independence for the Neurologically Impaired (CINI) is the only not-for-profit organization solely devoted to improving the quality of life of people with ALS/MND (Lou Gehrig's Disease), by disseminating information about the communication technology that can help them.

Rehabilitation Engineering Research Center on Communication Enhancement (http://aac-rerc.com)

The AAC-RERC is a collaborative research group dedicated to the development of effective AAC technology. Augmentative and alternative communication (AAC) refers to ways (other than speech) that are used to send a message from one person to another.

International Society for Augmentative and Alternative Communication (ISAAC) (http://www.isaac-online.org)

The ISAAC is a worldwide alliance working to create opportunities for people who communicate with little or no speech. ISAAC supports and encourages the best possible communication methods for people who find communication difficult. It has chapters in 15 countries and members in 60 other countries.

Rehabilitation and Assistive Technology Society of North America (RESNA) (http://www.resna.org)

RESNA's purpose is to improve the potential of people with disabilities to achieve their goals through the use of technology. It serves that purpose by promoting research, development, education, advocacy, and provision of technology; and by supporting the people engaged in these activities. RESNA's membership ranges from rehabilitation professionals, including speech-language pathologists, to consumers to students.

All members are dedicated to promoting the exchange of ideas and information for the advancement of assistive technology.

ADVOCACY GROUPS

The following list identifies select speech-language pathology advocacy groups. Both groups can be found on the ASHA Web site.

- SLP Associations outside of the United States: http://www.asha. org/about/membership-certification/international/intl_assoc. htm
- NonProfit Groups with an International Focus: http://www.asha. org/about/membership-certification/international/intNonProf Res.htm

REFERENCES

Accreditation Review Commission on Education for the Physician Assistant. (2001). *Accreditation standards for physician assistant education* (2nd ed., p. 5). Retrieved December 8, 2008, from http://www.arc-pa.org/Standards/ STANDARDScurrentap proved2ndedition1_3_02.pdf

Accreditation Review Commission on Education for the Physician Assistant. (2008). *Program data.* Retrieved December 10, 2008, from http://www.arc-pa.org/Acc_Pro grams/program_data.htm

Accreditation Review Commission on Education for the Physician Assistant. (2009). Retrieved May 30, 2009, from http://www.arc-pa.org/

American Academy of Audiology. (2004). *Audiology: Scope of practice.* Retrieved July 29, 2009, from http://www.audiology.org/resources/documentlibrary/Pages/ScopeofPrac tice.aspx

American Academy of Audiology. (2005). *Strategic plan, 2005–2011.* Retrieved July 29, 2009, from http://www.audiology.org/advocacy/priorities/Documents/ASAP.pdf

American Academy of Audiology. (2008a). *What is an audiologist?* Retrieved July 29, 2009, from http://www.audiology.org/resources/consumer/Documents/FSAudiolo gist08.pdf

American Academy of Audiology. (2008b). *Code of ethics [of the American Academy of Audiology].* Retrieved July 29, 2009, from http://www.audiology.org/publications/ documents/ethics/default.htm?PF=1

American Academy of Audiology. (2008c). *Choosing an audiology program.* Retrieved July 29, 2009, from http://www.audiology.org/aboutaudiology/studentinfo/Choosing/

American Academy of Physician Assistants. (2008a). *Facts at a glance.* Retrieved December 10, 2008, from http://www.aapa.org/glance.html

American Academy of Physician Assistants. (2008b). *Regional report of the 2007 new PA student census survey.* Retrieved December 12, 2008, from http://www.aapa.org/rese arch/2007StudentCensusRegionalReport.pdf

American Academy of Physician Assistants. (2008c). *Physician assistant education: Preparation for excellence issue brief.* Retrieved December 10, 2008, from http://www.aapa.org/gandp/issuebrief/education.pdf

American Academy of Physician Assistants. (2008d). *2008 AAPA physician assistant census report.* Retrieved December 10, 2008, from http://www.aapa.org/research/High lights08/2008AAPACensusNationalReport.pdf

American Academy of Physician Assistants. (2008e). *Guidelines for the ethical conduct for the physician assistant profession.* Retrieved December 8, 2008, from http://www.aapa.org/manual/22-EthicalConduct.pdf

American Board of Audiology. (2005). *Application handbook.* Retrieved July 29, 2009, from http://www.americanboardofaudiology.org/NR/rdonlyres/AA267E51-79AA-4080-B219-061E6DD78014/0/HandbookwithAddendum.pdf

American Board of Audiology. (2008a). *Purpose.* Retrieved July 29, 2009, from http://www.americanboardofaudiology.org/about/Purpose/

American Board of Audiology. (2008b). *What is ABA certification?* Retrieved July 29, 2009, from http://www.americanboardofaudiology.org/FAQs/Boardcert/

American Board of Audiology. (2008c). *Cochlear implants specialty certification.* Retrieved July 29, 2009, from http://www.americanboardofaudiology.org/specialtycert/cochlear/default.htm?PF=1

American Occupational Therapy Association, Inc. (2005). Occupational therapy code of ethics (2005). *American Journal of Occupational Therapy, 59*(6), 639–642.

American Occupational Therapy Association, Inc. (2006a). 2006 American Occupational Therapy Association workforce and compensation survey: Occupational therapy salaries and job opportunities continue to improve. [Electronic Version]. *OT Practice, 11*(117), 10–12.

American Occupational Therapy Association, Inc. (2006b). Guidelines to the occupational therapy code of ethics. *American Journal of Occupational Therapy, 61*(6), 652–658.

American Occupational Therapy Association, Inc. (2007). American Occupational Therapy Association's centennial vision and executive summary. *American Journal of Occupational Therapy, 61*(6), 613–614.

American Occupational Therapy Association, Inc. (AOTA). (2008). *The reference manual of the official documents of the American Occupational Therapy Association, Inc.* (13th ed.). Bethesda, MD: American Occupational Therapy Association Press.

American Physical Therapy Association. (2001). Guide to physical therapist practice. *Physical Therapy, 81,* 9–744.

American Physical Therapy Association. (2008a). *Code of ethics.* Retrieved September 8, 2009, from http://www.apta.org/AM/Template.cfm?Section=Core_Documents1&Tem plate=/CM/HTMLDisplay.cfm&ContentID=25854

American Physical Therapy Association. (2008b). *HOD standards, policies, positions and guidelines.* Retrieved December 8, 2008, from http://www.apta.org/AM/Template.cfm?Section=Core_Documents1&Template=/CM/HTMLDisplay.cfm&Content ID=25854

American Psychiatric Association. (2000). *Diagnostic and statistical manual of mental disorders* (4th ed., text revision). Washington, DC: American Psychiatric Association.

American Speech-Language-Hearing Association. (2003a). *Code of ethics.* Retrieved June 1, 2009, from http://www.asha.org/docs/html/ET2003–00166.html

American Speech-Language-Hearing Association. (2003b). *Conflicts of professional interest.* Retrieved July 29, 2009, from http://www.asha.org/docs/html/ET2004–00169.html

American Speech-Language-Hearing Association. (2004a). *Scope of practice in audiology.* Retrieved July 29, 2009, from http://www.asha.org/docs/html/SP2004–00192.html

American Speech-Language-Hearing Association. (2004b). *Support personnel [Issues in ethics].* Retrieved June 1, 2009, from www.asha.org/policy

American Speech-Language-Hearing Association. (2004c). *Training, use, and supervision of support personnel in speech-language pathology [Position statement].* Retrieved June 1, 2009, from www.asha.org/policy

American Speech-Language-Hearing Association. (2005). *Standards for the certificate of clinical competence/handbooks/slp/slp_standards.htm.* Retrieved June 1, 2009, from www.asha.org/about/membership-certification/handbooks/slp/slp_standards.htm

American Speech-Language-Hearing Association. (2007a). *2006 audiology survey— clinical focus patterns.* Retrieved July 29, 2009, from http://www.asha.org/NR/rdonlyres/5A8F29FE-47D8–4DCA-91F9–2094AD1E126F/0/06AudSurveyfocus patterns.pdf

American Speech-Language-Hearing Association. (2007b). *Doctoral program search.* Retrieved July 29, 2009, from http://hes.asha.org:8080/EdFind/Doctoral/DoctSearch.aspx

American Speech-Language-Hearing Association. (2007c). *Clinical specialty recognition: Introduction.* Retrieved July 29, 2009, from http://www.asha.org/about/ credentialing/specialty/

American Speech-Language-Hearing Association. (2007d). *Scope of practice in speech-language pathology.* Retrieved July 29, 2009, from http://www.asha.org/docs/html/SP2007-00283.html

American Speech-Language-Hearing Association. (2008a). *Membership profile: Highlights and trends.* Retrieved July 29, 2009, from http://www.asha.org/ about/membership-certification/member-data/member-counts.htm

American Speech-Language-Hearing Association. (2008b). *2007 standards and implementation procedures for the Certificate of Clinical Competence in Audiology* (rev. July, 2008). Retrieved July 29, 2009, from http://www.asha.org/about/membership-certification/certification/aud_standards_new.htm

American Speech-Language-Hearing Association. (2008c). *CAA accredited program listing.* Retrieved July 29, 2009, from http://www.asha.org/NR/rdonlyres/D99B1ABA-A314–4235-B862-F2407C06DCB4/0/2008CAAprograms.pdf

American Speech-Language-Hearing Association. (2008d). *Information about clinical doctoral programs in audiology.* Retrieved July 29, 2009, from http://www.asha.org/students/academic/doctoral/clinical_dr_audiology.htm

American Speech-Language-Hearing Association. (2008e). *Strategies for entry into graduate schools in communication sciences and disorders.* Retrieved July 29, 2009, from http://www.asha.org/students/academic/graduate/default.htm

American Speech-Language-Hearing Association. (2008f). *ASHA state-by-state.* Retrieved July 29, 2009, from http://www.asha.org/about/legislation-advocacy/state/

American Speech-Language-Hearing Association. (2008g). *Summary membership and affiliation counts by certification status January 1 through December 31, 2007.* Retrieved July 29, 2009, from http://www.asha.org/NR/rdonlyres/11DDE74E-5027–4BB1-BAE1-C89811B20A22/0/07memcountsTbl1.pdf

American Speech-Language-Hearing Association. (2008h). *Special interest divisions news and events.* Retrieved July 29, 2009, from http://www.asha.org/about/Membership-Certification/divs/

American Speech-Language-Hearing Association. (2008i). *International resources.* Retrieved July 29, 2009, from http://www.asha.org/about/membership-certification/international/

Bureau of Labor Statistics. (2009a). *Occupational outlook 2008–2009 edition: Occupational therapists.* Retrieved June 1, 2009, from http://www.bls.gov/oco/pdf/ocos078.pdf

Bureau of Labor Statistics. (2009b). *Occupational outlook 2008–2009 edition: Occupational therapy assistants.* Retrieved June 1, 2009, from http://www.bls.gov/oco/pdf/ocos166.pdf

Bureau of Labor Statistics. (2009c). *Occupational outlook 2008–2009 edition: Physical therapists.* Retrieved May 30, 2009, from http://www.bls.gov/oco/ocos080.htm

Bureau of Labor Statistics. (2009d). *Occupational outlook 2008–2009 edition: Physician Assistants.* Retrieved May 30, 2009, from http://www.bls.gov/oco/ocos081.htm

Bureau of Labor Statistics. (2009e). *Occupational outlook 2008–2009 edition: Speech-language pathologist.* Retrieved November 14, 2008, from http://www.bls.gov/oco/ocoso99.htm

Campinha-Bacote, J. (2007). The process of cultural competence in the delivery of health-care services: A model of care. *Journal of Transcultural Nursing, 13*(3), 181–184.

Cawley, J. F. (2007). Physician assistant education: An abbreviated history. *Journal of Physician Assistant Education, 18*(3), 6–15.

CGFNS International. (2008a). *VisaScreen data.* Retrieved December 2, 2008, from http://www.cgfns.org/sections/tools/data/vs/vs_data.shtml

CGFNS International. (2008b). *Welcome to CGFNS International.* Retrieved December 8, 2008, from http://www.cgfns.org

Commission on Accreditation in Physical Therapy Education (CAPTE). (2008a). *CAPTE mission and scope.* Retrieved December 8, 2008, from http://www.apta.org/AM/Template.cfm?Section=CAPTE3&Template=/TaggedPage/TaggedPageDisplay.cfm&TPLID=65&ContentID=49490

Commission on Accreditation in Physical Therapy Education. (2008b). *Accreditation update.* Retrieved December 7, 2008, from http: http://www.apta.org/AM/Template.cfm?Section=Accreditation_Update2&TEMPLATE=/CM/ContentDisplay.cfm&CONTENTID=54667

Council on Academic Accreditation. (2008). Retrieved December 1, 2008, from http://www.asha.org/about/credentialing/accreditation

Crepeau, E. B., Cohn, E. S., & Schell, B. A. (2009). *Willard and Spackman's Occupational Therapy* (11th ed.). Philadelphia: Lippincott Williams & Wilkins.

Federation of State Boards of Physical Therapy. (2008). Retrieved December 8, 2008, from http://www.fsbpt.org/index.asp

Fisher, G., & Keehn, M. (2007). *Workforce needs and issues in occupational and physical therapy.* University of Illinois at Chicago: Midwest Center for Health Workforce Studies.

Foreign Credentialing Commission on Physical Therapy (FCCPT). (2008a). *Summary of credential review results for 2006.* Retrieved November 30, 2008, from http://www.fccpt.org/aboutus.html

Foreign Credentialing Commission on Physical Therapy. (2008b). Retrieved December 8, 2008, from http://www.fccpt.org/questions.html

Joslin, V. H., Cook, P. A., Ballweg, R., Cawley, J. F., Miller, A. A., Sewell, D., et al. (2006). Value added: Graduate-level education in physician assistant programs. *Journal of Physician Assistant Education, 17*(2), 16–30.

Leininger, M., & McFarland, M. R. (2002). *Transcultural nursing: Concepts, theories, research and practice* (3rd ed.). New York: McGraw-Hill.

Licht, S. (1983). Early history of occupational therapy: An outline. *Occupational Therapy in Mental Health, 3*(1), 67–88.

National Board for Certification in Occupational Therapy (NBCOT). (2008). *Report to the profession: Visa credential verification year end review for 2006 & 2007, spring/ summer 2007 & 2008.* Retrieved December 7, 2008, from http://www.nbcot.org

National Board for Certification in Occupational Therapy. (2009a). *Welcome to NBCOT online.* Retrieved December 12, 2008, from http://www.NBCOT.org

National Board for Certification in Occupational Therapy. (2009b). *Applicant handbook.* Retrieved June 12, 2009, from http://www.nbcot.org/webarticles/articlefiles/FORM_ CertificationExaminationHandbook_2009.pdf

Pagliarulo, M. A. (2007). *Introduction to physical therapy.* (3rd ed.). St. Louis: Elsevier Mosby.

Physician Assistant Education Association. (2008). *Twenty-third annual report on physician assistant educational programs in the United States, 2006–2007.* Retrieved May 30, 2009, from http://www.paeaonline.org/index.php?ht=d/sp/i/254/pid/254

Sahrmann, S. A. (1988). Diagnosis by the physical therapist—a prerequisite for treatment: A special communication. *Physical Therapy, 68,* 1703–1706.

Schwartz, K. B. (2003). The history of occupational therapy. In E. B. Crepeau, E. S. Cohn, & B. B. Schell (Eds.), *Willard and Spackman's occupational therapy* (pp. 5–14). Philadelphia: Lippincott Williams & Wilkins.

South-Paul, J. E., & Like, R. C. (2008) Cultural competence for the health workforce. In D. E. Holmes (Ed.), *From education to regulation: Dynamic challenges for the health workforce* (pp. 123–152). Washington, DC: Association of Academic Health Centers.

Stone, R. I. (2008). The long term care workforce: Current and future trends, challenges, and potential solutions. In D. E. Holmes (Ed.), *From education to regulation: Dynamic challenges for the health workforce* (pp. 153–178). Washington, DC: Association of Academic Health Centers.

U.S. Census Bureau. (2004). *Table 1a: Projected population of the United States by race and Hispanic origin: 2000–2050.* Retrieved May 6, 2009, from http://www.census. gov/ipc/www/usinterimproj/natprojtab01a.pdf

Veatch, R. M., & Flack, H. E. (1997). *Case studies in allied health ethics.* Upper Saddle River, NJ: Prentice Hall.

7

Communicating in the U.S. Health Care System

CATHERINE R. DAVIS AND DONNA R. RICHARDSON

In This Chapter

Keywords

Acculturation program: A system of procedures or activities that has the specific purpose of training individuals to understand another culture and its practices.

Assertiveness: The ability to state one's position positively and in a self-confident manner.

Cross-cultural communication: Interactions between two or more individuals of different cultures.

Cultural conflicts: Disagreements that arise due to misunderstandings in communication and personal interpretations of words and actions.

Focus group: A small group of people who are questioned about their opinions as part of research.

Idiom: An expression of speech whose meaning is translated figuratively rather than literally.

Jargon: An informal language used by people who work together within a specific occupation or profession or within a common interest group.

Role-playing: Practicing how you will respond in a situation by playing the part you will take or that of another person, for example, practicing your interaction with a physician who has written an order that you must question.

Slang: Highly informal words or expressions that are not considered standard in the language.

The ability to communicate effectively in the health care setting is a skill that is not only critical to safe practice but also highly valued. This chapter will focus on the interpersonal and language challenges that many foreign-educated health care professionals face as they enter practice in the United States.

Communication—the exchange of ideas or information through spoken words, writing, or gestures—is important to safe health care practice. In the United States, English is the language used in health care settings and in health care practice. The perception of foreign-educated health care professionals as competent providers of care in the United States has been linked, in part, to their ability to communicate in English and to understand verbal and written English communication in order to ensure safe patient care.

LEGAL BASIS FOR U.S. LANGUAGE PROFICIENCY REQUIREMENTS

The United States relies on foreign-educated health care professionals to supplement its workforce in times of shortage. However, previous shortages and their corresponding recruitment patterns have not prepared the health care community for the magnitude of diverse backgrounds of health care professionals who migrate today. Most health care professionals who came to the United States during previous shortages were from the Philippines, the United Kingdom, or Canada. Today, as migration patterns evolve and health care education expands globally, health care professionals come to the United States from all over the world.

With health care professionals entering the U.S. health workforce from such diverse backgrounds, the U.S. government, through the 1996 Illegal Immigration Reform and Immigrant Responsibility Act, mandated that health care professionals seeking to practice in the United States demonstrate a certain level of proficiency in written and spoken English. The regulations implementing the 1996 Act identified the accepted English language tests and score requirements for the health care professions. The required English language proficiency examinations and their score requirements may be found in chapter 3, Table 3.1, or on the CGFNS International Web site: http://www.cgfns.org/files/pdf/req/vs-requirements.pdf.

One of the requirements of the CGFNS VisaScreen® Program—and of the federal screening programs of the National Board for Certification in Occupational Therapy (NBCOT®) and the Foreign Commission for Certification in Physical Therapy (FCCPT)—is the successful demonstration of English language proficiency as required by the 1996 law. Currently, foreign-educated health care professionals coming to work in the United States must achieve the government-mandated scores on one of the sets of English language proficiency examinations in order to obtain either the VisaScreen Certificate or the Health Care Worker Certificate required for the visa. One of these certificates must be presented at the embassy or consular office at the time of your visa interview.

In addition to the federal government's English language mandate, state licensure boards are requiring more documentation of English language proficiency to ensure that foreign-educated health care professionals can provide the health care team, patients, and families with the health information they need to make important health decisions. Patient complaints and poor patient outcomes are reinforcing the need for improved skills in communication, which can be an especially challenging issue for health care professionals whose first language is other than English. In fact, some states believe that lack of language proficiency contributes to medication errors and failures in multidisciplinary communication. For that reason, many states are requiring health care professionals to take and pass English language proficiency examinations or to submit a Health Care Worker Certificate (see chapter 3, section entitled "Immigration Requirements for Health Care Professionals").

INTERPERSONAL SKILLS

Health communication has recently received increased visibility in the United States with many health organizations conducting research and producing literature related to this topic. One objective of *Healthy People 2010*, a set of national health goals published by the U.S. Department of Health and Human Services (2008), is to "increase the proportion of persons who report that their health care providers have satisfactory communication skills." Effective communication of health care information is especially important because the U.S. health care system places increased responsibility on individuals for their own health and wellness.

Cross-Cultural Conflicts

Increasing globalization and global mobility are bringing new immigrants to the United States from a wide array of countries. As a result, health care professionals in the United States are interacting with people—both patients and colleagues—from many different cultures. Culture helps to shape an individual's values, beliefs, and identity. However, **cultural conflicts** can arise from misunderstandings in communication and personal interpretations. In the workplace some of these differences can relate to the perception of time, to the way work is organized and completed, and to the way in which communications and interactions are managed.

Cross-cultural conflicts in health care can be minimized or prevented by learning more about the individual cultures of coworkers and patients. Conflicts also may be minimized by a willingness and openness in sharing personal and professional experiences and practices. Many hospitals are providing opportunities for such interaction, which can help to reduce cultural conflict if U.S.-educated and foreign-educated health care professionals are willing to share their stories, discuss their similarities and differences, and develop a relationship built on respect.

Cross-Cultural Communication

It seems that in the workplace, at least, people are often more comfortable interacting with others who share the same cultural or ethnic background, especially where language is involved. This may provide a comfort zone or safe environment, especially for newly arrived immigrants. The way in which we communicate is probably influenced most by the culture in which we were reared; therefore, the foundation of *successful* **cross-cultural communication** is having some degree of understanding of each other's culture and its norms. This basic understanding can reduce the anxiety of living, working, and communicating in a culturally diverse country, such as the United States. One foreign-educated health care professional very eloquently addressed the topic of cultural challenges and communication during a CGFNS (2000) **focus group:**

> No one ever told me about in North America, the diversity. Here in North America there is a very wide diversity of cultures. The gays, the single mothers, teen pregnancies, those with addiction—they are accepted here. But in many countries and cultures, like India, Asia, the Middle East, these are not accepted. I'm not saying they don't exist, but they're not brought to light.

Tips to Promote Cross-Cultural Communication

The facility in which you work, and even the unit or department to which you are assigned, also will have its own culture, its own norms, and its own values and rules. Cross-cultural interaction has its challenges, and it is important to remember that you may not always be successful in communicating. However, you can minimize the stress of cross-cultural communication by:

- *Taking the initiative to ask* if you are unsure of what is expected of you, or what a colleague, supervisor, physician, or patient is trying to explain to you.
- *Making sure you understand* what was said by summarizing what you heard for clarification and accuracy. For example, you might say to a colleague or patient, "This is what I understood you to have said . . . Am I correct?" You should confirm the intended meaning of both verbal and nonverbal communication to prevent misunderstandings.
- *Finding an intermediary* who can interact with you and your patient or colleagues if messages are unclear. Your mentor/preceptor, or some other person you trust, might serve in this role.
- *Requesting feedback* by asking a colleague or patient, "Can you understand clearly what I'm saying?" Feedback can help to correct misconceptions so that both parties have the same understanding.

In a study of foreign-educated health care professionals in the U.S. workforce, CGFNS (2002) found that many of the professionals had communication difficulties in the workplace but were taking steps to increase their language proficiency. The most common issues were talking on the telephone, talking with physicians, and talking with patients and their families. Talking on the telephone was particularly challenging when speaking with a physician for whom English also was a second language.

Role-Playing

One of the suggestions for remedying the language challenges of foreign-educated health care professionals was **role-playing.** Many of the professionals reported practicing communicating with a "physician," both in person and on the telephone, during their orientation to the facility. Many also role-played situations in which they had to communicate with "patients" and their "families." The more they practiced, the easier the communication became when the health care professionals experienced these simulated communications in the actual practice setting.

ASSERTIVENESS

Assertiveness is the ability to honestly express your opinions, feelings, concerns, and attitudes in a way that does not infringe on another's rights and does not cause you and others undue anxiety. Assertive communication allows both parties to maintain self-respect.

Physician Interactions

In the United States, health care professionals see themselves as being colleagues of physicians, rather than as being subservient to them, because developing this attitude is an integral part of their education. Health care professionals interact frequently with physicians, discussing patient conditions, treatment options, and personal observations. Health care professionals are required to confirm physician orders and will question physician orders if they believe they are in error.

In fact, health care professionals in the United States are legally and ethically accountable for their own actions. Health care professionals must question the actions of doctors and other professionals if they pose a danger to patient care. This even includes refusing to carry out a physician's orders and notifying the appropriate supervisor if the health care professional believes the orders are unsafe. Such actions require assertiveness, tact, and negotiation, all of which necessitate proficiency in the use of the English language.

Patient Interactions

Interacting with patients also may require assertiveness. In the United States, the health care professional is not only a provider of care, but also a teacher, an intermediary between patient and physician, and many times, a patient advocate. To fulfill these roles, the health care professional must have not only good verbal communication skills but also good documentation skills to ensure continuity of care, patient understanding of care, and maintenance of legal records, such as the patient's chart.

As health care professionals work in more intense and complex situations, the need for assertiveness increases. Health care professionals who are not assertive in their communications often feel as if they have little or no control over a situation. Becoming more assertive can lead to more respect—and more positive responses to your health care knowledge and experience—from patients and coworkers.

Nonassertive Communication

Assertiveness is a skill that requires practice. It can be difficult to give your opinion, to express your needs, and to confront the behavior of others if you have not been encouraged to do so. Being assertive will take you out of your comfort zone, especially when you first attempt it. That is why many health care professionals move from being passive in their interactions to being aggressive in making their needs known—and then finally become assertive, with practice.

What are some of the signs that you are *not* being assertive? You are considered nonassertive in the United States if you:

- Consider yourself to be less knowledgeable or less capable than others, despite your education
- Avoid eye contact
- Don't take a position on issues—even when a situation dictates that you should
- Try to prevent conflict at all costs
- Try not to be the decision maker

- Are unable to say no
- Try not to be noticed in work or social situations

Assertive Communication

Assertiveness requires that you express your thoughts, opinions, and feelings without offending others. You can develop your assertiveness by following these recommendations:

- Use "I" statements instead of "You" statements when interacting. For example, when you disagree with someone, instead of saying, "You are not correct," try saying, "I appreciate your opinion—and I have a different perspective." Then calmly state that perspective.
- Use assertive body language. Face the person with whom you are attempting to communicate, keep your voice calm, stand up straight, and be aware of your facial expressions.
- Be factual and not judgmental. Do not apologize for your opinion.
- Make clear and direct requests that do not encourage the other person to say no. For example, if a patient tries to avoid participating in therapy, instead of saying, "Would you like to go to therapy today?" say, "I'll be taking you to therapy at 10 o'clock this morning."

Support Systems

Sometimes becoming assertive requires a support system. Practice with trusted friends and family. Start with small steps. If you find that you hesitate to speak up in meetings at work, find out what the meeting agenda is beforehand and decide to speak on a topic that is of interest to you. Try to choose a topic early in the agenda so that you don't have to think about your response during the entire meeting. Formulate your opinion, then practice speaking it out loud so that when you are in the meeting, you will feel less nervous and will be able to voice your opinion. Act confidently—even if you do not feel confident.

NONVERBAL COMMUNICATION

Communication is composed of two interrelated dimensions: verbal communication and nonverbal communication. The key components of verbal communication are sound, words, speaking, and language.

Nonverbal communication includes such attributes as facial expression, eye contact, touching, tone of voice, posture, and physical distance maintained during communication. Even silence can be a form of nonverbal communication, and it often can have a greater impact than the spoken word. Nonverbal communication tends to express inner feelings, is more genuine, and is less likely to be as controlled as the spoken word.

It is important for the health care professional to be aware of the role of nonverbal communication in the work setting because others make judgments about competence and character by observing nonverbal behaviors. Body posture can be an indicator of your self-confidence, your energy, or your fatigue. Facial expressions can intentionally or unintentionally convey emotions, attitudes, and internal feelings. Your eyes can indicate positive or negative relationships.

Eye Contact

People tend to look longer and more often at those whom they trust, respect, and care about than at those whom they dislike or mistrust. In some cultures, including the United States, direct eye contact conveys confidence and sincerity. Too little eye contact can indicate poor self-esteem, while too much eye contact can indicate aggression and an attempt to control.

It is important to understand cultural differences regarding eye contact because not being aware of the norm in the new culture can lead to misconceptions. For example, the health care professional who does not maintain eye contact during interactions often is considered untrustworthy, when, in fact, such eye contact actually may be considered rude and disrespectful in the individual's native culture.

Physical Distance

Appropriate physical distance during communication and interactions can vary among cultures. In some cultures, acceptable personal and social distance is much closer than it is in the United States. Observe the distance your colleagues maintain when interacting among themselves, with patients and families, and with other health team members. Remember that appropriate physical distance is determined by the situation, the nature of the relationship, the topic under discussion, and your physical surroundings.

Touching

Touching, such as putting your arm around someone or putting your hand on another's arm or shoulder, can be used to convey caring, sympathy, encouragement, and praise—as well as anger, control, and restraint. It is very important to remember that the norms that govern touching behavior differ among cultures.

In the United States, a certain amount of distance usually is maintained when interacting with others, unless the situation requires close physical contact, for example, comforting a grieving patient or family member. If your culture is one in which touching or physical closeness is the norm, you may have to adjust your personal space to accommodate the norms of your new work environment.

Tone of Voice

When speaking, the tone of your voice can indicate a range of feelings and emotions, from calm approval to angry disapproval. Often it is not what is said, but *how* you say it, that can make a difference in the outcome of an interaction with a patient, colleague, or health team member. For example, when you are stressed or anxious, your voice often is high pitched or loud, and your words are spoken at a rapid pace. In this way, you transmit your stress to others. By taking a deep breath or two before speaking, and by consciously slowing your breathing, your voice will become lower pitched and calmer, the pace of your words will slow, and patients and colleagues will relax.

Time

The way in which we perceive and structure our time is also a form of nonverbal communication. Time perceptions include punctuality, willingness to wait, speed of speech, and how long people are willing to listen.

Time in the United States often is viewed as a commodity, and fairly rigid time constraints are practiced in the workplace. Arriving for work on time and leaving work on time are the expected norms—and U.S. labor laws require strict adherence to work hours. Being on time for meetings and appointments is seen as a matter of respect, and it is expected that patient care will be carried out quickly and efficiently and in an organized manner. The United States is considered a fast-paced culture. If the pace of your native culture is slower, you will have to be aware of the perception of time in the United States because you may have to adjust your pace accordingly.

All health care professionals should be aware of the messages they are sending with their nonverbal communication and should carefully observe the nonverbal cues that others may be sending—intentionally or unintentionally.

IDIOMS, SLANG, AND ABBREVIATIONS

Proficiency in communication also includes an understanding of the **idioms, jargon,** and **slang** of the new country and new work setting. Failure to understand may create a barrier to communication.

Idioms

An *idiom* is an expression of speech whose meaning is translated figuratively rather than literally. The meaning of an idiom is only known through common usage; therefore idioms present a particular challenge for health care professionals entering a new culture—both a new host culture and a new employment culture. For example, in the United States you might hear a colleague say, "Well, I guess Mr. Jones will pull through." Translated, this means that Mr. Jones will recover from his illness—not that he will pull an object. A patient may say to you, "I have to use the facilities." This means that he/she has to go to the bathroom or restroom.

Jargon

Jargon is a form of language used by people who work together within a specific occupation or profession or within a common interest group. It is a kind of shorthand for the group. For example, Digoxin is a common medication used in the United States. However, when health care professionals talk about the medication, they often refer to it as "Dig" (using the first syllable of the word) rather than Digoxin as is seen in textbooks.

Slang

Slang is the use of highly informal words or expressions that are not considered standard in the language. You will encounter slang expressions both in the workplace and in the community. For example, when you first meet someone, that person might say to you, "What's up?" or "How're you doing?" What the individual really is asking is, "How are you?"

A list of the common slang, jargon, and idioms used in the United States and identified in focus groups with foreign-educated health care professionals may be found in Appendix E. A list of slang terms, idioms, and jargon commonly heard in practice situations may also be found in Appendix E. Both appendices give the terms and phrases and their common meanings.

Communication Challenges

Lack of experience with such terms can result in misunderstandings and even errors. Foreign-educated health care professionals often find that other people's perception of them as competent professionals is directly related to their ability to speak English like a native English speaker. In focus groups conducted with CGFNS applicants (2000), one participant described her experience:

> Anybody coming to the U.S. needs American-spoken English because here they have their own way of speaking, so they need to understand spoken English the way it is spoken here. We like America, obviously, because we all moved here, but it's just the way they treated us. I'm not saying we're better, but we are professionals and we just weren't treated as such.

Another focus group participant indicated that she had encountered a patient asking another health care provider, "What did she say?" because the patient could not understand her accent and pronunciation. This individual further indicated that such situations made her feel awkward and inadequate as a working professional. Yet another participant confirmed this perspective by adding, "It is difficult to communicate with patients and doctors, even simple words, because of pronunciation." Pronunciation, according to participants in the focus group, was considered a challenge—especially knowing what syllable to accent in a word—as was understanding the idioms and slang used not only in U.S. English but also as part of the language of health care.

The focus group shared several examples of how idioms and slang (often substituted for universal clinical terms) had confused them. Examples were the use of *puffer* for inhaler, when discussing asthma medication; *pickups* for forceps; *okie-dokie* for okay; *call the patient* or *pronounce the patient* for time of death; and the use of the terms *mad* (in some cultures a term for crazy) and *angry* interchangeably. In each of these examples, participants said that they had no idea what the slang terms meant when they first heard them. They felt they would have been better prepared for the workplace if they were more familiar with the idioms and slang commonly used in U.S. health care settings before they began to practice their profession in the United States.

Abbreviations

Some participants in the focus group also reported difficulty reading charts and doctors' orders because of the various ways written English is used in the U.S. health care setting and because of the frequent use of abbreviations. In fact one individual shared, "I read the chart and it said ABT, and I was embarrassed to ask what ABT means. But later I found that it means antibiotic treatment but I didn't know, and I felt bad. They use shortened forms for everything. Abbreviations are everywhere." A list of the abbreviations that focus group participants identified and their explanations may be found in Appendix E.

The use of abbreviations, however, is becoming less common in the United States. In an effort to promote patient safety, The Joint Commission reaffirmed its "Do Not Use" list of abbreviations in health care in May of 2005. The Do Not Use list identifies the abbreviations that can be misinterpreted and result in errors and that should not be used in the health care setting (see Exhibit 7.1). The Joint Commission is a nonprofit organization that evaluates and accredits over 15,000 health care organizations and programs in the United States, including hospitals, long-term care facilities and nursing homes, hospice services, and rehabilitation centers, to name a few. You can access The Joint Commission's Web site at http://www.jointcommission.org.

WHICH LANGUAGE TO USE

There have been reports of foreign-educated health care professionals regularly using their native, non-English language in the health care setting when there are coworkers from their home country also working or present on the unit. English-speaking health care professionals have complained about verbal reports sometimes being in a language other than English, and patients have expressed dissatisfaction when health

Exhibit 7.1

THE "DO NOT USE" LIST

Applies to all orders and all medication-related documentation that is handwritten (including free-text computer entry) or on preprinted forms.
[a]*Exception:* A "trailing zero" may be used only where required to demonstrate the level of precision of the value being reported, such as for laboratory results, imaging studies that report size of lesions, or catheter/tube sizes. It may not be used in medication orders or other medication-related documentation.

THE JOINT COMMISSION

May 2005
Official "Do Not Use" List[a]

Do Not Use	Potential Problem	Use Instead
U (unit)	Mistaken for "O" (zero), the number "4" (four) or "cc"	Write "unit"
IU (International Unit)	Mistaken for IV (intravenous) or the number 10 (ten)	Write "International Unit"
Q.D., QD, q.d., qd (daily) Q.O.D., QOD, q.o.d., qod (every other day)	Mistaken for each other Period after the Q mistaken for "I" and the "O" mistaken for "I"	Write "daily" Write "every other day"
Trailing zero (X.0 mg)[a] Lack of leading zero (.X mg)	Decimal point is missed	Write X mg Write 0.X mg
MS MSO4 and MgSO4	Can mean morphine sulfate or magnesium sulfate Confused for one another	Write "morphine sulfate" Write "magnesium sulfate"

Additional Abbreviations, Acronyms, and Symbols
(For *possible* future inclusion in the Official "Do Not Use" List)

Do Not Use	Potential Problem	Use Instead
> (greater than) < (less than)	Misinterpreted as the number "7" (seven) or the letter "L" Confused for one another	Write "greater than" Write "less than"
Abbreviations for drug names	Misinterpreted due to similar abbreviations for multiple drugs	Write drug names in full
Apothecary units	Unfamiliar to many practitioners Confused with metric units	Use metric units
@	Mistaken for the number "2" (two)	Write "at"
cc	Mistaken for U (units) when poorly written	Write "ml" or "milliliters"
µg	Mistaken for mg (milligrams) resulting in a one-thousandfold overdose	Write "mcg" or "micrograms"

care professionals caring for them have engaged in conversations with each other in another language.

Some employers have reacted to these reports by going so far as to prohibit employees from speaking languages other than English in the workplace, even in staff lounges and cafeterias. Such reports have been cited by state policy makers as they seek to have English declared the official language of their state.

Acculturation Programs

Transition and **acculturation programs** for foreign-educated health care professionals generally support and reinforce the use of English in the workplace because it is necessary to ensure comprehensive and safe patient care. Employers are attempting to make both foreign- and U.S.-educated health care professionals who speak more than one language aware that non-English conversations around patients and coworkers who do not understand that language can be viewed as disrespectful. They are attempting to do this without minimizing the value of diversity in the U.S. workforce and the U.S. patient population.

It should be noted that health care professionals from other countries bring not just ethnic and cultural diversity to the U.S. workforce, but also language diversity—and may be able to communicate with patients and families who do not speak English when other members of the health care team cannot do so.

Foreign-educated health care professionals report speaking such diverse languages as Spanish, French, Russian, Tagalog, Hindi, and Arabic, to name a few. The most common non-English language used by foreign-educated health care professionals in practice in the United States is Spanish. Knowing the appropriate time to use a language other than English in the workplace is critical to being seen as a valuable member of the health care team.

SUMMARY

English language proficiency has been cited by health care executives as critical to providing safe health care in the United States. As autonomous and accountable professionals, health care professionals are expected to advocate for their patients and to safely manage their patient's care. Proficiency in the English language, knowledge of the idioms and slang used in U.S. health care settings, assertiveness, good interpersonal skills, and being able to communicate effectively in the dominant language of the health care team are essential to accomplishing these roles.

As the U.S. population becomes more diversified, employers, government agencies, and businesses desire, and look for, professionals who are proficient in more than one language. The multilingual health care professional is, and will continue to be, a valuable asset in the health care setting.

REFERENCES

Commission on Graduates of Foreign Nursing Schools [CGFNS]. (2000). *Focus group report on the needs of foreign-educated health professionals.* Unpublished report.

Commission on Graduates of Foreign Nursing Schools [CGFNS]. (2002). *Characteristics of foreign nurse graduates in the United States workforce 2000–2001.* Philadelphia: Author.

U.S. Department of Health and Human Services, Office of Disease Prevention and Health Promotion. (2008). *Healthy People 2010.* Retrieved January 11, 2009, from http://www.health.gov/healthypeople/

8

Adjusting to a New Community

VIRGINIA C. ALINSAO

In This Chapter

Keywords

Automated teller machine (ATM): A street-side computerized device that provides bank customers with access to their accounts and the ability to withdraw money from a remote location.

Check card purchase: Buying an item that reduces the balance in your bank account using a bank debit card.

Credit history: Record of an individual's past borrowing and repayment of money. Includes history of late payment and bankruptcy.

Credit rating: An estimate of somebody's ability to repay money given on credit based on credit history.

Credit union: Owned and controlled by its members, a cooperative bank association that provides loans and other financial services to its members.

Debit card: A plastic card that provides an alternative payment method to cash when making purchases; also known as a bank card or check card.

Default clause: Section in a document; part of a contract that explains the consequence if someone fails to pay a debt or other financial obligation.

Direct deposit: Electronic delivery of a paycheck directly into an individual's bank account by the individual's employer.

Electronic transfer: Computer-based system used to perform financial transactions electronically.

Homeless shelter: Last resort in temporary housing for people in need who do not have a place to live.

Human resource department: Section of an organization responsible for coordinating the recruitment and hiring of employees as well as maintaining the organization's adherence to labor laws.

Identity theft: Theft of personal information such as someone's bank account or credit card details.

Scam: A scheme for making money by dishonest means.

Security deposit: A sum of money required by somebody selling something or leasing property as security against the buyer's or tenant's failure to fulfill the contract.

Whether you have already arrived in the United States or are still planning your journey, this chapter provides useful information for making your initial stay as comfortable as possible. Some health care professionals plan to stay temporarily and others for long-term employment, but both will be in need of advice on how to manage within U.S. society. This chapter discusses several key topics that are useful for newly arriving health care professionals as they adjust to a new community in the United States.

HOUSING

No matter where you decide to settle in the United States, you will have many options for housing. The most common initial housing options available include living with friends or family, renting a room in a house, sharing an apartment or house with coworkers or others, or renting an apartment by yourself or with your family. Some recruitment agencies or employers may coordinate housing arrangements for foreign-educated health care professionals, while others may not. If your housing is being selected for you prior to your arrival in the United States, you may wish to discuss housing options with the hiring agency and voice your preferences or requirements. If housing is not being selected for you, you should consider four factors when selecting housing: location, price, size, and privacy. If this is your first time living in the United States, it is a good idea to look for a residence convenient to your place of work, if possible.

To decide which housing option is best for you, ask yourself these questions:

- Do I prefer to live close to my place of work? Will I have a car, or will I rely on public transportation?
- How much of my income do I want to spend on housing costs? Are apartments near my place of work considerably more expensive than apartments in another part of the city?
- Do I have family members or friends who live in the same city, and do I prefer to live near them? Is there a community in this city where many other people from my country live, and do I prefer to live there?
- How much space do I need—or want—to live in? Am I coming to the United States with my family or alone? Will renting a bedroom and sharing a bathroom and kitchen be sufficient, or do I need to rent a house to accommodate my family?
- Do I want to live alone or with others? Do I mind living with strangers, friends, or coworkers? Do I prefer to live in an apartment community or in a private residence?

Finding Housing

If you are responsible for finding your own housing, there are several ways in which to search. One popular way to search for housing—from abroad or within the United States—is by using a search engine. One widely used site is called "Craigslist." It is an easy-to-use online resource that lets you locate housing within any of the 50 states and U.S. territories. To use it, log on to http://www.craigslist.com and click on the state and city in which you wish to search for housing. Craigslist allows you to search for roommates, shared apartments, and rooms for rent, as well as private apartments that are either furnished or unfurnished. If this is your initial trip abroad, you can also use Craigslist to find new and used furniture, appliances, community services, events, and other valuable information. However, remember to limit the amount of personal information you provide online for safety purposes and to prevent **identity theft.** Always advise someone of your intended appointments or meetings with strangers met through Internet sites.

Other methods for finding housing or roommates include looking in the classifieds section of local newspapers (which may be available on the Web), searching online communities from your country of origin (e.g., http://www.sulekha.com for Indian health care professionals), looking on bulletin boards at local coffee shops or grocery stores, or asking your employer's **human resource department.** Often large hospitals have partnerships with apartment communities where discount rates may be available.

Renting an Accommodation

Selecting an apartment or house to rent is not always an easy task. Photos of accommodations placed online can be deceiving; it is always better to view housing in person. If you are not confident in your English-speaking skills, it is a good idea to take a friend with you when you go to look at the rental accommodation. Carefully examine all of the rooms, making sure that the appliances and utilities (stove, refrigerator, toilet, shower, lights, heat, and air conditioning) are working properly. In addition, it may be helpful to visit the neighborhood at night before making a decision about renting there.

If you rent a house or an apartment within a house, the property owner is commonly referred to as the *landlord,* and the renter is referred to as the *tenant.* If you rent an apartment that is part of an apartment building or community, you might not deal directly with the landlord; instead, you may be dealing with a property management company or an individual property manager. In some areas, the property manager may be known as the building superintendent, commonly referred to as the "super."

The Cost of Rentals

Rental costs vary and may depend on the residence's location, size, and amenities. Typically, it is cheaper to rent from a private landlord than from an apartment community because large communities offer amenities, such as swimming pools and fitness centers, which can increase the price of renting. In the United States, it is considered reasonable to spend about 25% of one's income on housing costs (U.S. Citizenship and Immigration Services, 2007), but in areas with especially high rents, such as New York City or San Francisco, it is often common for people to spend a higher percentage of their income on rent.

If utilities such as gas, electricity, and water are not included in the monthly fee, the renter will have to pay for these expenses separately each month. The cost of renting also depends on the duration of the rental period. It is usually less expensive to rent an apartment for 1 year than it is to rent for 3 months or on a month-to-month basis. Additionally, the time of year in which you move may impact the price. Parts of the country experience seasonal high and low temperatures when people are less likely to move, and during these times rental companies offer lower rates to attract customers.

The Rental Process

Once you find and select a rental accommodation, there are several steps that may be required before you can move in. These steps include applying for occupancy, paying a **security deposit,** and signing a residential tenancy agreement (lease).

Laws regarding housing rentals vary greatly from state to state and sometimes vary even between cities in the same state. The information included here is for general information only.

Rental Application. The first step in obtaining a rental accommodation is to fill out an application form. This form requires you to demonstrate your financial ability to pay the rent, which is usually based on your salary, your previous rental history, and your credit report. In addition, there also may be a criminal background check included. Many health care professional migrants working in the United States for the first time will not have a rental or **credit history** and, therefore, will have to supply employment documentation and income verification. You will need to request such documents from your employer. Most property management companies require applicants to pay for the processing of the rental application; the application fee is usually $25 or $50. Always request receipts for monies you have paid.

Security Deposit. Once you apply for a rental accommodation, the landlord or property manager may ask you to pay a security deposit. A security deposit is a sum of money you pay before moving in. It is typically the amount of 1 month's rent. Once the security deposit is paid, the landlord cannot rent the house or apartment to anyone else. The landlord keeps the security deposit in case you damage the property, fail to pay the rent, or leave without cleaning the rental properly. As long as you do no damage, pay the rent, and clean the rental after vacating it, you will receive your security deposit back after you move out. New immigrants may have to pay a security deposit in the amount of 2 or 3 months' rent if they do not have a rental history or a credit history to show as proof of good financial standing.

Signing the Lease. A lease is a legal contract between the landlord/property manager and the renter/tenant that outlines the responsibilities of each party. The lease states the rules and responsibilities of both parties and mainly includes the monthly rental price, the number of months the renter is required to pay, the date of the month the rent is due, the number of people allowed to reside in the unit, the number, if any, and size of pets allowed to reside in the unit, and specific property rules. Any repairs or changes to the property promised by the landlord or property manager also should be included in the lease.

Leases for the duration of 1 year are most common, but other lease options also exist, such as 3-, 6-, 9-, and 18-month terms. Month-to-month rental agreements also exist, but often for much higher rent.

The lease or rental agreement should also specify the number of days' notice required before moving out of the apartment. If your lease is scheduled to expire on December 31, for example, you may need to give 60 days' notice to the landlord/property manager before vacating. In this case, you would need to specifically document, in writing, by October 31 that you wish to vacate the property on December 31.

Additionally, the lease will tell you the date by which you must pay your monthly rental fee. For example, the rent is normally due on the first of each month. However, the lease will usually specify a day (for example, the fifth of the month) by which the rent must be paid before late fees are assessed.

Terminating a Lease. Because the lease is a legally binding document, the renter is held by law to pay the entire term of the lease. However, there are ways to cancel—or "break"—a lease if you need to move out of the property before the contract has expired. Landlords will vary on the specific methods of breaking a lease. One example of a lease **default clause** is that the person responsible for renting the accommodation must pay 2 months' rent if vacating the property prior to the expiration of the contract.

If you need to move out of the apartment immediately, you may ask permission from the landlord/property manager to *sublet* the apartment. Subletting allows you to rent your apartment to a third party for the duration of the lease.

Renter's Insurance

You may wish to purchase renter's insurance to protect the contents of your home—your furniture, clothing, books, and other possessions— against damage or theft. The cost of renter's insurance varies, but it usually averages $10 to $20 per month.

Paying for Utilities

Common utilities include water, electricity, natural gas, trash disposal, recycling, telephone, Internet, and cable television. In some apartments, the landlord will pay for water, electricity, and/or gas and will include these utilities in the monthly rental fee. Otherwise, tenants will pay for their own utilities. In this case, the landlord or management company usually will provide you with a list of service providers, which you must then call and ask to activate new service. Some utility companies may charge an activation fee for initiating the service. Others charge a small deposit fee, which you can pay by check, money order, or credit card. Most household bills and other transactions in the United States are paid for using one of these methods rather than cash (see section on banking in this chapter).

Household Appliances

Rental property almost always will be equipped with necessities, such as a cooking stove, an oven, and a refrigerator. Some apartments have electric stoves, while others use gas. Electric and gas stoves operate differently. If you are not familiar with how to operate the stove, ask the landlord or property manager for assistance.

Some rental properties come with additional kitchen equipment, such as a garbage disposal (located in the sink drain for shredding food waste), dishwasher, or microwave. Make sure the landlord or property manager shows you how to operate these appliances safely. For example, you need to know which switch turns the garbage disposal on and off; it can easily be confused with a light switch. *Never* stick your hand in the disposal while it is running. The disposal has sharp blades that can severely cut your hand and fingers. If you are unsure how to operate an appliance, ask the landlord to demonstrate its use.

Other appliances, such as a washing machine and clothes dryer, may not be included in your apartment. Many older apartment buildings have a common laundry facility that may require you to pay to use the washing machine and dryer. If no laundry facilities are available, then you may need to do your laundry at a public laundromat.

Furnished Versus Unfurnished Rentals

Your apartment may be rented as a "furnished" apartment—with living room, dining room, and bedroom furniture provided by the property owner—or as an "unfurnished" apartment. If the apartment is unfurnished, you will need to either rent or purchase the necessary furniture. If you are interested in renting furniture, there are companies that provide this service. If you are interested in purchasing furniture, you can either look for used furniture or buy new.

TRANSPORTATION

Public Transportation

Many, but not all, major cities in the United States provide public transportation services. The most common types of public transport are buses, subway, train, and streetcar services. Taxis are also common but cost more than public transportation.

City Buses

Public buses run along designated routes and have fixed stops to get on or off the vehicles. Bus schedules are available at bus stops, online, and in public libraries. Most bus systems require riders to pay the exact fare, meaning that you should always have change with you if you are riding the bus. Bus drivers generally cannot make change. In some cities, you can buy daily, weekly, or monthly bus passes for frequent use.

Intercity Buses

Intercity buses provide transportation to the general public across U.S. cities and states. Intercity buses, also called coach buses, are generally less expensive than other commercial modes of transportation. A number of discount bus lines offering service along specific routes (New York to Washington, D.C.; New York to Boston; and, more recently, between some West Coast cities) recently have grown in popularity. Schedules and fares can be viewed online, and tickets can be purchased either online or at the bus station.

Subway

The subway is an electronic, heavy rail service that provides frequent and rapid passenger transport in urban areas. The subway system can be operated either underground in tunnels or elevated above street level. The subway may be called various names depending on the city. Some, such as the New York subway, charge a flat fee per episode of travel. Other systems, such as the one in Washington, D.C., charge a fee based on the distance you travel.

Train

The United States has one of the lowest intercity rail usages in the developed world. Amtrak is the sole nationwide passenger rail carrier in the United States and offers regional train service throughout the country. Other companies offer regional rail service (particularly for commuters traveling from suburban areas into cities) in metropolitan areas around the country.

Streetcars

Streetcars are an electronic rail system used for urban public transportation. They function at the street level and, therefore, at a lower capacity and lower speed than a heavy rail metro system. Streetcars are sometimes also called trams, trolleys, or light rail.

Air Travel

Travel by air is significantly more common in the United States than in some other parts of the world, largely due to the size of the country and the lack of widespread rail service. Flights in and out of major cities are frequent and can be found relatively easily. Depending on which part of the country you are flying from, certain airline carriers are less expensive than others. Other factors, including the time of year and how far in advance you purchase your tickets, can have a significant impact on cost. There are many search engines that allow you to compare airfares and purchase tickets online. Another option is to use a travel agent when booking a flight or trip, but this option can be more costly.

Private Transportation

Car Rental

Car rental is a common service in most U.S. cities, with a wide variety of companies in the industry. Some car rental agencies require you to have a major credit card to rent a vehicle, while others accept **debit cards** or cash deposits (see the banking section in this chapter). Most car rental agencies have minimum age requirements (typically between 18 and 25) to rent a vehicle.

Obtaining a Driver's License

If you plan to drive an automobile after moving to the United States, you must obtain a driver's license in the state in which you live. Information on how to obtain a license is available from your state's Department of Motor Vehicles (DMV). Even if you do not plan to drive, it is a good idea to get either a driver's license or a nondriver identification card from your state's DMV because these are commonly used forms of identification throughout the United States.

Motor vehicle laws and procedures will vary from state to state. Generally, to get a driver's license you will first need to apply for a learner's permit at the local DMV. In order to receive this permit, you will be required to take and pass a written examination on your state's traffic laws. In most states, a driver's handbook, containing a summary of the state's traffic laws, is available through the DMV. Following the test, you will take a driving test to obtain a driver's license.

BANKING

As soon as you arrive in the United States, you should open a bank account. For convenience, choose a bank with branches (offices) close to your work or home. Just as with any business transaction, banks have certain conditions on opening an account. You will need an acceptable form of identification—a valid passport or alien registration card, driver's license, or state identification card. Most banks also require a minimum deposit to open an account. Other financial institutions, such as **credit unions,** offer the same services as a commercial bank, but they are not-for-profit organizations that cater to specific groups of people, such as employees of a large university or state government. Ask your employer if they are affiliated with a credit union where you can become a member.

Insured Banks

Make sure that the bank you choose is insured by the Federal Deposit Insurance Corporation (FDIC). This is indicated by an FDIC decal at the front entrance of the bank. You also can check to see if a bank is FDIC-insured by going to http://www.fdic.gov. This is important because if an FDIC-insured bank closes its business for any reason, the federal government will reimburse the funds in your bank deposit accounts up to a maximum amount set by federal law. That amount is temporarily set at $250,000 until December 31, 2009, after which it will be $100,000. The National Credit Union Share Insurance Fund (NCUSIF) offers similar insurance for Credit Union deposits.

Checking and Savings Accounts

You should consider opening both a checking and a savings account at the bank you select. A savings account is for saving money for emergencies and large expenses, such as vacations, holiday gifts, or the down payment on a car. If you lose your job, for example, you can use the money you have saved to pay for rent, utilities, food, or transportation. The general advice is to have the equivalent of at least 3 months' salary in your savings account for unexpected expenses.

Use your checking account to pay your bills or to get cash from the bank. When you open a checking account, the bank will order you a booklet of checks that can be printed with your name and address.

Before writing checks, make sure you have enough funds deposited in your checking account to cover the amount of the check that you write. An *overdraft* can occur if you do not have enough money to cover checks or withdrawals from your account. This a common mistake, and depending on the circumstances, the bank *may* or *may not* pay the check, **check card purchase,** or withdrawal; the bank will usually fine you an additional fee, sometimes daily, until you pay for the overdraft. However, intentionally *bouncing* (or writing bad checks) is a federal offense, and you can ruin your credit at stores and banks, in addition to possibly being fined, going to jail, or even being deported. In most cases, if you accidentally bounce a check and contact the payee as soon as you realize the error, they will allow you to pay them the value of the bounced check, along with any nominal service charges that may have resulted because of your mistake.

Monthly Statements

Each month, your bank will mail you a written statement or provide you with an online record showing you every transaction made in the previous month. Transactions include deposits, checks you wrote to others, cash withdrawals, earned interest, and any fees or penalties. Get in the habit of reviewing your bank statement as soon as you receive it. If you find an error in the statement, there are written instructions on the back of the document telling you what you should do to report it. It is important to follow these instructions carefully because there is a time limit for filing such complaints.

Depositing Funds

The most convenient way to deposit or to withdraw cash from your account is through one of your bank's **automated teller machines (ATMs).** ATMs can usually be found throughout the area in a number of different locations. Your bank will issue you an ATM card at the time you open your account. The bank can also issue a debit card, which can be used both as an ATM card and to make purchases, but you must ask for it. At that time, you will be asked to provide a 4-digit number, called a personal identification number (PIN), which is necessary to use the card. Make sure it is a memorable number, and *never* share it with anyone. Be aware that if you use your ATM card to withdraw money from an ATM belonging to an institution other than your bank, you may have to pay an additional service charge for each transaction.

Direct Deposit

To avoid having to go to the bank or ATM to deposit each paycheck, you can authorize your employer to use a transaction called **direct deposit.** As the term implies, on paydays your paycheck automatically is deposited electronically into your account. You can designate a portion of your paycheck to be deposited to your checking account and a portion to your savings account.

Electronic Banking

Another convenient way to do your banking is electronically through on-line banking. Using the Internet, you can visit your bank's personal and secure Web site to check your account information and **electronically transfer** funds. Beware of **scams,** however. Never share your banking information online, on the telephone, or through the mail without using great caution. If you have any questions or doubts about e-mails, telephone calls, or mailings that ask you for personal banking information, call your bank directly and confirm.

Remittances

At some point, you may wish to send money back to your home country. Family and friends may refer you to one of several overseas money wiring services, but be sure to ask about fees for this service and the safeguards that will protect your money. Make sure that you know exactly when the recipient will retrieve the funds in either local currency or in U.S. dollars, and don't forget to check with your local bank, which may offer a similar service at a lower cost.

Credit Cards

Many U.S. residents use credit cards to purchase items or services. This is a convenient way to pay for goods and services when you may not have cash with you or sufficient funds in your checking account on a particular day. However, it is also an easy way to acquire significant debt.

Credit Card Payments

Failing to pay your credit card bill completely at the end of a billing cycle will result in interest charges on the amount you still owe. Make sure you understand the terms and interest rate of your credit card, as they vary widely. All credit card companies assess a finance charge for late payment or if you exceed your credit limit. The credit card company may also increase your interest rate for late payment.

Always pay at least the minimum amount or more (preferably the full balance) by the due date on the statement you receive from the credit card company. It is good practice to mail your payment at least a week before the due date to avoid a late payment. Online payments, if made by a certain time, usually are credited the same day.

Credit History

Your interest rate may be higher on your credit card if you do not have a credit history in the United States. One way to prove your creditworthiness is to provide a copy of your job offer letter with salary information and the length of the contract. Most banks honor this documentation and may issue a credit card with a lower credit limit.

In the United States, a good credit history is essential. You can usually get a good **credit rating** if you pay all of your bills on time and keep your balances (how much you owe) low. In addition to paying your credit card bills on time, you should pay your gas and electric bill, land line and mobile telephone service, cable service, rent or mortgage, and car payments on time. Keep your credit card balances low or at zero, and do not apply for too many loans and credit cards. A good credit rating will make it easier to get a lower credit card interest rate and obtain a loan with a favorable interest rate to buy a car or a home.

Credit Card Security

Carry your credit cards in a safe place to avoid misplacing them or having them stolen. Write down your credit card numbers and the company contact information, and keep these pieces of information separate from your credit cards. This way, if you lose your wallet with your credit cards in it, you can immediately report the loss to the credit card company and cancel your credit cards. In most cases, you will not be responsible for fraudulent charges if you notify the company right away.

COMMUNITY INVOLVEMENT

Getting involved in your new community may be hard at first, but making the effort to get to know your neighbors will help you feel more connected to your community so you can better enjoy your new life in the United States. Simple gestures, such as introducing yourself and greeting your neighbors whenever you see them, are a good start.

Community Organizations

Visit the city or town hall in your community to inquire about community organizations and recreational activities that you and your family can join, or volunteer for projects that benefit your community. When you arrive in the United States, you should visit your home country's consulate or embassy. This office also can provide information about various hometown associations and volunteer projects. Informal immigrant organizations, known as *Hometown Associations* (HTA), also can play a critical role in an immigrant's integration into the community. HTAs offer support services such as language classes, day care, and resources to other community services.

Government Services

Most U.S. state governments have offices for "New Americans" that offer services for recent immigrants. There also are nongovernmental organizations (NGOs), such as the Foreign Born Information and Referral Network (FIRN; http://www.firnon-line.org), that work to ensure equal access to community resources and opportunities for all foreign-born individuals. These organizations welcome volunteers.

Religious Organizations

Other ways to get involved in your new community is through your place of worship, the schools your children attend, or through your work. Your place of worship may initiate a special project for the poor, or provide opportunities for members to volunteer at a **homeless shelter.** Your child's school may need volunteers to accompany students on school trips or participate in parent–teacher association (PTA) activities. At work, your coworkers may ask you to volunteer or donate to a special community project.

Public Libraries

Finally, the public library is open to everyone and provides mostly free and valuable resources and library staff that can help you. The public library is also a great place to review materials and literature about events happening in your community. There are many opportunities for community involvement. You can do your part and feel connected to your new community by participating in local, state, and national projects and initiatives.

SAFETY

From popular television programs, newspapers, magazines, and the Internet, you may already have an impression of safety issues in the United States. Sometimes the reality can be quite different from what is magnified through the media, but being in a new and different culture, far from family and friends, can foster a sense of vulnerability and helplessness. Unfortunately, immigrants can be easy targets for dishonest individuals. Criminals may take advantage of immigrants because immigrants may be less likely to report a crime.

Law Enforcement Agencies

Law enforcement agencies in the United States exist to protect all members of a community from harm. If you come in contact with a police officer, there are certain things that you should know. When an officer approaches you, you should be polite and cooperative. If an officer stops you while driving, immediately pull your vehicle to the side of the road and stop. When the officer approaches you, do not make any sudden movements. Do not reach for your identification until the officer instructs you to do so. Additionally, do not get out of the car unless the police officer instructs you to do so. Keep your hands where the officer can see them, and do not attempt to reach into your pockets or other areas of the car. *Never* attempt to bribe a police officer, as this is a crime in the United States. You can ask the officer to show you his/her identification and badge.

Emergency Systems

Emergencies do happen, and everyone must plan for them. In the United States, the emergency number is 911. You can call this number from any landline or mobile telephone. Only call 911 for life-threatening medical emergencies, to report a fire, or to report a crime in progress or suspicious activities, such as screams or calls for help.

All 911 calls are recorded, and operators are trained to handle emergencies. Nonemergency phone numbers can be found by looking in your local telephone book.

When you call 911, stay calm. Remember your location (your home address or present location), and be prepared to describe the emergency. Do not hang up until you have answered all the questions posed by the operator. If you do not speak English well, let the operator know. This is the time to practice one basic sentence: "I do not speak English well. I speak [Cantonese or Vietnamese, etc.]." The operator will get an interpreter on the line to help you communicate.

Also, become acquainted with the police department near your house or apartment. Keep the telephone numbers of your local emergency service providers visible and accessible at all times in your home. That includes the police department, the fire and emergency rescue department, the poison control center, as well as the local animal control office.

SUMMARY

Generally, the concerns of foreign-educated health care professionals when they first come to the United States are about housing, transportation, and personal safety. Addressing these concerns as early as possible in the immigration process will help you to adapt more quickly to a new country and a new work environment.

There are many resources available to everyone in the United States. Our citizens welcome and value the contribution of all international workers. We realize that all people add to the tapestry of this great land of opportunity!

Preparation is one key to your success as a new resident of the United States. By knowing what to expect when you arrive, you will spend less time wondering and worrying and more time enjoying your new life and community.

RESOURCES

Foner, N., & Alba, R. (2006). *The second generation from the last great wave of immigration: Setting the record straight. Migration Policy Institute.* Retrieved October 6, 2008, from http://www.immigrationinformation.org/issue_Oct06.cfm

Hopkins Medicine. http://www.hopkinsmedicine.org/security/CS/crimeprev.htm

Maryland Department of Transportation. http://www.sha.state.md.us/safety

Migration Policy Institute. (2008). *Hometown associations: An untapped resource for immigrant integration?* Retrieved October 31, 2008, from http://migrationpolicy.org/news/2008_07_15.php

REFERENCE

U.S. Citizenship and Immigration Services. (2007). *Welcome to the United States: A guide for new immigrants.* Retrieved October 17, 2008, from http://www.uscis.gov/portal/site/uscis

9 Furthering Your Education

JULIA TO DUTKA

In This Chapter

Keywords

Articulation agreements: Agreements between academic institutions that facilitate the transition of a student from one academic institution to another, or from one level of education to the next, with minimum duplication of coursework.

Community colleges: Two-year public institutions of higher education; once commonly called junior colleges.

Junior colleges: Two-year, postsecondary schools that provide academic, vocational, and professional education.

Postsecondary education: Education that occurs following completion of high school (secondary school) in the United States. Colleges and universities are examples of postsecondary institutions.

Proprietary colleges: For-profit academic institutions operated by their owners or investors, rather than a not-for-profit institution, religious organization, or government.

Opportunities to further your education in the United States abound. Whether you are pursuing an additional academic degree, taking courses to supplement your basic education, or seeking to maintain or improve your clinical competence, you will find educational offerings to meet your needs.

Once you start applying for an employment-based visa, you may find that you need information with regard to furthering your education for a variety of reasons. This chapter will provide you with an analysis of the opportunities for continuing your education in the United States as a health professional. The complexity of this topic makes it difficult to present the details and nuances of every health profession covered in this book. The goal, therefore, is to focus on general principles, directions, observations, and practices commonly shared among the professions, rather than on the particulars of a specific field.

HIGHER EDUCATION IN THE UNITED STATES

Higher education is a term used to describe all levels of education beyond the 12 years of schooling offered to people across the United States. This term is used broadly to cover a variety of institutional types that offer different levels of education and grant a range of degrees. Your understanding of the structure of higher education in the United States will help you to determine how to go about choosing educational options that satisfy professional requirements and advance your career. In general, it is appropriate to divide higher education into two levels: undergraduate and graduate.

Undergraduate Education

Undergraduate education refers to **postsecondary education** taken prior to gaining a first degree. One way of classifying undergraduate academic institutions is by degree type.

Associate Degrees

There are institutions that grant 2-year degrees, which are commonly termed associate degrees and can be earned by successful completion of a 2-year curriculum in a chosen field of study. Students generally are required to complete 60 undergraduate credits to earn an associate degree. Depending on the field chosen, the degree can be designated as an Associate of Arts (AA) degree, an Associate of Science (AS) degree, or an Associate of Applied Science (AAS) degree.

Generally speaking, the AA and the AS degrees are intended for students who plan to continue with their program of study at a 4-year institution. The AAS degree, however, is usually designed as a professionally oriented degree and is intended primarily for employment purposes rather than for degree completion at a 4-year institution. Most states have **articulation agreements** in place to ensure that all the credits earned at a 2-year institution can be applied toward a 4-year degree when students transfer to a 4-year institution to complete a baccalaureate degree in the same field.

Associate degrees generally are offered through **community colleges** supported by public funds. The tuition is set relatively low in order to support public access to higher education. Because of their distinct mission and affordability, community colleges currently account for about 46% of all college students in the United States (National Center for Education Statistics, 2008). In order to manage their resources, some students may choose to enroll in a community college for the first 2 years and then transfer to a 4-year institution for the subsequent 2 years.

In the private sector, there are **junior colleges** and **proprietary colleges** offering programs leading to an associate degree to meet the career needs of students. However, tuition is generally set higher due to the institution's reliance on fees paid directly by students.

Baccalaureate Degrees

Programs leading to a baccalaureate degree are offered by colleges and universities, both public and private. Public colleges are funded primarily by resources from the state to keep tuition affordable, especially for students residing in that state. Private colleges, however, rely on tuition as a major source of income and are, therefore, more expensive. Programs leading to a baccalaureate degree grant either a Bachelor of Arts (BA) degree or a Bachelor of Science (BS) degree. The degree awarded is based on the completion of 120 credits in accordance with a specified curriculum over a period of 8 semesters in 4 years. These 4 years of full-time study are named the freshman, sophomore, junior, and senior years. The basic tenet of this intellectual framework is that of a degree in the liberal arts, broadly defined.

In the past several decades, the need for preprofessional education within the undergraduate curriculum created a new breed of institution—the comprehensive college and university. This type of institution has allowed students to enroll in a professional major and to graduate with a baccalaureate degree that satisfies the entry-level requirements of a profession, such as medical technology, nursing, accounting, and teaching, while at the same time, meeting the mandates of a liberal education. In most programs of study, students have one-third to one-half of their education devoted to general education in the arts, humanities, sciences, social sciences, and in quantitative reasoning, the goal of which is to develop the student's capacity for critical thinking and moral reasoning.

Most curricula require students to take these general education courses in the first 2 years—before they concentrate on their academic major, which can be in a professional field. It is this fundamental value placed on liberal learning as a requisite in U.S. education that poses a significant challenge for many foreign-educated health care professionals who must demonstrate educational comparability when they have been prepared in systems that do not share this philosophy. Analysis of the academic transcripts of foreign-educated health professionals indicates that, in general, fewer liberal arts courses are part of the curriculum; thus, the comparability to U.S. education, which must be demonstrated to obtain an occupational visa, may pose some challenges.

Graduate Education

Graduate education is pursued by students who have successfully completed a course of study on the undergraduate level and have received a baccalaureate degree. Graduate programs are generally administered under the oversight of the graduate school of a university. The most common degree on the graduate level is the master's degree, pursued by 74% of all graduate students. Those pursuing a traditional Doctor of Philosophy (PhD) degree with a research focus comprise about 26% of the graduate population (Redd, 2007).

Master's Degrees

A significant percentage of those pursuing a master's degree are teachers seeking permanent certification or career advancement in jurisdictions that require such stipulations for licensure, promotion, and salary increases. The relationship between graduate education and professional advancement is therefore quite evident. In the past decade there has been a significant trend toward graduate, and in some instances doctoral, education as an entry-level requirement for certain allied health professions. The recent increase in entry-level degree requirements in the health professions at the graduate level has created a new set of professional degrees as well as a new set of dynamics in the graduate education community. The health professions have become active participants in the graduate community.

The master's degree is generally a 2-year program that requires a range of 30 to 40 credits for completion depending on the program of study. It may be pursued on a full-time or part-time basis. Some colleges and universities require a comprehensive examination for completion of the degree, some require a master's thesis, and some simply require completion of the program of study. You should check descriptions of the program of study carefully to determine what is required.

Doctoral Degrees

The doctoral degree covers many fields of study. Most doctoral degrees are conferred in the form of a PhD (Doctor of Philosophy) degree, with some applied or professional doctorates being offered in the fields of education, science, medicine, and law including the EdD, ScD, MD, and JD respectively.

A doctoral degree typically requires 3 to 4 years of formal study beyond the baccalaureate degree, followed by subject matter relevant requirements in the form of research, internship, and practicum. For most PhD programs, there is a qualifying comprehensive examination of subject matter knowledge, a dissertation based on original research, an oral defense of this research, and in some fields, a foreign language requirement. Consequently, these programs usually take an average of 5 to 7 years beyond the bachelor's degree for completion.

Clinical Doctorates.   Doctoral degrees for entry into the health professions generally are referred to as the clinical doctorate or the professional doctorate, and programs leading to these degrees are generally housed under professional schools. Depending on the institution, the program may or may not be administered under the oversight of the graduate school. Clinical doctoral programs generally are 6 years in length, requiring 3 to

4 years of undergraduate study followed by 2 or 3 years of professional education in a specific field. The 3+3 model (3 years of undergraduate followed by 3 years of study at the graduate level) and the 4+2 model (4 years of undergraduate education followed by 2 years of study on the graduate level) appear to be most common.

Professional Education

Education for health professionals was, for many years, placed at the undergraduate level. The entry-level requirement for health professionals has traditionally been a bachelor's degree, which is commonly described as the first professional degree. In the past decade or so, several health professions have increased their entry-level requirement to that of the master's degree and more recently, to that of the doctorate.

The increase in degree requirements across the health professions is motivated by a variety of factors, most critically, the emerging complexity of meeting the demands of patient care in a rapidly evolving health care system. Other factors include raising the prestige of the profession, improving autonomy and earning power, and being an effective member of a health care team. The Institute of Medicine (IOM) advocated that "all health professionals should be educated to deliver patient-centered care as members of an interdisciplinary team, emphasizing evidence-based practice, quality improvement approaches and informatics in order to improve patient care delivery quality" (Montoya & Kimball, 2007).

EDUCATIONAL COMPARABILITY

Credentials Evaluation

Foreign-educated health professionals applying for a visa to enter the United States to seek employment or applying for licensure to practice in a given jurisdiction generally must have their education evaluated to determine comparability to U.S. education. Often they find themselves needing to complete certain educational requirements by enrolling in specific courses or programs of study. This need for additional course work to meet U.S. standards is largely created by the differences between the educational systems in which foreign-educated health professionals have been prepared and the educational systems through which health professionals are being prepared in the United States.

One likely area of difference is in the concept of liberal learning, which is usually manifested in the United States in the general education component of the undergraduate curriculum, regardless of the profession. Health professionals who have graduated from an academic program that focuses almost exclusively on professional education may find that they have insufficient credits to satisfy the breadth of general education requirements commonly associated with an undergraduate education in the United States. Curricula that reflect this professional focus are quite common among European countries as well as countries that have been influenced by these educational philosophies and practices owing to historical contexts.

Meeting U.S. Educational Standards

Residing Within the United States

After your credentials have been assessed for eligibility for certification for an employment-based visa, you will be informed if you need additional course work. You have a number of educational options available to you to meet U.S. educational standards. For additional course work in general education, if you are already in the United States, a rather cost-effective option is to enroll in specific courses in a community college. You also can take College Level Examination Program (CLEP) examinations to earn college credits in specific subject domains. Information on CLEP examinations may be found at http://www.college board.com/student/testing/clep/about.html. You also may be able to take Excelsior College Exams (ECEs) to earn college credits in various subjects. Information on the ECEs may be found at https://www. excelsior.edu/Excelsior_College/Excelsior_College_Examinations. However, before you pursue additional course work, make sure that these credits will be accepted by the requesting authority to satisfy their requirements.

Residing Outside the United States

If you are residing outside the United States, you may avail yourself of online courses offered via the Internet. You also may enroll in courses in your local universities, if such courses are offered. Regardless of your approach, it would be prudent to verify that these institutions are government approved and/or accredited, and that the specific courses in which you plan to enroll provide the necessary content to remedy the identified deficiencies.

For insufficient credits in professional education, you will need to examine the specific syllabus of the course you plan to take to verify that the specified content assessed to have been missing from your education is in fact taught in the course. This careful scrutiny is necessary to ensure an appropriate match.

GRADUATE EDUCATION FOR HEALTH PROFESSIONALS

The graduate education scene for health professionals is complex. There are many professions clustered together under the broad category of health professions, yet each has its distinct requirements for education, licensure, and continuing practice. Academic programs in the United States are governed by a set of standards against which they are evaluated for accreditation purposes. It is important that you look for academic programs that are accredited by the respective professional organizations and enroll only in those that have been accredited.

Educational Trends

The trend in education for health professionals is that more and more professions are moving in the direction of requiring a higher level of education to satisfy entry-level requirements. These requirements are usually set by profession and the accrediting bodies will not accredit academic programs beyond a specified date if they fail to meet the degree or coursework requirements.

State licensure is a different matter. Graduate education is not required for licensure in all health professions in all jurisdictions. It is the jurisdiction in which an individual seeks to practice that determines the requirements for a given profession in that jurisdiction. Some states may continue to license individuals for practice without the requisite degrees and some states may not. It is this assertion of the respective rights and responsibilities in protecting the public on the part of all parties—the academic community, the state licensure authority, and the organization representing the profession—that has heightened the complexity of the requirements for individuals seeking to enter their respective health professions for practice.

As a foreign-educated health professional, it is important for you not only to understand but also to demonstrate that you meet the specific entry-level requirements for the particular state in which you seek your licensure. Being attentive to these requirements will save you valuable time and resources and will yield a positive outcome to support your career goal.

Rationale for Increase in Degree Requirement

It is instructive to examine the trends established by some health professions in increasing the degree requirements. The development of professional doctorates in any health care field will follow similar pathways and require related skills as well as discipline-specific skills (Montoya & Kimball, 2007). While the manner in which each profession has pursued the argument in support of an increase in degree attainment may differ, the premise for this trend is motivated by several shared factors.

Primary Factors. The most significant rationale for increasing degree requirements is the increasing level of the complexity of practice itself—with increased knowledge in the field, expansion in the use of interdisciplinary approaches, and demand for teamwork across the professions in rendering patient-centered care often being cited as keys to this phenomenon. It also is argued that it is not feasible to provide a high-quality education without an advanced degree. The time necessary to cover the breadth and depth of the curriculum would make it virtually impossible to house the program within a traditional baccalaureate education, particularly in light of the liberal education expectations of the undergraduate degree in U.S. higher education.

Secondary Factors. Secondary factors influencing the increase in degree requirements have to do with the increased prestige or recognition of the profession and the independence of practice required for care delivery. The parity of status across the health professions, accorded through a comparable degree designation for all the health professions, often is cited as critical to achieving quality patient care. Independence of practice ensures direct access to patients and allows for direct billing for services provided within the health care system.

Meeting Higher Education Entry-Level Requirements

The degree offered to satisfy this higher entry-level requirement in the health professions can be in the form of either a master's degree or a clinical doctorate depending on the profession. For example, in the field of physical therapy, CAPTE, the Commission on Accreditation of Physical Therapy Education, stopped accrediting academic programs on the undergraduate level on December 31, 2001, after 83% of programs already had transitioned to the master's degree level (Commission on Accreditation in Physical Therapy Education, 2004, p. 4). While some programs have stayed at the master's degree level, many have continued to evolve and have moved to the Doctor of Physical Therapy (DPT) level. This doctoral degree is now the preferred standard for entry into the profession. Students enrolled in this first professional degree program, starting as an undergraduate, can complete this course of study in 6 or more years and will earn a clinical doctorate, the DPT, upon graduation.

Another example can be found in occupational therapy. As of January 1, 2007, the Accreditation Council for Occupational Therapy Education (ACOTE), the accrediting body of the American Occupational Therapy Association (AOTA), stopped accrediting programs that did not meet the threshold requirement of being a master's degree program (American Occupational Therapy Association, 2007). Some universities now offer the clinical doctorate in occupational therapy (OTD), although most programs are still at the master's level. This mandate for graduate education puts an end to accrediting undergraduate programs for the occupational therapy profession.

Since January 2009 the first professional degree in the field of audiology is a clinical doctorate (American Academy of Audiology, 2009). In the field of speech-language pathology, the first professional degree is currently a master's degree (American Speech-Language-Hearing Association, 2008), and in the field of physician assistant, the first professional degree is currently a master's degree. There has been discussion to move in the direction of the clinical doctorate requirement but that has not been approved by the profession (American Academy of Physician Assistants, 2008).

In the field of medical technology, discussion is being pursued to advance the clinical laboratory science (CLS) profession by requiring a master's degree as the entry-level requirement for clinical laboratory scientists, who are also known as medical technologists (Doig, 2005). This increase in degree requirement is viewed as important in more clearly distinguishing the medical technologist, who currently is required to hold a bachelor's degree, from the medical technician, who currently is required to hold an associate degree. The case for a clinical doctorate in laboratory science, the DLS, also is gaining momentum.

The Transitional Doctorate

With many of the licensed practitioners in the field not holding advanced degrees at the time of transition, clinical doctorates have been introduced with their fair share of controversy, despite strong arguments from the academic community in support of increased academic preparation for future professionals. Some professional organizations have pushed for the clinical doctorates despite concerns from their members who were educated before these new guidelines were put in place. A common approach in responding to these concerns is a transitional doctorate degree. By taking some additional courses, practitioners who already are licensed are awarded a transitional doctorate.

Specialty Master's Degrees

The master's degrees for subject matter specialty education continue to be offered by some universities. Practitioners interested in pursuing specialty training should understand that these graduate programs are not entry-level programs and will not satisfy the entry-level requirements for professional practice in specific states. For example, holding a master's degree in pediatric physical therapy may meet the academic requirement for certification in the specialty but it may not necessarily satisfy the requirements for entry-level licensure for a physical therapist in a specific state. While not being certified may make it more difficult for you to find employment in a specific specialty, it is unlawful for you to work without a license in the profession if a license is required.

Meeting Graduate Degree Requirements

For foreign-educated health professionals, the challenge in navigating these graduate degree requirements is considerable. This is particularly the case given that graduate programs in the allied health professions are uncommon or not available in many regions of the world. A general word of advice is to be vigilant regarding specific requirements for the state in which you intend to practice and your career goals. The state regulatory authority usually posts its requirements on its Web site. If the information is not clear or is not directly applicable to your situation, contact the authority to have the requirements clarified so that you can meet entry-level specifications.

For some professions, the assessment of comparability of education may be based on degree equivalency. In those instances, foreign-educated health professionals may find it hard to demonstrate educational comparability if no such graduate degree has been earned. For other professions, there are evaluative tools that have been developed and adopted for assessing the content of the education you received in your home country and for determining if that education is substantially equivalent or comparable to the education that students graduating from accredited programs in the United States would have received. The Physical Therapy Course Work Tool (CWT) is one such example. This tool focuses on content analysis and does not invoke the concept of degree equivalency. Students educated in countries in which professional education is the core of the physical therapy program may be able to demonstrate substantial educational comparability in course content in professional education despite the difference in degree earned. They may, however, still have to remedy deficiencies in general education or professional education to match the specificities of a CAPTE-accredited curriculum.

Selecting an Academic Program

If you are interested in pursuing graduate education for a specific purpose, it is your responsibility to study the options and quality of the programs and then use the findings to guide your program selection. Given that clinical doctorates and transitional doctorates are entry-level degrees and not designed in the same way that traditional PhD programs are, you will need to carefully examine these programs and come to an appropriate decision regarding their suitability in meeting your needs.

As wise consumers, it is important to bear in mind that neither the clinical doctorate nor the transitional doctorate in the health professions is designed to develop the research capabilities or teaching capacities of program graduates, as commonly expected of doctoral programs in other fields of studies. It is equally important to know that there is no evidence that holders of these doctoral degrees would command higher compensation for their services. If you plan to apply to these programs, you should first familiarize yourself with the nature and purpose of the education offered. You should then use this information to determine if these programs would satisfy your career objectives and support your professional goals.

Distance and Online Education

Distance or online education is different from traditional education in that classes are taken from a person's home rather than attending classes at a college, school, or university. Online education, rather than distance education, is the preferred term to use in describing this form of educational program. Online education involves providing classes and courses using Web-based programs and the Internet. Online educational programs can lead to a degree or a certificate indicating special knowledge, or they can provide continuing education for professional development. It is recommended, however, that you check the validity of all online programs with the state licensure board and the Better Business Bureau. Some programs may not be authentic and may be considered "diploma mills," organizations that award academic degrees and diplomas with little or no academic study (usually for monetary gain) and without recognition by official educational accrediting bodies.

How Do Online Programs Work?

Many institutions of higher education offer online programs. These programs are accredited by university and profession-specific accrediting bodies and offer financial aid. Schools also offer tuition assistance programs, and the federal government offers assistance in the forms of loans and grants.

Online education programs vary from school to school and are generally hosted on the school's own Web site. The instructors for particular classes post lecture materials and assignments to the site, and there is usually a bulletin board or other discussion forum where students may post comments and questions. Assignments are e-mailed to the instructor usually on designated due dates. For many online classes, written course work takes the place of traditional examinations.

In these online courses, generally, the nonclinical component of the course work is done online. Because there are no schools that allow students to fulfill the clinical requirements online, the clinical requirements are usually arranged at a medical facility near the individual's home.

While some online classes or degree programs allow students to complete course work at their own pace, many programs affiliated with traditional universities require online students to maintain the same quarter or semester schedule as on-campus students. Many online classes are structured around a series of assignments and examinations, and online course content generally is the same as that of traditional courses.

What Are the Costs of Online Education Programs?

Costs of online education offerings vary widely by school and degree program. Applicants should check the school's Web site for tuition and fees. Students enrolled in online degree programs are eligible for the same types of scholarships and financial aid as students enrolled in traditional programs.

There are many grants, loans, scholarships, work-study, and loan forgiveness programs available for qualifying candidates. The financial aid office at the school to which you apply can assist you with this information.

Also, many workplaces offer tuition reimbursement for both online and traditional programs. This reimbursement may cover all or part of the cost of your courses. Generally, the employee must remain with that employer for at least 180 days following completion of the final course. You should check with your employer to see if tuition reimbursement is offered.

What Type of Computer Equipment Is Needed?

The computer equipment needed varies from program to program, but students planning to enroll in online classes should expect to have regular access to a computer with an Internet connection and a personal e-mail account. Schools will identify their specific requirements.

In summary, an increasing demand for health professionals of all skill levels makes the accessibility and convenience of online education a suitable choice to advance one's education.

OPPORTUNITIES FOR FURTHERING YOUR EDUCATION

Opportunities for you to continue your education are likely to occur in two ways: through academic programs for degree attainment or through credit or noncredit continuing education offerings. Both may be guided by individual choice, shaped by career objectives, and driven by personal goals for professional advancement, for intellectual satisfaction, or both. Regardless of the reason for pursuing your education, you must confirm if the programs, courses, or experiences that you plan to undertake will yield the results that you seek. You can do this by verifying the statutory requirements of the state and by examining the quality of the academic programs and course offerings.

Graduate Degrees

U.S. graduate education is arguably one of the most successful systems of education in the world, both in terms of its scope and the inherent opportunities for advancing and creating knowledge, regardless of the field of study. If you wish to pursue your graduate education in the United States, you will need to decide which academic program offered by which institution will best meet your needs. It will be to your advantage to determine which graduate programs are more able to meet the needs of professionals who hold academic credentials from another country.

Some of you may decide to take the academic route and pursue a master's degree or a doctoral degree in the United States before applying for an employment-based visa. This option can be attractive to some, given that programs leading to these degrees may not be available in your home country. If this is your choice, you may need to consider applying to an academic institution that can assist you with obtaining a student visa. Most universities offer graduate assistantships in one form or another and these programs are usually open to international students.

Some of you may decide to first secure an employment-based visa to enable you to seek work in the United States and then continue with your graduate education at a later time. Regardless of the sequence or the approach, you need to be mindful of the specific requirements and follow the necessary steps to reach your goal.

Types of Educational Institutions

Graduate education is offered by a wide range of institutions in the United States. Some are publicly funded institutions; others are privately funded. Some are situated in urban centers; others are in the suburbs or rural communities. Some are large universities with a large graduate population; others are small colleges with graduate programs only in select fields. Some offer a combination of online and in-person courses; others are more restrictive in their use of technology. Some are adept in meeting the needs of working professionals; others are geared toward full-time students. Some offer programs with a strong theoretical base and a research focus; others offer programs that are applied. It is important for you to evaluate which of these factors are important to your career path when choosing an academic program at a particular institution.

Accreditation of Educational Institutions

In addition to accessibility and affordability, you should pay special attention to whether the academic program is accredited by the professional accrediting body entrusted to perform this evaluation. The institution in which this program is housed is equally important. Institutions of higher education in the United States are accredited by their respective regional accrediting organizations, depending on the location of the institution in the country. All institutions of higher education in Pennsylvania, for example, are under the accreditation authority of the Middle States Commission on Higher Education. You can find the status of accreditation of a specific institution through the Web site of the respective agencies. For information on accreditation, please see: http://ope.ed.gov/accreditation/.

This voluntary submission by institutions to accreditation review is unique to U.S. education and is different from the concept of governmental approval administered in many countries in the world. Choosing a professionally accredited program offered by a regionally accredited institution will afford you a high level of quality assurance. There also are rankings of graduate programs for different professional fields for you to review. The *U.S. News and World Reports* is one source for this purpose (see: http://grad-schools.usnews.rankingsandreviews.com/grad/health.html). You can then further evaluate other factors you deem important to arrive at a decision that works for you.

Obtaining Academic Guidance

If your decision is to pursue a clinical doctorate, a transitional doctorate, or a master's degree in a specialty area in a health profession, you should seek guidance from the school to determine if you have met all the requirements for admission into these programs or if you have prerequisites to fulfill because of differences between the education you received in your home country and the requirements of the degree program in the United States. If your decision is to pursue a PhD, you should seek guidance from the university's Office of Graduate Studies to learn about requirements for admission into the graduate program of your choice. You may also be required to take the Graduate Record Examination (GRE) and the Test of English as a Foreign Language (TOEFL) to meet established standards for graduate admissions. The Office of Graduate Studies can also provide you with information about fellowships, scholarships, financial aid, and graduate assistantships.

Getting the Most Out of Your Academic Education

Depending on the institutional type and the degree program you have chosen, the educational experience may vary. On the master's degree level, there is still a heavy reliance on course work to address the theoretical components of the degree. This is augmented by clinical work and practicum to afford opportunities for application. On the doctoral level, there is usually strong emphasis on individual inquiry and, in some programs, research. Regardless of the type of program in which you are enrolled, you are expected to exercise critical analysis and independent judgment on the subject matter under study. Your ability to use library resources can be critical to your success.

Verbal Communication Skills

Your success in your graduate studies depends to a large extent on your understanding of what is expected of you as a graduate student. In a learning community in which participation is not only expected but often required, your ability to speak up in class and to engage in discourse with your professors and your peers may impact your learning. This type of interactive and collaborative learning may not be particularly comfortable for students coming from cultural backgrounds in which there exists a clear demarcation between the role of the teacher and that of the learner. Students studying under such cultural contexts often are not expected to actively participate in discussion.

However, U.S. professors do expect their students to be active learners and to contribute to the learning community regardless of whether it is in a classroom or in a clinical setting. Furthermore, U.S. professors encourage open dialogue and healthy debate and regard these approaches as critical to the formation of knowledge. Attaining a high level of comfort and proficiency in oral communication to support full participation in learning is therefore vitally important for academic purposes. These communication skills will likewise be important for the delivery of health care services to patients in your chosen profession.

Written Communication Skills

Writing often presents a major challenge for graduate students whose first language is not English. The challenge often presents itself in the form of logic of reasoning and clarity of thought rather than in the mechanics of language use. It is not uncommon for international students to find themselves needing to break away from their cultural communicative mode and embrace inductive and deductive logic to effectively present their arguments. Directly stating your point of view is not considered confrontational and is commonly expected in an academic environment. Circular argument in which you fail to define the relationship between the main point and its supportive evidence will not earn you high marks.

Professors in U.S. academic institutions usually keep office hours for students to visit with them. It is your responsibility to speak with your professors to clarify concepts that you find confusing. Many universities also offer tutorial services for students who desire improvement in writing. It is important for you to visit the university's Writing Center and other similar services to obtain the needed help to facilitate your learning.

Style of Writing. In addition to being able to handle the language with fluency, a clear understanding of format and style expected of written discourse in a particular discipline is important. For example, the American Psychological Association (APA) style is commonly used in professional writing in the health professions (see: http://www.apastyle.org/). Following the specifics in the APA manual will save you time and effort in the long run. Students from countries and cultures that do not share the same academic traditions may find it helpful to familiarize themselves with the format and style of the discipline through reading articles in reputable journals in the field.

Outcome of Graduate Education

The goals of U.S. graduate education are to prepare students for lifelong learning, active participation in the profession, leadership, and contribution to knowledge creation and practice development in the field. It is this broad framework for professional and intellectual engagement that will serve as a useful reference for foreign-educated health professionals in their pursuit of graduate education.

International Student Bill of Rights

There are two organizations that are particularly relevant to international students pursuing graduate work in the United States. NAFSA: Association of International Educators (see http://www.nafsa.org/) and AACRAO, the American Association of Collegiate Registrars and Admissions Officers (see http://www.aacrao.org/) both serve international students in different ways. Your institution is likely to have staff members who are active in these organizations and can serve as a point of contact for you regarding your needs as an international student.

AACRAO has an International Student Bill of Rights that explains the roles and responsibilities of both the international student and of the institution (see: http://www.aacrao.org/international/rights/bill.cfm). Understanding your rights as a student can assist you in achieving success as a graduate student. Although you may not be on a student visa, you may still find the services extended to international students useful as you navigate the academic world.

CONTINUING EDUCATION OFFERINGS

Continuing Education for Continued Competence

Continuing education courses and certificate programs may be offered through academic institutions, such as community colleges, and through continuing education providers, organizations approved to offer continuing education credits for completion of the course of study. Generally, continuing education credits may not be used for academic admission and may not be transferable to other institutions (Lederman, 2007). Such courses, designed to meet the needs of working professionals and nontraditional students, are usually found in the Division of Continuing Education in both public and private institutions regardless of institutional types. Continuing education courses may be required to maintain continued competence in the practice setting and to keep abreast with current developments in your chosen field.

Continuing Education for Licensure

Continuing education courses also may be mandated for licensure renewal depending on your U.S. state of practice. Licensure is a formal governmental activity specified in the Practice Act of the health profession and undertaken by the designated authority to protect the public from potential harm. Although the components of licensure may differ from state to state, they generally include an annual, biannual, or triannual licensing fee, a provision for continuing education for licensure renewal, and minimum education and professional competency requirements.

Medical Technology

The continuing education requirements of the medical technology field can serve as a useful model to illustrate the role of continuing education in meeting licensure renewal requirements. Currently there are 12 states with laboratory personnel licensure, namely California, Hawaii, Florida, New York, North Dakota, Rhode Island, Tennessee, Louisiana, Nevada, West Virginia, Montana, and Georgia. Puerto Rico also has a licensure requirement for practice (American Society for Clinical Laboratory Science, 2007). A clinical laboratory scientist (CLS) or clinical laboratory technician (CLT) must comply with the specificity for continuing education to meet licensure renewal requirements for a particular state. Most states require a defined number of contact hours for continuing education, ranging from 10 to 14 hours per year. Some states may specify the requirements on an annual basis; others on a biannual basis.

The manner through which these contact hours for continuing education are accepted may vary from state to state. New York State, for example, distinguishes between licensure and registration. Some states grant reciprocity or endorsement of licensure; others do not. Most states require some kind of certification from an acceptable certification agency for this profession. It is important to learn about the regulatory standards for the state of intended practice. California, for example, has its own requirements, and you must meet these stipulations if you intend to practice in this state. Each state regulatory authority has a Web site dedicated to communicating its requirements for initial licensure as well as for renewal for the medical technology profession. It is your responsibility to gather the information pertaining to your specific needs.

Physical Therapy

In the field of physical therapy, the emerging construct is one of continuing competence for practice rather than continuing education. This shift is influenced by the increasing reliance on assessment of learning outcomes through performance-based measures as a more effective means to document what is learned in order to continually develop one's practice competence.

Currently all 50 states and the District of Columbia regulate the practice of physical therapy. At this time, 37 of these jurisdictions require that continuing education be completed during a prescribed licensure renewal period. The number of continuing education hours required during the renewal period ranges from 10 to 40 hours, with the majority of jurisdictions requiring 30 hours or more. Furthermore, in 22 jurisdictions, the continuing education courses must be preapproved. Eight jurisdictions require that a jurisprudence exam be passed for renewal, seven require an ethics course be taken, and two require an HIV course for renewal (Federation of State Boards of Physical Therapy, 2008). Each state regulatory authority has a Web site dedicated to communicating its requirements for initial licensure and for renewal.

SUMMARY

Continuing your education as a health professional is both a challenge and an opportunity. It is a challenge in that the education you received prior to coming to the United States, while deemed comparable, may not necessarily have prepared you for the next level of education in the American system. It is an opportunity in that you will be introduced to a different way of thinking about what you know and to use this reflection as the basis for new learning. You are likely to arrive at a level of cognitive awakening that can be energizing as you establish yourself as a professional in a different cultural context.

Through your journey to migrate to the United States to work as a health professional, your credentials will have been evaluated against U.S. standards. Your ability to satisfy these requirements bears testimony to your qualifications. As you seek to advance your education, it is important that you keep in mind the range of options and the variety of models that are available. It is now your turn to evaluate these opportunities and to determine what best meets your needs. Given that state licensure requirements and academic requirements may not necessarily align consistently across jurisdictions and job types, it is important that you identify your needs carefully and study the information thoroughly to find for yourself a program that works for you.

I wish you every success in your personal and professional journey!

REFERENCES

American Academy of Audiology. (2009). *Three versus four year AuD educational programs.* Retrieved May 5, 2009, from http://www.audiology.org/resources/document library/Pages/ProgramLength.aspx

American Academy of Physician Assistants. (2009). *PA clinical doctorate summit: Final report and summary.* Retrieved May 5, 2009, from http://www.aapa.org/clinissues/PAClinicalDoctorateSummiFinalReportSummary.pdf

American Occupational Therapy Association. (2007). *ACOTE adopts doctoral standards.* Retrieved November 12, 2008, from http://www.aota.org/Educate/Accredit/StandardsReview/guide/38110.aspx

American Society for Clinical Laboratory Science. (2007). *Personnel licensure.* Retrieved May 5, 2009, from http://www.ascls.org/jobs/grads/personnel_licensure.asp

American Speech-Language-Hearing Association. (2008). *Strategies for entry into graduate schools.* Retrieved November 13, 2008, from http://www.asha.org/students/academic/graduate/

Commission on Accreditation in Physical Therapy Education [CAPTE]. (2004). *Evaluative criteria for accreditation of education programs for the preparation of physical therapists.* Alexandria, VA: Commission on Accreditation in Physical Therapy Education.

Doig, K. (2005). The case for the clinical doctorate in laboratory science. *Clinical Laboratory Science, 18*(3), 132.

Federation of State Boards of Physical Therapy. (2008). *Jurisdiction licensure reference guide topic: Continuing competence.* Retrieved May 6, 2009, from https://www.fsbpt.org/download/JLRG_ContinuingCompetency_200806.pdf

Lederman, D. (2007, February 26). Tussling over transfer credit. *Inside Higher Ed.* Retrieved November 11, 2008, from http://insidehighered.com/news/2007/02/26/transfer

Montoya, I. D., & Kimball, O. M. (2007). Marketing clinical doctorate programs. *Journal of Allied Health, 36*(2), 107–112.

National Center for Education Statistics. (2008). *Special analysis 2008—community colleges.* Retrieved November 11, 2008, from http://nces.ed.gov/programs/coe/2008/analysis/

Redd, K. E. (2007). *Graduate enrollment and degrees: 1997–2007.* Washington, DC: Office of Research and Policy Analysis, Council of Graduate Schools.

Appendix A
Discussion of the Professions

This appendix presents an overview of the health care professions in the United States. It provides a description of the nature of the work in which the health care professions are engaged, the work environment, employment opportunities, and, in some cases, earnings potential. It is excerpted from the Bureau of Labor Statistics' *Occupational Outlook Handbook, 2009* edition. A more in-depth discussion of the health care professions may be found at the Bureau of Labor Statistics' Web site, www.bls.gov.

AUDIOLOGISTS

- More than half work in health care facilities; many others are employed by educational services.
- A master's degree in audiology (hearing) is the standard level of education required; however, a doctoral degree is becoming more common for new entrants.
- Few openings are expected because of the small size of the occupation.
- Job prospects will be favorable for those possessing the doctoral (AuD) degree.

Nature of the Work

Audiologists work with people who have hearing, balance, and related ear problems. They examine individuals of all ages and identify those with the symptoms of hearing loss and other auditory, balance, and related sensory and neural problems. They then assess the nature and extent of the problems and help the individuals manage them. Using audiometers, computers, and other testing devices, they measure the loudness at which a person begins to hear sounds, the ability to distinguish between sounds, and the impact of hearing loss on an individual's daily life. In addition, audiologists use computer equipment to evaluate and diagnose balance disorders. Audiologists interpret these results and may coordinate them with medical, educational, and psychological information to make a diagnosis and determine a course of treatment.

Hearing disorders can result from a variety of causes including trauma at birth, viral infections, genetic disorders, exposure to loud noise, certain medications, or aging. Treatment may include examining and cleaning the ear canal, fitting and dispensing hearing aids, and fitting and programming cochlear implants. Audiologic treatment also includes counseling on adjusting to hearing loss, training on the use of hearing instruments, and teaching communication strategies for use in a variety of environments. For example, they may provide instruction in listening strategies. Audiologists also may recommend, fit, and dispense personal or large area amplification systems and alerting devices.

In audiology clinics, audiologists may independently develop and carry out treatment programs. They keep records on the initial evaluation, progress, and discharge of patients. In other settings, audiologists may work with other health and education providers as part of a team in planning and implementing services for children and adults. Audiologists who diagnose and treat balance disorders often work in collaboration with physicians, and physical and occupational therapists.

Some audiologists specialize in work with the elderly, children, or hearing-impaired individuals who need special treatment programs. Others develop and implement ways to protect workers' hearing from on-the-job injuries. They measure noise levels in workplaces and conduct hearing protection programs in factories and in schools and communities.

Work Environment

Audiologists usually work at a desk or table in clean, comfortable surroundings. The job is not physically demanding but does require attention to detail and intense concentration. The emotional needs of patients and their families may be demanding. Most full-time audiologists work about 40 hours per week, which may include weekends and evenings to meet the needs of patients. Some work part-time. Those who work on a contract basis may spend a substantial amount of time traveling between facilities.

All states require audiologists to be licensed or registered. Licensure or registration requires at least a master's degree in audiology; however, a first professional, or doctoral, degree is becoming increasingly necessary.

Employment

Audiologists held about 12,000 jobs in 2006. More than half of all jobs were in health care facilities—offices of physicians or other health practitioners, including audiologists; hospitals; and outpatient care centers. About 13% of jobs were in educational services, including elementary and secondary schools. Other jobs for audiologists were in health and personal care stores, including hearing aid stores; scientific research and development services; and state and local governments.

A small number of audiologists were self-employed in private practice. They provided hearing health care services in their own offices or worked under contract for schools, health care facilities, or other establishments (BLS, 2009a).

CLINICAL LABORATORY (MEDICAL) TECHNOLOGISTS AND TECHNICIANS

- Faster than average employment growth and excellent job opportunities are expected.
- Clinical laboratory technologists usually have a bachelor's degree with a major in medical technology or in one of the life sciences; clinical laboratory technicians generally need either an associate degree or a certificate.
- Most jobs will continue to be in hospitals, but employment will grow faster in other settings.

Nature of the Work

Clinical laboratory testing plays a crucial role in the detection, diagnosis, and treatment of disease. Clinical laboratory technologists—also referred to as clinical laboratory scientists or medical technologists—and clinical laboratory technicians, also known as medical technicians or medical laboratory technicians, perform most of these tests.

Clinical laboratory personnel examine and analyze body fluids, and cells. They look for bacteria, parasites, and other microorganisms; analyze the chemical content of fluids; match blood for transfusions; and test for drug levels in the blood that show how a patient is responding to treatment. Technologists also prepare specimens for examination, count cells, and look for abnormal cells in blood and body fluids. They use microscopes, cell counters, and other sophisticated laboratory equipment. They also use automated equipment and computerized instruments capable of performing a number of tests simultaneously. After testing and examining a specimen, they analyze the results and relay them to physicians.

With increasing automation and the use of computer technology, the work of technologists and technicians has become less hands-on and more analytical. The complexity of tests performed, the level of judgment needed, and the amount of responsibility workers assume all depend largely on the amount of education and experience they have. Clinical laboratory technologists usually perform more complex tasks than clinical laboratory technicians.

Work Environment

Clinical laboratory personnel are trained to work with infectious specimens. When proper methods of infection control and sterilization are followed, few hazards exist. Protective masks, gloves, and goggles often are necessary to ensure the safety of laboratory personnel. Working conditions vary with the size and type of employment setting.

Work hours of clinical laboratory technologists and technicians vary with the size and type of employment setting. In large hospitals or in independent laboratories that operate continuously, personnel usually work the day, evening, or night shift and may work weekends and holidays. Laboratory personnel in small facilities may work on rotating shifts, rather than on a regular shift. In some facilities, laboratory personnel are on call several nights a week or on weekends, in case of an emergency.

Employment

Rapid job growth and excellent job opportunities are expected. Although hospitals are expected to continue to be the major employer of clinical laboratory workers, employment is expected to grow faster in medical and diagnostic laboratories, offices of physicians, and all other ambulatory health care services.

Earnings

Median annual wage-and-salary earnings of medical and clinical laboratory technologists were $49,700 in May 2006. The middle 50% earned between $41,680 and $58,560. The lowest 10% earned less than $34,660, and the highest 10% earned more than $69,260.

Median annual wage-and-salary earnings of medical and clinical laboratory technicians were $32,840 in May 2006. The middle 50% earned between $26,430 and $41,020. The lowest 10% earned less than $21,830, and the highest 10% earned more than $50,250 (BLS, 2009b).

OCCUPATIONAL THERAPISTS

- Employment is expected to grow much faster than average and job opportunities should be good, especially for therapists treating the elderly.
- Typically, occupational therapists must be state licensed, requiring a master's degree in occupational therapy, 6 months of supervised fieldwork, and passing scores on national and state examinations.
- Occupational therapists are increasingly taking on supervisory roles, allowing assistants to work more closely with clients under the guidance of a therapist.
- More than a quarter of occupational therapists work part time.

Nature of the Work

Occupational therapists help patients improve their ability to perform tasks in living and working environments. They work with individuals who suffer from a mentally, physically, developmentally, or emotionally disabling condition. Occupational therapists use treatments to develop, recover, or maintain the daily living and work skills of their patients. The therapist helps clients not only to improve their basic motor functions and reasoning abilities, but also to compensate for permanent loss of function. The goal is to help clients have independent, productive, and satisfying lives.

Occupational therapists help clients to perform all types of activities, from using a computer to caring for daily needs such as dressing, cooking, and eating. Physical exercises may be used to increase strength and dexterity, while other activities may be chosen to improve visual acuity or the ability to discern patterns. For example, a client with short-term memory loss might be encouraged to make lists to aid recall, and a person with coordination problems might be assigned exercises to improve hand-eye coordination. Occupational therapists also use computer programs to help clients improve decision-making, abstract-reasoning, problem-solving, and perceptual skills, as well as memory, sequencing, and coordination—all of which are important for independent living.

Some occupational therapists treat individuals whose ability to function in a work environment has been impaired. These practitioners might arrange employment, evaluate the work space, plan work activities, and assess the client's progress. Therapists also may collaborate with the client and the employer to modify the work environment so that the client can successfully complete the work.

Occupational therapists in hospitals and other health care and community settings usually work a 40-hour week. Those in schools may participate in meetings and other activities during and after the school day. In 2006, more than a quarter of occupational therapists worked part time.

Employment

Occupational therapists held about 99,000 jobs in 2006. About 1 in 10 occupational therapists held more than one job. The largest number of jobs was in hospitals. Other major employers were offices of other health practitioners (including offices of occupational therapists), public and private educational services, and nursing care facilities. Some occupational therapists were employed by home health care services, outpatient care centers, offices of physicians, individual and family services, community care facilities for the elderly, and government agencies.

A small number of occupational therapists were self-employed in private practice. These practitioners treated clients referred by other health professionals. They also provided contract or consulting services to nursing care facilities, schools, adult day care programs, and home health care agencies.

Employment of occupational therapists is expected to grow much faster than the average for all occupations. The increasing elderly population will drive growth in the demand for occupational therapy services. The baby boom generation's movement into middle age, a period when the incidence of heart attack and stroke increases, will spur demand for therapeutic services. Growth in the population 75 years and older—an age group that suffers from high incidences of disabling conditions—also will increase demand for therapeutic services. In addition, medical advances now enable more patients with critical problems to survive—patients who ultimately may need extensive therapy. Hospitals will continue to employ a large number of occupational therapists to provide therapy services to acutely ill inpatients. Hospitals also will need occupational therapists to staff their outpatient rehabilitation programs.

Job opportunities should be good for licensed occupational therapists in all settings, particularly in acute hospital, rehabilitation, and orthopedic settings because the elderly receive most of their treatment in these settings.

Earnings

Median annual earnings of occupational therapists were $60,470 in May 2006. The middle 50% earned between $50,450 and $73,710. The lowest 10% earned less than $40,840, and the highest 10% earned more than $89,450 (BLS, 2009c).

PHYSICAL THERAPISTS

- Employment is expected to increase much faster than average.
- Job opportunities should be good, particularly in acute hospital, rehabilitation, and orthopedic settings.
- Physical therapists need a master's degree from an accredited physical therapy program and a state license, requiring passing scores on national and state examinations.
- About 6 out of 10 physical therapists work in hospitals or in offices of physical therapists.

Nature of the Work

Physical therapists provide services that help restore function, improve mobility, relieve pain, and prevent or limit permanent physical disabilities of patients suffering from injuries or disease. They restore, maintain, and promote overall fitness and health. Their patients include accident victims and individuals with disabling conditions such as low-back pain, arthritis, heart disease, fractures, head injuries, and cerebral palsy.

Therapists examine patients' medical histories and then test and measure the patients' strength, range of motion, balance and coordination, posture, muscle performance, respiration, and motor function. Next, physical therapists develop plans describing a treatment strategy and its anticipated outcome.

Treatment often includes exercise, especially for patients who have been immobilized or who lack flexibility, strength, or endurance. Physical therapists encourage patients to use their muscles to increase their flexibility and range of motion. More advanced exercises focus on improving strength, balance, coordination, and endurance. The goal is to improve how an individual functions at work and at home.

Physical therapists also use electrical stimulation, hot packs or cold compresses, and ultrasound to relieve pain and reduce swelling. They may use traction or deep-tissue massage to relieve pain and improve circulation and flexibility. Therapists also teach patients to use assistive and adaptive devices, such as crutches, prostheses, and wheelchairs. They also may show patients how to do exercises at home to expedite their recovery.

As treatment continues, physical therapists document the patient's progress, conduct periodic examinations, and modify treatments when necessary.

Physical therapists often consult and practice with a variety of other professionals, such as physicians, dentists, nurses, educators, social workers, occupational therapists, speech-language pathologists, and audiologists.

Some physical therapists treat a wide range of ailments; others specialize in areas such as pediatrics, geriatrics, orthopedics, sports medicine, neurology, and cardiopulmonary physical therapy.

Work Environment

Physical therapists practice in hospitals, clinics, and private offices that have specially equipped facilities. They also treat patients in hospital rooms, homes, or schools. In addition, physical therapists move heavy equipment and lift patients or help them turn, stand, or walk.

Employment

About 6 out of 10 physical therapists worked in hospitals or in offices of physical therapists in 2006. Other jobs were in the home health care services industry, nursing care facilities, outpatient care centers, and offices of physicians.

Employment of physical therapists is expected to grow much faster than average. Job opportunities will be good, especially in acute hospital, rehabilitation, and orthopedic settings. The increasing elderly population will drive growth in the demand for physical therapy services. The elderly population is particularly vulnerable to chronic and debilitating conditions that require therapeutic services. Also, the baby boom generation (1946–1964) is entering the prime age for heart attacks and strokes, increasing the demand for cardiac and physical rehabilitation.

Future medical developments also should permit a higher percentage of trauma victims to survive, creating additional demand for rehabilitative care. In addition, growth may result from advances in medical technology that could permit the treatment of an increasing number of disabling conditions that were untreatable in the past. Widespread interest in health promotion also should increase demand for physical therapy services. A growing number of employers are using physical therapists to evaluate worksites, develop exercise programs, and teach safe work habits to employees.

Earnings

Median annual earnings of physical therapists were $66,200 in May 2006. The middle 50% earned between $55,030 and $78,080. The lowest 10% earned less than $46,510, and the highest 10% earned more than $94,810 (BLS, 2009d).

PHYSICIAN ASSISTANTS

- Physician assistant programs usually last at least 2 years; admission requirements vary by program, but many require at least 2 years of college and some health care experience.
- All states require physician assistants to complete an accredited education program and to pass a national exam in order to obtain a license.
- Employment is projected to grow much faster than average as health care establishments increasingly use physician assistants to contain costs.
- Job opportunities should be good, particularly in rural and inner-city clinics.

Nature of the Work

Physician assistants (PAs) practice medicine under the supervision of physicians and surgeons. PAs are formally trained to provide diagnostic, therapeutic, and preventive health care services, as delegated by a physician. Working as members of the health care team, they take medical histories, examine and treat patients, order and interpret laboratory tests and x-rays, and make diagnoses. They also treat minor injuries, by suturing, splinting, and casting. PAs record progress notes, instruct and counsel patients, and order or carry out therapy. In 48 states and the District of Columbia, physician assistants may prescribe some medications. In some establishments, a PA is responsible for managerial duties, such as ordering medical supplies or equipment and supervising technicians and assistants.

Physician assistants work under the supervision of a physician. However, PAs may be the principal care providers in rural or inner-city clinics where a physician is present for only one or two days each week. In such cases, the PA confers with the supervising physician and other medical professionals as needed and as required by law. PAs also may make house calls or go to hospitals and nursing care facilities to check on patients, after which they report to the physician.

The duties of physician assistants are determined by the supervising physician and by state law. Many PAs work in primary care specialties, such as general internal medicine, pediatrics, and family medicine. Other specialty areas include general and thoracic surgery, emergency medicine, orthopedics, and geriatrics. PAs specializing in surgery provide preoperative and postoperative care and may work as first or second assistants during major surgery.

Work Environment

Work schedules vary according to the practice setting, and often depend on the hours of the supervising physician. The workweek of hospital-based PAs may include weekends, nights, or early morning hospital rounds to visit patients. These workers also may be on call. PAs in clinics usually work a 40-hour week.

Employment

Physician assistants held about 66,000 jobs in 2006. According to the American Academy of Physician Assistants, about 15% of actively practicing PAs worked in more than one clinical job concurrently in 2006. More than half of jobs for PAs were in the offices of physicians. About a quarter were in hospitals, public or private. The rest were mostly in outpatient care centers, including health maintenance organizations, the federal government, and public or private colleges, universities, and professional schools. A few were self-employed.

Employment is expected to grow much faster than the average as health care establishments increasingly use physician assistants to contain costs. Job opportunities for PAs should be good, particularly in rural and inner-city clinics, as these settings typically have difficulty attracting physicians.

Besides working in traditional office-based settings, PAs should find a growing number of jobs in institutional settings such as hospitals, academic medical centers, public clinics, and prisons. PAs also may be needed to augment medical staffing in inpatient teaching hospital settings as the number of hours physician residents are permitted to work is reduced, encouraging hospitals to use PAs to supply some physician resident services.

Earnings

Median annual earnings of wage-and-salary physician assistants were $74,980 in May 2006. The middle 50% earned between $62,430 and $89,220. The lowest 10% earned less than $43,100, and the highest 10% earned more than $102,230.

According to the American Academy of Physician Assistants, median income for physician assistants in full-time clinical practice was $80,356 in 2006; median income for first-year graduates was $69,517. Income varies by specialty, practice setting, geographical location, and years of experience. Employers often pay for their employees' liability insurance, registration fees with the Drug Enforcement Administration, state licensing fees, and credentialing fees (BLS, 2009e).

SPEECH-LANGUAGE PATHOLOGISTS

- About half work in educational services; most others are employed by health care and social assistance facilities.
- A master's degree in speech-language pathology is the standard credential required for licensing in most states.
- Excellent job opportunities are expected.

Nature of the Work

Speech-language pathologists, sometimes called *speech therapists,* assess, diagnose, treat, and help to prevent disorders related to speech, language, cognitive communication, voice, swallowing, and fluency.

Speech-language pathologists work with (a) people who cannot produce speech sounds or cannot produce them clearly; (b) those with speech rhythm and fluency problems, such as stuttering; (c) people with voice disorders, such as inappropriate pitch or harsh voice; (d) those with problems understanding and producing language; (e) those who wish to improve their communication skills by modifying an accent; and (f) those with cognitive communication impairments, such as attention, memory, and problem-solving disorders. They also work with people who have swallowing difficulties.

Speech, language, and swallowing difficulties can result from a variety of causes including stroke, brain injury or deterioration, developmental delays or disorders, learning disabilities, cerebral palsy, cleft palate, voice pathology, mental retardation, hearing loss, or emotional problems. Problems can be congenital, developmental, or acquired. Speech-language pathologists use special instruments and qualitative and quantitative assessment methods, including standardized tests, to analyze and diagnose the nature and extent of impairments.

Speech-language pathologists develop an individualized plan of care, tailored to each patient's needs. For individuals with little or no speech capability, speech-language pathologists may select augmentative or alternative communication methods, including automated devices and sign language, and teach their use. They teach patients how to make sounds, improve their voices, or increase their oral or written language skills to communicate more effectively. They also teach individuals how to strengthen muscles or use compensatory strategies to swallow without choking or inhaling food or liquid. Speech-language pathologists help patients develop, or recover, reliable communication and swallowing skills so patients can fulfill their educational, vocational, and social roles. Speech-language pathologists keep records on the initial evaluation, progress, and discharge of clients. Their records help pinpoint problems, track client progress, and justify the cost of treatment when applying for reimbursement. Speech-Language pathologists counsel individuals and their families concerning communication disorders and how to cope with the stress and misunderstanding that often accompany a disorder. They also work with family members to recognize and change behavior patterns that impede communication and treatment and show them communication-enhancing techniques to use at home.

Most speech-language pathologists provide direct clinical services to individuals with communication or swallowing disorders. In medical facilities, they may perform their job in conjunction with physicians, social workers, psychologists, and other therapists. Speech-language pathologists in schools collaborate with teachers, special educators, interpreters, other school personnel, and parents to develop and implement individual or group programs, provide counseling, and support classroom activities. Some speech-language pathologists conduct research on how people communicate. Others design and develop equipment or techniques for diagnosing and treating speech problems.

Work Environment

Speech-language pathologists usually work at a desk or table in clean comfortable surroundings. In medical settings, they may work at the patient's bedside and assist in positioning the patient. In schools, they may work with students in an office or classroom. Some work in the client's home.

Although the work is not physically demanding, it requires attention to detail and intense concentration. The emotional needs of clients and their families may be demanding. Most full-time speech-language pathologists work 40 hours per week. Those who work on a contract basis may spend a substantial amount of time traveling between facilities.

Employment

Speech-language pathologists held about 110,000 jobs in 2006. About half were employed in educational services, primarily in preschools and elementary and secondary schools. Others were employed in hospitals; offices of other health practitioners, including speech-language pathologists; nursing care facilities; home health care services; individual and family services; outpatient care centers; and child day care centers.

A few speech-language pathologists are self-employed in private practice. They contract to provide services in schools, offices of physicians, hospitals, or nursing care facilities, or work as consultants to industry.

Earnings

Median annual earnings of wage-and-salary speech-language pathologists were $57,710 in May 2006. The middle 50% earned between
$46,360 and $72,410. The lowest 10% earned less than $37,970, and
the highest 10% earned more than $90,400. Some employers may reim-
burse speech-language pathologists for their required continuing education credits (BLS, 2009f).

REFERENCES

Bureau of Labor Statistics. (2009a). *Occupational outlook 2008–2009 edition: Audiologists.* Retrieved June 1, 2009, from http://www.bls.gov/oco/ocos085.htm
Bureau of Labor Statistics. (2009b). *Occupational outlook 2008–2009 edition: Clinical
laboratory technologists and technicians.* Retrieved June 1, 2009, from http://www.
bls.gov/oco/ocos096.htm
Bureau of Labor Statistics. (2009c). *Occupational outlook 2008–2009 edition: Occupational therapists.* Retrieved June 1, 2009, from http://www.bls.gov/oco/ocos078.htm
Bureau of Labor Statistics. (2009d). *Occupational outlook 2008–2009 edition: Physical
therapists.* Retrieved June 1, 2009, from http://www.bls.gov/oco/ocos080.htm
Bureau of Labor Statistics. (2009e). *Occupational outlook 2008–2009 edition: Physician
assistants.* Retrieved June 1, 2009, from http://www.bls.gov/oco/ocos081.htm
Bureau of Labor Statistics. (2009f). *Occupational outlook 2008–2009 edition: Speech-
language pathologists.* Retrieved June 1, 2009, from http://www.bls.gov/oco/ocos099.htm

SAMPLE COVER LETTER

Rhonda P. Jackson
1855 West Patterson Street
Philadelphia, PA 19104
(123) 456-7890
rpjackson@yahoo.com
May 2, 2009

Fred Clarkson, MBA
Director of Human Resources
Prince George's Medical Center
323 South Franklin Drive
Baltimore, MD 21075

Dear Mr. Clarkson:

Please accept this letter of application for your advertised position of clinical laboratory scientist. I have more than five years of experience in clinical laboratory science and am currently working in the laboratory at All Saints Community Hospital in Philadelphia, PA. During the past two years of my career I have obtained a Master's degree in Healthcare Management and have taken on increasing management responsibilities in the laboratory.

I will be relocating to the Baltimore area in July of this year and am interested in moving into a laboratory management position in a large, acute care hospital. I look forward to hearing from you regarding an interview at your convenience. You may contact me at: (123) 456-7890 or by e-mail at rpjackson@yahoo.com.

Respectfully,
Rhonda P. Jackson
Enclosure: Résumé

SAMPLE RÉSUMÉ

Rhonda P. Jackson
1855 West Patterson Street
Philadelphia, PA 19104
(123) 456-7890
E-mail: rpjackson@yahoo.com

Objective: Seeking an entry-level management position in an acute care hospital where my extensive professional and practical experience will be fully utilized.

Employment History
2004–Present
All Saints Community Hospital, Philadelphia, PA
Clinical Laboratory Scientist

- Performed and interpreted laboratory tests. Maintained meticulous attention to detail on test-result validity, recording/reporting results, troubleshooting, and documentation.
- Conducted quality control and quality assurance measures.
- Ensured compliance with government regulations and laboratory policies and procedures.
- Supervised full- and part-time laboratory personnel in the areas of hematology, clinical chemistry, urinalysis, and phlebotomy.
- Evaluated staffing requirements and developed monthly on-call assignments.

Education
2007–2009: Boston College, Boston, MA: MSc in Health Care Management
2000–2004: Philadelphia University, Philadelphia, PA: Bachelor of Science in Clinical Laboratory Science

Certification
Board of Registry of the American Society for Clinical Pathology (BOR)

References
Available upon request.

SAMPLE THANK-YOU LETTER

Rhonda P. Jackson
1855 West Patterson Street
Philadelphia, PA 19104
(123) 456-7890
May 18, 2009

Fred Clarkson, MBA
Director of Human Resources
Prince George's Medical Center
323 South Franklin Drive
Bladensburg, MD 20072

Dear Mr. Clarkson:

Thank you for the opportunity to meet with you and to see your facilities last Wednesday. Both the interview and the tour made for an exciting and complete day. I was particularly impressed with the laboratory and the workflow model that you have instituted. It was very apparent that your staff enjoys working within this model.

Again, thank you for your kindness during my visit and for your efforts in arranging my interview and tour. I look forward to your decision.

Sincerely,
Rhonda P. Jackson

GLOSSARY OF SELECTED VISA TERMS

Accompanying: A type of visa in which family members travel with the principal applicant (in immigrant visa cases, within six months of issuance of an immigrant visa to the principal applicant).

Adjust Status: (1) To change from a nonimmigrant visa status or other status, (2) To adjust the status of a permanent resident (green card holder).

Admission: Entry into the United States is authorized by a Department of Homeland Security, Customs and Border Protection (CBP) officer. When you come from abroad and first arrive in the United States, the visa allows you to travel to the port of entry and request permission to enter the United States. Admission, or entering the United States, by non-U.S. citizens must be authorized by a CBP officer at the port of entry, who determines whether you can enter and how long you can stay here, on any particular visit. If you are allowed to enter, how long you can stay and the immigration classification you are given is shown as a recorded date or Duration of Status (D/S) on Form I-94, Arrival Departure Record, or Form I-94W, if arriving on the Visa Waiver Program. If you want to stay longer than the date authorized, you must request permission from the Department of Homeland Security, U.S. Citizenship and Immigration Services (USCIS).

Advance Parole: Permission to return to the United States after travel abroad granted by DHS prior to leaving the United States. The following categories of people may need advance parole: people on a K-1 visa, asylum applicants, parolees, people with Temporary Protected Status (TPS), and some people trying to adjust status while in the United States. If these categories of people do not apply for advance parole before they leave the United States, they may be unable to return.

An alien in the United States and applying for an Advance Parole document for him- or herself must attach: (1) a copy of any document issued to the alien by USCIS or former INS showing present status in the United States; and (2) an explanation or other evidence demonstrating the circumstances that warrant issuance of Advance Parole.

If the alien is basing his or her eligibility for Advance Parole on a separate application for adjustment of status or asylum, he must also attach a copy of the filing receipt for that application. If the alien is traveling to Canada to apply for an immigrant visa, he or she must also attach a copy of the consular appointment.

Agent: In immigrant visa processing the applicant selects a person who receives all correspondence regarding the case and pays the immigrant visa application processing fee. The agent can be the applicant, the petitioner, or another person selected by the applicant.

Alien: A foreign national who is not a U.S. citizen.

Applicant (Visa): A foreign citizen who is applying for a nonimmigrant or immigrant U.S. visa. The visa applicant may also be referred as a beneficiary for petition-based visas.

Appointment package: The letter and documents that tell an applicant of the date of the immigrant visa interview. It includes forms that the applicant must complete before the interview and instructions for how to get everything ready for the interview.

Approval notice: A Department of Homeland Security, U.S. Citizenship and Immigration Services (USCIS) immigration form, Notice of Action, Form I-797 that says that USCIS has approved a petition, or request for extension of stay or change of status.

Arrival-departure card: Also known as Form I-94, Arrival-Departure Record. The Department of Homeland Security, Customs and Border Protection official at the port of entry gives foreign visitors (all non-U.S. citizens) an Arrival-Departure Record (a small white card) when they enter the United States. Recorded on this card are the immigrant classification and the authorized period of stay in the United States. This is either recorded as a date or the entry of D/S, meaning duration of status. It is important to keep this card safe because it shows the length of time you are permitted and authorized by the Department of Homeland Security to stay in the United States. It is best kept stapled with your passport, kept in a safe place. The visitors return the I-94 card when they leave the country. The I-94W, Nonimmigrant Visa Waiver Arrival-Departure Record (green card) is for travelers on the Visa Waiver Program.

Asylee: An alien in the United States or at a port of entry who is found to be unable or unwilling to return to his or her country of nationality, or to seek the protection of that country because of persecution or a well-founded fear of persecution. Persecution or the fear thereof must be based on the alien's race, religion, nationality, membership in a particular social group, or political opinion. For persons with no nationality, the country of nationality is considered to be the country in which the alien last habitually resided. Asylees are eligible to adjust to lawful permanent resident status after one year of continuous presence in the United States. These immigrants are limited to 10,000 adjustments per fiscal year.

Biometrics: A biometric or biometric identifier is an objective measurement of a physical characteristic of an individual which, when captured in a database, can be used to verify the identity or check against other entries in the database. The best known biometric is the fingerprint, but others include facial recognition and iris scans.

Case number: The National Visa Center (NVC) gives each immigrant petition a case number. This number has three letters followed by ten digits (numbers). The three letters are an abbreviation for the overseas embassy or consulate that will process the immigrant visa case (for example, GUZ for Guangzhou, CDJ for Ciudad Juarez).

Certificate of Naturalization: A document issued by the Department of Homeland Security as proof that the person has become a U.S. citizen (naturalized) after immigration to the United States.

Child: Unmarried child under the age of 21 years. A child may be natural born, step, or adopted. If the child is a stepchild, the marriage between the parent and the American citizen must have occurred when the child was under the age of 18. If the child is adopted, he/she must have been adopted with a full and final adoption when the child was under the age of 16, and the child must have lived with and been in the legal custody of the parent for at least two years. An orphan may qualify as a child if he/she has been adopted abroad by an American citizen or if the American citizen parent has filed an immediate-relative (IR) visa petition to go to the United States for adoption by the American citizen.

In certain visa cases a child continues to be classified as a child after he/she becomes 21, if the petition was filed for him/her when he/she was still under 21 years of age. For example, an IR-2 child of an American citizen remains a child after the age of 21 if a petition was filed for him/her on or after August 6, 2002, when he/she was still under 21 years old. The child must meet other requirements of a child as listed above.

Common-law marriage: An agreement between a man and woman to enter into marriage without a civil or religious ceremony. It may not be recognized as a marriage for immigration purposes.

Conditional residence visa: If you have been married for less than two years when your husband or wife (spouse) gets lawful permanent resident status (gets a green card), then your spouse gets residence on a conditional basis. After two years you and your spouse must apply together to the Department of Homeland Security to remove the condition to the residence.

The investor visa (EB5 or T5/C5) is also a conditional residence. It requires an application procedure after two years to remove the condition on the permanent residence.

Current/noncurrent: There are numerical limits on the number of immigrant visas that can be granted to aliens from any one foreign country. The limit is based on place of birth, not citizenship. Because of the numerical limits, this means there is a waiting time before the immigrant visa can be granted. The terms current/noncurrent refer to the priority date of a petition in preference immigrant visa cases in relationship to the immigrant cut-off date. If your priority date is before the cut-off date according to the monthly Visa Bulletin, your case is current. This means your immigrant visa case can now be processed. However, if your priority date is later/comes after the cut-off date, you will need to wait longer, until your priority date is reached (becomes current).

Cut-off date: The date that determines whether a preference immigrant visa applicant can be scheduled for an immigrant visa interview in any given month. The cut-off date is the priority date of the first applicant who could not get a visa interview for a given month. Applicants with a priority date earlier than the cut-off date can be scheduled. However, if your priority date is on or later than the cut-off date, you will need to wait longer, until your priority date is reached (becomes current).

Department of Labor: The Department of Labor fosters and promotes the welfare of the job seekers, wage earners, and retirees of the United States by improving their working conditions, advancing their opportunities for profitable employment, protecting their retirement and health care benefits, helping employers find workers, strengthening free collective bargaining, and tracking changes in employment, prices, and other national economic measurements. In carrying out this mission, the Department administers a variety of Federal labor laws including those that guarantee workers' rights to safe and healthful working conditions; a minimum hourly wage and overtime pay; freedom from employment discrimination; unemployment insurance; and other income support.

Duration of status: In certain visa categories such as diplomats, students, and exchange visitors, the alien may be admitted into the United States for as long as the person is still doing the activity for which the visa was issued, rather than being admitted until a specific departure date. This is called admission for "duration of status." For students, the time during which a student is in a full course of study plus any authorized practical training, and following that, authorized time to depart the country, is duration of status. The length of time depends upon the course of study. For an undergraduate degree this is commonly four years (eight semesters). Normally the immigration officer gives a student permission to stay in the United States for "duration of status." Duration of Status (or D/S) is recorded on Form I-94, Arrival-Departure Record. The Department of Homeland Security U.S immigration inspector at port of entry gives foreign visitors (all non-U.S citizens) an Arrival-Departure Record (a small white card) when they enter the United States. Recorded on this card are the visa classification and the authorized period of stay in the United States. This is either recorded as a date or the entry or D/S, meaning duration of status. The I-94 is a very important card to make sure you keep, because it shows the length of time you are permitted and authorized by the Department of Homeland Security to stay in the United States.

Green card: A wallet-sized card showing that the person is a lawful permanent resident (immigrant) in the United States. It is also known as a permanent resident card (PRC), an alien registration receipt card, and I-551. It was formerly green in color.

I-551 (green card): Permanent residence card or alien registration receipt card or "green card." *See* Lawful Permanent Resident.

Immigrant visa: A visa for a person who plans to live indefinitely and permanently in the United States.

Immigration and Nationality Act (INA): The Immigration and Nationality Act, or INA, was created in 1952. Before the INA, a variety of statutes governed immigration law but were not organized in one location. The McCarran-Walter bill of 1952, Public Law No. 82-414, collected and codified many existing provisions and reorganized the structure of immigration law. The Act has been amended many times over the years, but is still the basic body of immigration law.

The INA is divided into titles, chapters, and sections. Although it stands alone as a body of law, the Act is also contained in the United States Code (U.S.C.). The code is a collection of all the laws of the United States. It is arranged in fifty subject titles by general alphabetic order. Title 8 of the U.S. Code is but one of the fifty titles and deals with "Aliens and Nationality." When browsing the INA or other statutes you will often see reference to the U.S. Code citation. For example, Section 208 of the INA deals with asylum, and is also contained in 8 U.S.C. 1158. Although it is correct to refer to a specific section by either its INA citation or its U.S. code, the INA citation is more commonly used.

In status: It's important to understand the concept of immigration status and the consequences of violating that status. Being aware of the requirements and possible consequences will make it more likely that you can avoid problems with maintaining your status. Every visa is issued for a particular purpose and for a specific class of visitor. Each visa classification has a set of requirements that the visa holder must follow and maintain. Those who follow the requirements maintain their status and ensure their ability to remain in the United States. Those who do not follow the requirements violate their status and are considered "out of status." For more information see "Out of Status" below. In Status means you are in compliance with the requirements of your visa type under immigration law. For example, you are a foreign student who entered the United States on a student visa. If you are a full-time student and pursuing your course of study, and are not engaged in unauthorized employment, you are "in status." If you work full time in your uncle's convenience store and do not study, you are "out of status."

Labor Condition Application (LCA): A request to the Department of Labor for a foreign citizen to work in the United States.

Lawful Permanent Resident (LPR): A person who has immigrated legally but is not an American citizen. This person has been admitted to the United States as an immigrant and has a Permanent Resident Card, Form I-551, also known as *green card.* It is a wallet-sized card showing that the person is a lawful permanent resident (immigrant) in the United States. This person is also called a legal permanent resident, a green card holder, a permanent resident alien, a legal permanent resident alien (LPRA) and resident alien permit holder.

Lose status: To stay in the United States longer than the period of time which Department of Homeland Security (DHS) gave to a person when he/she entered the United States, or to fail to meet the requirements or violate the terms of the visa classification. The person becomes "out of status."

Machine Readable Passport (MRP): A passport that has biographic information entered on the data page according to international specifications. A machine readable passport is required to travel with a visa on the Visa Waiver Program.

Machine Readable Visa (MRV): A visa that contains biometric information about the passport holder. A visa that immigration officers read with special machines when the applicants enter the United States. It gives biographic information about the passport holder and tells the Department of Homeland Security (DHS) information on the type of visa. It is also called MRV.

National Visa Center (NVC): A Department of State facility located in Portsmouth, New Hampshire. It supports the worldwide operations of the Bureau of Consular Affairs Visa Office. The NVC processes immigrant visa petitions from the Department of Homeland Security (DHS) for people who will apply for their immigrant visas at embassies and consulates abroad. It also collects fees associated with immigrant visa processing.

Nonimmigrant Visa (NIV): A U.S. visa allows the bearer, a foreign citizen, to apply to enter the United States temporarily for a specific purpose. Nonimmigrant visas are primarily classified according to the principal purpose of travel. With few exceptions, while in the United States, nonimmigrants are restricted to the activity or reason for which their visa was issued. Examples of persons who may receive nonimmigrant visas are tourists, students, diplomats, and temporary workers.

Out of status: A U.S. visa allows the bearer to apply for entry to the United States in a certain classification, for a specific purpose. For example, student (F), visitor (B), temporary worker (H). Every visa is issued for a particular purpose and for a specific class of visitor. Each visa classification has a set of requirements that the visa holder must follow and maintain. When you arrive in the United States, a Department of Homeland Security (DHS) Customs and Border Protection (CBP) inspector determines whether you will be admitted, length of stay and conditions of stay in, the United States. When admitted you are given a Form I-94 (Arrival/Departure Record), which tells you when you must leave the United States. The date granted on the I-94 card at the airport governs how long you may stay in the United States. If you do not follow the requirements, you stay longer than that date, or you engage in activities not permitted for your particular type of visa, you violate your status and are considered be "out of status." It is important to understand the concept of immigration status and the consequences of violating that status. Failure to maintain status can result in arrest, and violators may be required to leave the United States. Violation of status also can affect the prospect of readmission to the United States for a period of time, by making you ineligible for a visa. Most people who violate the terms of their status are barred from lawfully returning to the United States for years.

Port of entry: Place (often an airport) where a person requests admission to the United States by the Department of Homeland Security, Customs and Border Protection officer.

Priority date: The priority date decides a person's turn to apply for an immigrant visa. In family immigration the priority date is the date when the petition was filed at a Department of Homeland Security (DHS), U.S. Citizenship and Immigration Services office or submitted to an Embassy or Consulate abroad. In employment immigration the priority date may be the date the labor certification application was received by the Department of Labor (DOL).

Sponsor: (1) A person who fills out and submits an immigration visa petition. Another name for sponsor is petitioner, *or* (2) a person who completes an affidavit of support (I-864) for an immigrant visa applicant.

Spouse: Legally married husband or wife. A cohabiting partner does not qualify as a spouse for immigration purposes. A common-law husband or wife may or may not qualify as a spouse for immigration purposes, depending on the laws of the country where the relationship occurs.

Temporary worker: A foreign worker who will work in the United States for a limited period of time. Some visas classes for temporary workers are H, L, O, P, Q, and R. If you are seeking to come to the United States for employment as a temporary worker (H, L, O, P, and Q visas), your prospective employer must file a petition with the Department of Homeland Security (DHS), USCIS. This petition must be approved by USCIS before you can apply for a visa.

Visa Waiver Program (VWP): The Visa Waiver Program (VWP) enables nationals of certain countries to travel to the United States for tourism or business [visitor (B) visa purposes] for stays of 90 days or less without obtaining a visa. The program was established in 1986 with the objective of eliminating unnecessary barriers to travel, stimulating the tourism industry, and permitting the Department of State to focus consular resources in other areas. VWP eligible travelers may apply for a visa, if they prefer to do so. Not all countries participate in the VWP, and not all travelers from VWP countries are eligible to use the program. VWP travelers are required to apply for authorization though the Electronic System for Travel Authorization (ESTA), are screened at their port of entry into the United States, and are enrolled in the Department of Homeland Security's US-VISIT Program.

Glossary of Selected Visa Terms From:

http://www.travel.state.gov/visa/frvi/glossary/glossary_1363.html
http://www.cbp.gov/xp/cgov/travel/id_visa/legally_admitted_to_the_u_s.xml
http://www.uscis.gov/portal/site/uscis/menuitem.eb1d4c2a3e5b9ac89243c6a75
43f6d1a/?vgnextoid=b328194d3e88d010VgnVCM10000048f3d6a1RCRD&
vgnextchannel=b328194d3e88d010VgnVCM10000048f3d6a1RCRD

FREQUENTLY ASKED QUESTIONS AND ANSWERS ABOUT ADMISSION INTO THE UNITED STATES

Q: What is the Inspection Process?
A: All persons arriving at a port of entry to the United States are subject to inspection by U.S. Customs and Border Protection (CBP) Officers. CBP Officers will conduct the Immigration, Customs and Agriculture components of the Inspections process. If a traveler has health concerns, he/she will be referred to a Public Health Officer for a separate screening.

Q: What Does the Law Say?
A: The legal foundation that requires the inspection of all persons arriving in the United States comes from the Immigration and Nationality Act (INA), see INA § 235 [8 U.S.C.]. Rules published in the Federal Register explain the inspection requirements and process. These rules are incorporated into the Code of Federal Regulations [CFR] at 8 CFR § 235.

Q: What Can I Expect to Happen at a Port of Entry?
A: **Airport**
When arriving at an airport, the airline will give all non-U.S. citizens a form to complete while still en route to the United States, either Form

I-94 (white), Arrival/Departure Record, or Form I-94W (green), Non-immigrant Visa Waiver Arrival/Departure Form and Customs Declaration form 6059B. The forms ask for basic identification information and the address where you will stay in the United States.

Upon arrival, the airline personnel will show you to the inspection area. You will queue up in an inspection line and then speak with a CBP officer. If you are a U.S. citizen, special lines may be available to you. If you are not a U.S. citizen, you should use the lanes marked for non-citizens. If you are a U.S. citizen, the officer will ask you for your passport and Customs Declaration form, verify your citizenship, and welcome you back to the United States. You may be asked to proceed to a second screening point with your belongings for additional questioning by CBP Officers. You will then proceed to the Customs inspection area.

If you are an alien, the CBP Officer must determine why you are coming to the United States, what documents you may require, if you have those documents, and how long you should be allowed to initially stay in the United States. These determinations usually take less than one minute to make. If you are allowed to proceed, the officer will stamp your passport and customs declaration form and issue a completed Form I-94 to you. A completed form I-94 will show what immigration classification you were given and how long you are allowed to stay.

Also, if you are an alien, CBP Officers may decide that you should not be permitted to enter the United States. There are many reasons why this might happen (see INA § 212(a)). You will either be placed in detention, or temporarily held until return flight arrangements can be made. If you have a visa, it may be cancelled. In certain instances, Officer(s) may not be able to decide if you should be allowed into the United States. In this case, your inspection may be deferred (postponed), and you will be instructed to go to another office located near your intended destination in the United States for further processing.

Land

At a land border port of entry you will undergo the same general process. One officer will conduct the primary inspection in the vehicle lane. That officer may send you for further review or issuance of needed papers to a secondary inspection area. Once a determination is made to allow you into the United States, you may be sent for further Customs inspection or immediately allowed to proceed on your trip. Alien truck drivers may qualify for admission as B-1 visitors for business to pick up or deliver cargo traveling in the stream of international commerce. Please see "How Do I Enter the United States as a Commercial Truck Driver?" for more information.

Sea

The inspection process at a sea port of entry is similar to the airport process if inspection facilities are available. Otherwise passengers will be instructed where to report for inspection on board the vessel.

Q: What Documents Must I Present?

A: U.S. citizens must present a passport when entering or departing the United States by air. If traveling by land or sea, any proof of U.S. citizenship that clearly establishes identity and nationality is permitted, such as a birth record or baptismal record, along with government-issued photo ID, such as a driver's license.

An alien who is a lawful permanent resident of the United States must present a Permanent Resident Card (Green Card, Form I-551), a Reentry Permit, or a Returning Resident Visa. For further information, see "How Do I Become a Lawful Permanent Resident While in the United States?" and "How Do I Get a Travel Document?"

Q: How Can I Appeal?

A: In certain circumstances, if you used a valid visa to apply for admission and your application for admission has been denied, you can request a hearing before the Immigration Court, where an immigration judge will determine your case. A judge's decision can be appealed to the Board of Immigration Appeals (BIA). You will receive instructions on where and how to appeal. If you apply for admission to the United States under the Visa Waiver Pilot Program, the decision of the officer is final. In cases involving fraud, willful misrepresentation, false claim to U.S. citizenship or lack of a valid immigrant visa for an intending immigrant, the officer's decision is final.

Appendix D
Speech-Language
Pathology Documents

SPEECH-LANGUAGE PATHOLOGY TREATMENT AREAS

Speech Sound Production

- Articulation
- Apraxia of speech
- Dysarthria
- Ataxia
- Dyskinesia

Resonance

- Hypernasality
- Hyponasality
- Cul-de-sac resonance
- Mixed resonance

Voice

- Phonation quality
- Pitch
- Loudness
- Respiration

Fluency

- Stuttering
- Cluttering

Language (Comprehension and Expression)

- Phonology
- Morphology
- Syntax
- Semantics
- Pragmatics (language use, social aspects of communication)
- Literacy (reading, writing, spelling)
- Prelinguistic communication
- Paralinguistic communication

Cognition

- Attention
- Memory
- Sequencing
- Problem solving
- Executive functioning

Feeding and Swallowing

- Oral, pharyngeal, laryngeal, esophageal
- Orofacial myology
- Oral-motor functions

POTENTIAL ETIOLOGIES OF COMMUNICATION AND SWALLOWING DISORDERS

- Neonatal problems (e.g., prematurity, low birth weight, substance exposure)
- Developmental disabilities (e.g., specific language impairment, autism spectrum disorder, dyslexia, learning disabilities, attention deficit disorder)
- Auditory problems (e.g., hearing loss or deafness)
- Oral anomalies (e.g., cleft lip/palate, dental malocclusion, macroglossia, oral-motor dysfunction)
- Respiratory compromise (e.g., bronchopulmonary dysplasia, chronic obstructive pulmonary disease)

COMPARISON OF ASHA CERTIFICATION, STATE LICENSURE, AND STATE DEPARTMENT OF EDUCATION CERTIFICATION

ASHA CERTIFICATION	STATE LICENSURE/ EDUCATION CERTIFICATION	ASHA CERTIFICATION, LICENSURE, AND EDUCATION CERTIFICATION
Voluntary professional credential	Mandatory for practice	
Based on validation studies of required knowledge, skills, and tasks for independent practice	Established by the state legislature and usually implemented by different state agencies	
Portable: national recognition of being a qualified professional	Possibly recognized by other states	Provides different levels of assurances to the public, other professionals, third-party payers, and employers
Verifies: a master's degree, accredited academic program, supervised clinical experience and mentorship, passing score on a national exam	Dictates: minimal qualifications to practice, job titles, and supervision of support personnel, where applicable	License and education certification requirements differ from state to state. Requirements for a license and for an education certification in the same state are usually different.
Requires continuing education/professional development to maintain. Wide range of activities and content is accepted	Requires continuing education/professional development to renew licensure or education certification in most states; may require preapproval of sponsor of activities	
Accepts only official transcripts, test scores, and supervision by an individual who holds the Certificate of Clinical Competence (CCC) as validation to earn the credential.	Many states will accept ASHA CCC as documentation necessary to meet some or all requirements.	

(continued)

COMPARISON OF ASHA CERTIFICATION, STATE LICENSURE, AND STATE DEPARTMENT OF EDUCATION CERTIFICATION *(CONTINUED)*

ASHA CERTIFICATION	STATE LICENSURE/ EDUCATION CERTIFICATION	ASHA CERTIFICATION, LICENSURE, AND EDUCATION CERTIFICATION
Requires 30 contact hours of continuing education every 3 years for maintenance of the certificate	Continuing education required by most state licensing boards and some state education agencies; number of required contact hours and the length of renewal cycles vary from state to state and from license to education certificate	
Accepts contact hours for continuing education (CE) activities offered by many respected educational agencies	Generally requires that CE contact hours be from an educational agency that is preapproved by the state licensing board or by the state education agency; may also accept only certain content	What is acceptable for ASHA continuing education may not be acceptable to the state and vice versa.

- Pharyngeal anomalies (e.g., upper airway obstruction, velopharyngeal insufficiency/incompetence)
- Laryngeal anomalies (e.g., vocal fold pathology, tracheal stenosis, tracheostomy)
- Neurological disease/dysfunction (e.g., traumatic brain injury, cerebral palsy, cerebral vascular accident, dementia, Parkinson's disease, amyotrophic lateral sclerosis)
- Psychiatric disorder (e.g., psychosis, schizophrenia)
- Genetic disorders (e.g., Down syndrome, fragile X syndrome, Rett syndrome, velocardiofacial syndrome)

Speech-language pathologists provide clinical services that include prevention and prereferral, screening, assessment/evaluation, consultation, diagnosis, treatment, intervention, management, counseling, collaboration, documentation, and referral.

Appendix E
Communication Aids

SLANG TERMS, IDIOMS, AND JARGON FOR LIVING IN THE UNITED STATES

Slang Term or Idiom	*Actual Meaning*
"All in all ..."	Taking everything into consideration. For example, "All in all, it was a good day."
ASAP	As soon as possible
"He/she has an attitude problem."	Phrase used to describe someone who is antagonistic or argumentative.
"I'm having a bad hair day."	Phrase used to describe a day in which nothing seems to go right or the way you planned it.
Bye-bye	Shortened form of saying good-bye.
"I'm just chilling."	Phrase to describe a period when you are relaxing so that you don't feel stressed.
"Everything's cool."	Term used to mean that everything is all right.
"Correct!"	Term used to assure another that he/she understands what you have said. For example, the other person says, "So, you've completed all your work." Your response might be "Correct" instead of "Yes."
"I have to do the dishes."	Phrase indicating the need to wash and dry the dishes used during a meal.
"He/she is driving me nuts."	Phrase used to describe someone whose behavior is bothering you.

369

"I'm fixing to ..."	"I plan to ..."
"From now on"	From this moment forward.
FYI	For your information
"How you doing?"	Term used to ask another person how they are.
"Later."	Term used to close a conversation, meaning that the person will see you or talk to you at another time.
"Make up your mind."	Phrase used when telling someone to make a decision.
Messed up	Can be used to describe a mistake, e.g., "I messed up" or to describe a person who is having difficulty managing his/her life, e.g., "He's messed up."
"Never mind!"	Phrase used to tell someone not to do something you previously requested, e.g., "Never mind doing that assessment." Can also be used in a negative sense or tone when you become frustrated when another individual does not seem to understand what you are asking or saying, e.g., "Oh, never mind!"
Off the hook	Phrase used to describe no longer being required to do something or to be accountable for something, e.g., "I'm off the hook for that error."
Pocketbook	A purse or handbag
Pop, soda, or Coke	Three terms used to mean essentially the same thing—soda pop
Quarter of eight	Used as an expression of time, i.e., 7:45
"I'm screwed."	I'm in trouble
"Sorry? "	Way of asking someone to repeat what he/she said
STAT	Immediately

| "Take it easy." | Term used to end an interaction; it is used instead of good-bye. Can also be used to try to calm someone down. |

"What've you been up to?"
Form of greeting that doesn't require full disclosure of all activities in which you are involved. Usually a short answer, such as, "I've been working a lot of hours at the hospital," will suffice.

"What's up?"
Term used as a form of greeting, instead of hello. Does not require a lengthy explanation of what you have been doing. A simple response such as "Not much" or "I'm excited about starting work" followed by asking about the other person will suffice.

"Y'all"
Contraction for *you all*. Used when conversing with a group of people. For example, "How y'all doing?" Used more frequently in the southern part of the United States.

SLANG TERMS, IDIOMS, AND JARGON COMMONLY HEARD IN PRACTICE SITUATIONS

Slang Term or Idiom	*Actual Meaning*
"I'll give him a piece of my mind."	To give another your opinion, usually in anger.
Badge	Identification card
"I can't seem to get my wind."	Indicates that the person is short of breath
Code blue; Call a code	General terms used to indicate the need to mobilize the emergency team (physician, anesthesiologist or anesthetist, nurses, and other health care personnel) when a patient experiences cardiac arrest, respiratory arrest, or life-threatening cardiac arrhythmias.

Come down with	Phrase used to describe becoming ill, e.g., "I seem to be coming down with a cold."
"I can't seem to come out of it."	Can't seem to move on with one's life after an illness or depression.
"Will you crank up my bed?"	Term used to mean raise the head of the bed.
"I'm under the weather."	Term used to mean that the person is feeling ill.
Goof off	Term used to describe not working or doing something else when one should be working, e.g., "He's goofing off."
"He's a pain in the neck."	Phrase used to describe someone who annoys you.
"I'm tied up right now."	"I don't have time to help you."
"I need to have a BM."	"I need to make a bowel movement."
"We need to run fluids."	Need to give intravenous fluids to rehydrate a patient.
"I need to do number 1."	"I need to urinate."
"I need to do number 2."	"I need to move my bowels."
"She's out to lunch."	Phrase describing someone who is oblivious to what is happening.
The patient passed or passed away	The patient has died.
"Do you have to pee?"	Slang way of asking if a person has to urinate.
"Do you need to use the restroom?"	Refers to using the toilet or bathroom.
"I'm going to throw up."	"I'm going to vomit."
"It really tickled my fancy."	Something that appealed to you, e.g., "Seeing him really tickled my fancy."
"What's cooking?"	Form of greeting asking about what is going on in your life. Similar to "What's happening?"
"I'll push it through."	Making sure that what you are requesting is done, e.g., "I'll push through your request for additional staff."
Yo!	Form of greeting comparable to saying hello.

LISTING OF COMMON ABBREVIATIONS

Abbreviation	*Meaning*
ABD	Type of abdominal pad or dressing
ABGs	Arterial blood gases
ABT	Antibiotic therapy
ac	Before meals
AMA	Against medical advice
APAP	Automatic Positive Airway Pressure. An APAP machine automatically adjusts on a breath-by-breath basis to deliver the minimum pressure needed to keep an airway open while asleep.
ARDS	Acute respiratory distress syndrome
ASAP	As soon as possible
bid	Twice a day
bpm	Beats per minute
CA	Cancer
CABG	Coronary Artery Bypass Graft
CAD	Coronary Artery Disease
CCU	Critical Care Unit
CHF	Congestive Heart Failure
COPD	Chronic obstructive pulmonary disease
CPAP	Continuous Positive Airway Pressure (CPAP), a common treatment for obstructive sleep apnea. CPAP is produced by a machine that delivers pressurized air to a nasal mask. This airflow acts like a splint to the airway, keeping it open and enabling uninterrupted sleep.
C-section	Cesarean section
CSF	Cerebral spinal fluid
CVA	Cerebral vascular accident
Detox	Detoxification
Dig	Digoxin

DNR	Do not resuscitate
DOA	Dead on arrival
DOB	Date of birth
Drsg	Dressing
DSD	Dry sterile dressing
Dx	Diagnosis
ER	Emergency room or department
Foley	Foley catheter; a type of indwelling, urethral catheter
FYI	For your information
GERD	Gastroesophageal Reflux Disease
GVHD	Graft versus Host Disease, seen following organ transplantation; usually indicative of organ rejection
Hep-C	Hepatitis C
Hoh	Hard of hearing
Hs	Hour of sleep
Hx	History
I&O	Intake and output
IV	Intravenous
IVPB	IV piggyback; secondary intravenous connected to primary tubing
K	Potassium
KCl	Potassium chloride
KUB	An examination of the kidneys, ureters, and bladder
KVO	Keep vein open; intravenous fluids are run at a slow rate so that the vein is preserved for subsequent IVs.
Labs	Laboratory values
LOC	Level of consciousness
Lytes	Electrolytes
MOM	Milk of Magnesia (a laxative)
MRSA	Methicillin resistant staphylococcus aureus

MS	Multiple Sclerosis
MVA	Motor vehicle accident
NANDA	North American Nursing Diagnosis Association
NIDDM	Non–Insulin-Dependent Diabetes Mellitus; Type 2 Diabetes
Nitro	Nitroglycerin
NKA	No known allergies
NPO	Nothing by mouth
NSAID	Nonsteroidal anti-inflammatory drugs; used to relieve pain and inflammation
NVD	Nausea, vomiting, and diarrhea
OB	Obstetrics
od	once daily
OOB	Out of bed
os	Left eye
ou	Both eyes
PCA	Patient-controlled anesthesia
PD	Peritoneal dialysis
PEEP	Positive End Expiratory Pressure; parameter used as a measure of maintaining acceptable gas exchange and to minimize adverse effects in patients on ventilators
PICC	Peripherally inserted central catheter; used for long-term, intravenous administration of drugs, such as antibiotics
Pit	Pitocin
po	By mouth
prn	As needed
ptca	Percutaneous Transluminal Coronary Angioplasty; procedure used when coronary arteries are blocked.
ROM	Range of motion
stat	Right away/immediately

tid	Three times a day
Vanco	Vancomycin (an antibiotic)
Vent	Ventilator
VS	Vital Signs

Note: The Joint Commission has attempted to limit the use of abbreviations in health care settings. This list was identified by foreign-educated health care professionals as abbreviations they had seen on patient charts and could not understand. The editors of this book do not suggest that you use these abbreviations in your practice.

Glossary

Academy of Rehabilitative Audiology (ARA): An organization that promotes hearing care through the provision of comprehensive, rehabilitative, and habilitative services.

Accreditation Council for Occupational Therapy Education (ACOTE): The accrediting body of the American Occupational Therapy Association. ACOTE accredits approximately 275 occupational therapy and occupational therapy assistant educational programs.

Accreditation Commission for Audiology Education (ACAE): Organization whose mission is to assure the public that only those programs that have complied with this agency's standards and that graduate competent audiologists trained at the AuD level will be accredited.

Accreditation Review Commission on Education for Physician Assistants (ARC-PA): The accrediting agency that defines the standards for physician assistant education and evaluates physician assistant educational programs within the United States to ensure their compliance with those standards.

Accrediting Bureau of Health Education Schools (ABHES): An independent, nonprofit agency recognized by the U.S. Secretary of Education for the accreditation of private, postsecondary institutions in the United States offering predominantly allied health education programs, and the programmatic accreditation of medical assistant, medical laboratory technician, and surgical technology programs.

Acculturation program: A system of procedures or activities that has the specific purpose of training individuals to understand another culture and its practices.

Advocacy: Active support for a cause or position.

Affidavit: A sworn statement or a written declaration made in the presence of someone authorized to administer pledges.

Allied health professionals: Clinical health care professions distinct from medicine, dentistry, and nursing. Allied health professionals work as part of the health care team.

Alternative therapies: A variety of therapeutic or preventive health care practices, such as homeopathy, naturopathy, chiropractic, and herbal medicine, that complement generally accepted medical methods.

American Academy of Audiology (AAA): An organization that promotes quality hearing and balance care by advancing the profession of audiology through leadership, advocacy, education, public awareness, and support of research.

American Academy of Physician Assistants (AAPA): National professional society, founded in 1968, that represents physician assistants in all 50 states, the District of Columbia, Guam, and the Federal Services.

American Board of Audiology (ABA): An organization dedicated to enhancing audiologic services to the public by promulgating universally recognized standards in professional practice.

American Medical Technologists (AMT): Established in 1939, the American Medical Technologists (AMT) is a national, not-for-profit agency that certifies health care professionals, such as medical technologists and medical technicians.

American Occupational Therapy Association (AOTA): The national professional association established in 1917 to represent the interests and concerns of occupational therapy practitioners and students of occupational therapy and to improve the quality of occupational therapy services.

American Physical Therapy Association (APTA): The national professional organization for physical therapists representing more than 72,000 members. Its goal is to advocate for the advancement of physical therapy practice, research, and education.

American Speech-Language-Hearing Association (ASHA): The professional, scientific, and credentialing association for audiologists, speech-language pathologists, and speech, language, and hearing scientists.

Americans With Disabilities Act: The 1990 civil rights law that prohibits, under certain circumstances, discrimination based on disability.

Articulation agreements: Agreements between academic institutions that facilitate the transition of a student from one academic institution to another, or from one level of education to the next, with minimum duplication of coursework.

Assertiveness: The ability to state one's position positively and in a self-confident manner.

Associate degree: A degree earned on completion of a 2-year program of study at a community college, junior college, technical school, or other institution of higher education.

Asylum status: Protection and immunity from extradition granted by a government to a foreign political refugee.

Attestation: A statement that something is true, especially in a formal written document.

Audiologists: Professionals that work with people who have hearing, balance, and related ear problems, especially diagnosing and treating hearing loss. Audiology is regulated by licensure or registration in all 50 states.

Automated teller machine (ATM): A street-side computerized device that provides bank customers with access to their accounts and the ability to withdraw money from a remote location.

Baby boomer: Individual born during a period of extreme population increase due to high birth rates. Generally refers to those born in the period following the end of World War II.

Backlog: A quantity of unfinished business or work that has built up over a period of time and must be dealt with before progress can be made.

Bias: Term used to describe an action, judgment, or other outcome influenced by a prejudged perspective.

Biomedical research: Medical research and evaluation of new treatments for both safety and efficacy, in what are termed clinical trials, and all other research that contributes to the development of new treatments.

Board of Registry of the American Society for Clinical Pathology (BOR): The Board of Registry (BOR) was founded in 1928 by the American Society for Clinical Pathology (ASCP), 6 years after the society was founded in 1922. The BOR is a separate certifying body within the organizational structure of the ASCP. To date, over 430,000 individuals have been certified by the BOR, which is recognized as the preeminent certifying agency for clinical laboratory personnel.

Botanicals: Drugs or products made directly from plants.

Brain drain: The large emigration of individuals with technical skills and knowledge from one (usually developing) country to another (usually developed) country. It generally occurs when a professional is faced with lack of opportunity, political conflict and instability, and poor working conditions in the home country.

Breach of contract: A legal concept in which a binding agreement is not honored by one or more of the participants.

Bureau of Labor Statistics: The principal fact-finding agency for the federal government in the broad field of labor economics and statistics.

Canadian Association of Speech-Language Pathologists and Audiologists (CASLPA): The national body that supports and represents the professional needs of speech-language pathologists, audiologists and supportive personnel inclusively within one organization. The organization supports and empowers its members to maximize the communication and hearing potential of the people of Canada.

Career mobility: Progress in a chosen profession or during a person's working life.

Centers for Medicare & Medicaid Services (CMS): The federal agency responsible for administering the Medicare, Medicaid, SCHIP (State Children's Health Insurance), HIPAA (Health Insurance Portability and Accountability Act), CLIA (Clinical Laboratory Improvement Amendments), and several other health-related programs. Formerly known as the Health Care Financing Administration (HCFA).

Certification: A process indicating that an individual or institution has met predetermined standards.

Certificate of Clinical Competence (CCL): ASHA offers the Certificate of Clinical Competence in two areas: speech-language pathology (CCC-SLP) and audiology (CCC-A). All applicants must possess an earned graduate degree (master's or doctoral degree) in order to meet application qualifications.

Certificate of Clinical Competence in Audiology (CCC-A): The American Speech-Language-Hearing Association, ASHA, offers the Certificate of Clinical Competency in two areas: Speech-Language Pathology and Audiology. All applicants must possess an earned graduate degree (master's or doctoral degree) in order to meet application qualifications.

Certification: A process for verifying that an individual or institution has met predetermined standards.

CGFNS International: CGFNS International is an internationally recognized authority on credentials evaluation and verification pertaining to the education, registration, and licensure of nurses and health care professionals worldwide. Named in the 1996 immigration law to screen all health professionals (except physicians) seeking an occupational visa to practice in the United States.

Check card purchase: Buying an item that reduces the balance in your bank account using a bank debit card.

Clinical practice acuity: The complexity of care required to meet patient care needs and goals.

Codes of Conduct: A set of rules outlining the responsibilities of, or proper practices for, an individual, a profession, or an organization.

Cohort: Statistically, a group of subjects defined by their common experience of an event in a particular time span.

Collective bargaining: Negotiations between management and a union about pay and conditions of employment on behalf of all the workers in the union.

Commission on Accreditation in Physical Therapy Education (CAPTE): The accreditation agency recognized by the U.S. Department of Education and the Council for Higher Education Accreditation to accredit entry-level physical therapist and physical therapist assistant education programs.

Community-based care: Services provided in one's own home or other community settings that supply a variety of health care options. These options allow people to stay in their homes, while still providing important health care support.

Community colleges: Two-year public institutions of higher education; once commonly called junior colleges.

Compliance: A state in which someone or something is in accordance with established guidelines, specifications, or legislation. The adjective form is *compliant* and indicates readiness to conform to or agree to do something.

Coordinated care: Strategies to make health care systems more cost-effective and responsive to the needs of people with complex chronic illnesses.

Consul: An official appointed by the government to reside in a foreign country in order to represent the commercial interests of foreign citizens from the official's home country.

Continuing education: Regular courses or training designed to bring professionals up to date with the latest developments in their particular field.

Council for Clinical Certification: ASHA council that defines the standards for clinical certification and applies those standards in the certification of individuals; may also develop and administer a credentialing program for speech-language pathology assistants.

Council for Clinical Specialty Recognition (CCSR): An agency that implements, monitors, and revises as may become necessary the specialty recognition standards in audiology and in speech-language pathology.

Council of State Association Presidents (CSAP): An organization that provides leadership training for state speech-language-hearing association presidents and provides a forum for collaborating and networking.

Council on Academic Accreditation in Audiology and Speech-Language Pathology (CAA): Accreditation board responsible for evaluating and accrediting master's programs in speech-language pathology and clinical doctoral programs in audiology.

Credentials evaluation: An analysis of an individual's qualifications, such as education and licensure, to ensure that they are comparable to U.S. qualifications.

Credit history: Record of an individual's past borrowing and repayment of money. Includes history of late payment and bankruptcy.

Credit rating: An estimate of somebody's ability to repay money given on credit based on credit history.

Credit union: Owned and controlled by its members, a cooperative bank association that provides loans and other financial services to its members.

Cross-cultural communication: Interactions between two or more individuals of different cultures.

Cultural competence: An ability to interact effectively with people of different cultures, often in the context of health care.

Cultural conflicts: Disagreements that arise due to misunderstandings in communication and personal interpretations of words and actions.

Curative care: Refers to treatment and therapies provided to a patient with intent to improve symptoms and cure the patient's medical problem.

Debit card: A plastic card that provides an alternative payment method to cash when making purchases; also known as a bank card or check card.

Default clause: Section in a document; part of a contract that explains the consequence if someone fails to pay a debt or other financial obligation.

Department of Homeland Security (DHS): A government agency created in 2003 to handle immigration and other security-related matters. A component of DHS is the Citizenship and Immigration Services, the government agency that oversees lawful immigration to the United States of America.

Direct deposit: Electronic delivery of a paycheck directly into an individual's bank account by the individual's employer.

Disaster preparedness: Process of ensuring that an organization is prepared in the event of a forecasted disaster to minimize loss of life, injury, and damage to property; and can provide rescue, relief, rehabilitation, and other services after the disaster.

Electronic transfer: Computer-based system used to perform financial transactions electronically.

Endorsement: Acceptance by one state of a professional license issued to an individual by another U.S. state or jurisdiction. Also, an amendment to a contract or license allowing a change in the original terms.

Entitlement: Guarantee of access to benefits because of right or by agreement through law. Also refers to one's belief that he or she deserves some particular reward or benefit.

Federation of State Boards of Physical Therapy (FSBPT): Organization that develops and administers the National Physical Therapy Examinations for both physical therapists (PT) and physical therapist assistants (PTA).

Focus group: A small group of people who are questioned about their opinions as part of research.

Foreign Credentialing Commission on Physical Therapy (FCCPT): A nonprofit organization created to assist the U.S. Citizenship and Immigration Services (USCIS) and U.S. jurisdiction licensing authorities by evaluating the credentials of foreign-educated physical therapists who wish to immigrate and work in the United States.

Garnished wages: Monies taken from payroll or royalty checks, or from investment checks, to pay a debt.

Grandfathering: To exempt a person involved in an activity, business, or profession from new regulations.

Health Care Worker Certificates: Health care worker certification provides documentary proof that the education, training, licensure, and English language proficiency of a foreign health care worker has met U.S. comparability standards.

Homeless shelter: Last resort in temporary housing for people in need who do not have a place to live.

Hospice: A usually small residential institution for terminally ill patients where treatment focuses on the patient's well-being rather than a cure and includes drugs for pain management. It often includes spiritual counseling.

House staff: Individual employed directly by a health care institution, usually a hospital.

Human resource department: Section of an organization responsible for coordinating the recruitment and hiring of employees as well as maintaining the organization's adherence to labor laws.

Identity theft: Theft of personal information such as someone's bank account or credit card details.

Idiom: An expression of speech whose meaning is translated figuratively rather than literally.

Internship: The program through which an individual can work as a trainee to gain practical, on-the-job experience for a specified amount of time.

Jargon: An informal language used by people who work together within a specific occupation or profession or within a common interest group.

Junior colleges: Two-year, postsecondary schools that provide academic, vocational, and professional education.

Mandatory overtime: Term for overtime that is required by an employer rather than being optional for the employee.

Meals on Wheels: Provides home-delivered meals to people in need, usually the elderly or the disabled.

Medical technicians: Medical technicians, or clinical laboratory technicians, perform less complex tests and laboratory procedures than medical technologists, typically have a 2-year specialized education, and are supervised by a medical technologist.

Medical technologists: Health care professionals who perform chemical, hematological, immunologic, microscopic, and bacteriological diagnostic analyses on body fluids. Medical technologists, also known as clinical laboratory scientists, have at least a baccalaureate degree and work in clinical laboratories at hospitals, doctor's offices, and biotechnology laboratories.

Mentor: A senior or experienced person in a company or organization who gives guidance and training to a junior colleague; a wise and trusted teacher and counselor.

Municipal hospitals: Hospitals controlled by the city government.

Mutual Recognition Agreement: An international agreement by which two or more countries agree to recognize one another's education, programs, licensure, and so forth, in an effort to increase mobility between and among the nations that sign the agreement.

National Accrediting Agency for Clinical Laboratory Sciences (NAACLS): An agency for the accreditation and approval of educational programs in the clinical laboratory sciences and related health care professions.

National Board for Certification in Occupational Therapy, Inc. (NBCOT®): A not-for-profit credentialing agency that provides certification for the occupational therapy profession and federal screening for international occupational therapists seeking a visa to practice in the United States.

National Commission on Certification of Physician Assistants (NCCPA): The credentialing organization for physician assistants in the United States that administers the Physician Assistant National Certifying Exam (PANCE).

National Credentialing Agency for Laboratory Personnel (NCA): A voluntary, nonprofit, nongovernmental organization that conducts certification of medical laboratory personnel.

National Labor Relations Board: An independent federal agency created by Congress in 1935 to administer the National Labor Relations Act, the primary law governing relations between unions and employers in the private sector. The statute guarantees the right of employees to organize and to bargain collectively with their employers, and to engage in other protected concerted activity with or without a union, or to refrain from all such activity.

National Physical Therapy Examinations: Examinations that assess the basic, entry-level competence for first-time licensure or registration as a physical therapist (PT) or physical therapist assistant (PTA) within 53 U.S. states and jurisdictions.

Networking: Making connections among people or groups of a like kind.

North American Free Trade Agreement (NAFTA): A trade agreement that allows for the exchange of products and services in North America, involving the United States, Canada, and Mexico.

Occupation: The means through which a client achieves therapeutic goals for maximum independence and life satisfaction.

Occupational Therapist Registered (OTR): Designation for an individual who has passed the national certification examination for occupational therapy.

Occupational therapists: Occupational therapists use treatments to develop, recover, or maintain the daily living and work skills of their patients. They work with individuals, families, groups, and populations to facilitate health and well-being through engagement or reengagement in occupation.

Occupational therapy assistant (OTA): Occupational therapy assistants work under the direction of occupational therapists to provide rehabilitative services to persons with mental, physical, emotional, or developmental impairments.

On-the-job training (OJT): Employee training at the place of work. On-the-job training takes place in a normal working situation, using the actual tools, equipment, documents or materials that are part of the real-life job.

Palliative care: A specialized form of care focused on the pain, symptoms, and stress of serious illness.

Pen pals: Two people, usually in different countries, who become friends through an exchange of letters but who may never meet.

Petition: To appeal to or request something of a higher authority.

Phlebotomist: An individual trained to draw blood either for laboratory tests or blood banking.

Phlebotomy: The medical practice of opening a vein to draw blood, usually for diagnostic tests.

Physical therapists: Physical therapists provide services that help restore function, improve mobility, relieve pain, and prevent or limit permanent physical disabilities of patients suffering from injuries or disease. They restore, maintain, and promote overall fitness and health.

Physical therapist assistants: Physical therapist assistants and aides help physical therapists to provide treatment that improves patient mobility, relieves pain, and prevents or lessens physical disabilities of patients.

Physical therapy: A health care profession that provides services to clients in order to develop, maintain, and restore maximum movement and functional ability throughout life.

Physician assistants: Individuals formally trained to provide diagnostic, therapeutic, and preventive health care services, as delegated by a physician.

Physician Assistant National Certifying Exam (PANCE): Credentialing examination for physician assistants that entitles those who pass it to use the designation PA-C.

Physician Assistant National Recertifying Exam (PANRE): Examination required to maintain certification as a physician assistant.

Portfolio: A collection of items or documents outlining one's work experience, achievements, and skills that is organized in a binder, file, or electronic format.

Postsecondary education: Education that occurs following completion of high school (secondary school) in the United States. Colleges and universities are examples of postsecondary institutions.

Praxis examination: The national examination in speech-language pathology and audiology required for certification.

Preceptor: A specialist in a profession, especially health care, who gives practical training to a student or novice in the profession.

Prescriptive authority: Right granted by law to prescribe medications, usually under the supervision of a physician.

Professional autonomy: Responsible discretionary decision making by a profession or an individual within the profession; the quality or condition of being self-governing.

Professional fluency: The ability to discuss the motivation and reasoning behind research or general research trends in a particular field or profession.

Professional/practice doctorates: Practice-focused doctoral degree programs as opposed to a research-focused doctorate degree, such as a PhD.

Proprietary colleges: For-profit academic institutions operated by their owners or investors, rather than a not-for-profit institution, religious organization, or government.

Reciprocity: Recognition by a state or territory of a license acquired in another state or territory.

Refugee status: Protection granted by a government to someone who has fled another country, often because of political oppression or persecution.

Reimbursement: Payment by government or private insurers for services provided by certain allied health professionals.

Remittances: The portions of migrant income that, in the form of either funds or goods, go back into the home country.

Residency programs: Working for a specific period of time in a community or a facility to gain experience. In many U.S. facilities such programs are structured learning experiences.

Retribution: Something given or demanded in repayment, especially punishment.

Retrogression: The procedural delay in issuing an immigrant visa when there are more people applying for immigrant visas in a given year than the total number of visas available.

Role-playing: Practicing how you will respond in a situation by playing the part you will take or that of another person, for example, practicing your interaction with a physician who has written an order that you must question.

Scam: A scheme for making money by dishonest means.

Security deposit: A sum of money required by somebody selling something or leasing property as security against the buyer's or tenant's failure to fulfill the contract.

Self-learning modules: Activities designed for participants to do independently when they are unable to attend traditional education sessions.

Slang: Highly informal words or expressions that are not considered standard in the language.

Speech-language pathologists: Individuals with specialized education who assess, diagnose, treat, and help to prevent disorders related to speech, language, cognitive communication, voice, swallowing, and fluency.

Third-party authorization: Occurs when the individual for whose benefit a contract is created gives another person the right to act on that individual's behalf.

Third-party payers: Any insurer, nonprofit hospital service plan, health care service plan, health maintenance organization, self-insurer or any person or other entity that provides payment for medical and related services.

Trademark: A distinctive sign or indicator used by an individual to identify that the services provided by the individual are unique. The trademark distinguishes the services provided from those of other entities. Occupational Therapist Registered (OTR) and Certified Occupational Therapy Assistant (COTA) are examples of trademarks.

Unencumbered: Not held back or delayed because of difficulties or problems, for example, a professional license that is not revoked, suspended, or made probationary or conditional by a licensing or regulatory authority as a result of disciplinary action.

Union: A trade union or labor union is an organization run by and for workers who have banded together to achieve common goals in key areas and working conditions.

U.S. Citizenship and Immigration Services (USCIS): The government agency that oversees lawful immigration to the United States. It establishes immigration services, policies, and priorities, and adjudicates (decides upon) the petitions and applications of potential immigrants.

U.S. Department of Labor (DOL): The government department responsible for improving working conditions and promoting opportunities for profitable employment in the United States.

U.S. Department of State: The U.S. government department that sets and maintains foreign policies, runs consular offices abroad, and makes decisions about nonimmigrant visas and immigrant visas that are processed through U.S. consulates.

Videoconference: Live audio and visual transmission of meeting activities that enables people at different sites to interact remotely in real time.

World Federation of Occupational Therapists (WFOT): Key international representative for occupational therapists and occupational therapy around the world and the official international organization for the promotion of occupational therapy. Founded in 1952, WFOT currently has 66 member associations.

Index